The International Library of Bioethics

Volume 90

The *International Library of Bioethics* – formerly known as the International Library of Ethics, Law and the New Medicine comprises volumes with an international and interdisciplinary focus on foundational and applied issues in bioethics. With this renewal of a successful series we aim to meet the challenge of our time: how to direct biotechnology to human and other living things' ends, how to deal with changed values in the areas of religion, society, and culture, and how to formulate a new way of thinking, a new bioethics.

The *International Library of Bioethics* focuses on the role of bioethics against the background of increasing globalization and interdependency of the world's cultures and governments, with mutual influencing occurring throughout the world in all fields. The series will continue to focus on perennial issues of aging, mental health, preventive medicine, medical research issues, end of life, biolaw, and other areas of bioethics, whilst expanding into other current and future topics.

We welcome book proposals representing the broad interest of this series' interdisciplinary and international focus. We especially encourage proposals addressing aspects of changes in biological and medical research and clinical health care, health policy, medical and biotechnology, and other applied ethical areas involving living things, with an emphasis on those interventions and alterations that force us to re-examine foundational issues.

More information about this series at http://www.springer.com/series/16538

Allan J. Jacobs

Assigning Responsibility for Children's Health When Parents and Authorities Disagree: Whose Child?

Springer

Allan J. Jacobs
Gynecologic Oncology
Coney Island Hospital
Brooklyn, NY, USA

SUNY Downstate College of Medicine
Brooklyn, New York, USA

NIH

ISSN 2662-9186 ISSN 2662-9194 (electronic)
The International Library of Bioethics
ISBN 978-3-030-87697-5 ISBN 978-3-030-87698-2 (eBook)
https://doi.org/10.1007/978-3-030-87698-2

This Springer imprint is published by the registered company Springer Nature Switzerland AG
The registered company address is: Gewerbestrasse 11, 6330 Cham, Switzerland

This book is dedicated to

Pamela Ravin Jacobs, my wife;

the memory of my parents, Pauline and Arnold Jacobs

and

all of the other parents in my family and in Pam's

Acknowledgments

This book is the product of a lifetime of experience and study.

Richard L. O'Brien, M.D., M.S., and Norman Gant, M.D., remain my models for professionalism. Both set high intellectual and humanitarian standards, which I hope I have upheld. Dr. O'Brien did more to influence me as a person than anyone except my wife and my parents.

My wife, Pamela Jacobs, JD, Ph.D., was my muse, teacher, and supporter as I wrote this book. She did more than tolerate the time I lent to this effort. She introduced me to various fields of psychology. Our conversations provided me with many ideas and sharpened others. Pam has read the entire manuscript critically. Every page of this book bears her imprint. This would have been a far different and worse book without her input.

Kavita Shah Arora, M.D., MBE, helped me refine my ideas regarding the State Intervention Test, as did Hillel Levin, JD. Several of our collaborations are cited in this book. Other scholars who have read and provided useful suggestions about portions of this book include Johan C. Bester, M.D., Ph.D., Raphael Cohen-Almagor, Ph.D., Jules Gleicher, Ph.D., Yakov Korach, M.D., and Maury Silver, Ph.D.

I also wish to thank two anonymous reviewers for reading the book and offering valuable suggestions.

I alone am responsible for the content of this book, of course.

I am grateful to Floor Oosting, the Editorial Director at Springer Humanities, for her confidence in me, and for patiently waiting for the manuscript, which was delayed by a change in authorship and by the coronavirus pandemic. I appreciate, too, the help of Christopher Wilby of the Springer editorial staff.

Finally, I thank my children, Tamara Block, Sarah Jacobs, and Ethan Jacobs for their support and inspiration.

Notes

The opinions expressed in this book are solely those of the author. They do not necessarily represent the opinions of the New York City Health + Hospitals Corporation, the Physician's Associate Group of New York, the State University of New York, or any other organization with which the author is affiliated.

Statements about laws and medical facts are believed to reflect the state of knowledge at the time the author wrote them. They are subject to change, however, and should not be construed as statements of legal or medical fact at the time this book is read. All statements about law or medicine are meant as general statements, and are not to be construed as legal or medical advice, or applicable to the personal circumstances of any individual.

Contents

Chapter 1
Introduction: What We Owe the Child

Abstract Parents and physicians do not always agree on how to care for a child. In such cases, the state may be asked to arbitrate. Alternatively, the state, for reasons of its own, may seek to restrict parental authority over matters pertaining to children's health and safety. Much work in this area has focused on the primacy of the child in question. Other work has focused on the parent–child dyad. The needs of other stakeholders, and of the state itself, have received inadequate attention. Furthermore, the appropriate limits of state power have not been sufficiently interrogated. Much liberal democratic thought has pointed out the potential for abuse of government power, but much ethical literature has not seriously considered the impact of government intervention into private relationships. In this chapter I begin to outline the problems the book will consider. I try to show that there is no principled way to settle many controversies over parental decisions. My argument is based on the doctrines of value pluralism and liberal pluralism. However, society owes children the opportunity to flourish. The elements of flourishing should be determined empirically to the greatest extent possible, rather than by armchair speculation.

Former Texas Senator Phil Gramm is said to have told a government official, "My educational policies are based on the fact that I care more about my children than you do." The official said, "No, you don't." Gramm replied, "Okay: What are their names?"

A. J. Jacobs, *Assigning Responsibility for Children's Health When Parents and Authorities Disagree: Whose Child?*, The International Library of Bioethics 90,
https://doi.org/10.1007/978-3-030-87698-2_1

Everyone reading this has been a child.[1] Many of us have taken care of children in a professional capacity. Many of us have been parents. Those who have not been parents might ask why anyone would want to be a parent. Table 1.1 lists some reasons that actual parents have recently provided in Internet blogs. Notably absent from these sources is the desire to raise an autonomous child, or the desire to raise a child who will hold values the state considers normative. It is the thesis of this book that

1. In a liberal democracy, parents should be allowed to raise children according to their beliefs, and their perceptions of what is good for the child.
2. Ideally, parents will consider the flourishing of their children as their goal, though concepts of flourishing vary.
3. The role of the state is to intervene with parents only when their child-raising practices are likely to cause serious damage to their children or a serious burden to society or its members.

I have tried to write this book so that it will be comprehensible to educated general readers as well as to those immersed in ethics or medicine. The first part of the book serves as an intellectual backdrop for my approach to specific health-related problems. This part should be clear to a general audience, though philosophers may find it oversimplified. The second portion of the book is meant to be comprehensible to non-physicians, though scientific information will be discussed. My references to Biblical and Classical sources do not imply endorsement of these views. Rather, they are meant to show the reader where we came from, and to demonstrate the universality of the issues discussed.

---

[1] For purposes of the entire book, the following definitions apply:

Adult: Someone old enough that her age will not be a factor in determining her has capacity to make medical decisions.

Child: Someone too young for categorical legal presumption that he has capacity to make medical decisions. This may be based on age, but the age of competence to make health care decisions differs among nations, usually 16–18 years.

Parent: An adult who is the default decision-maker for a child who does not have legal competence to make that decision.

State: An entity capable of enacting and enforcing legislation. States may be nations or subdivisions of nations.

Government: The organization(s) that enact and enforce legislation within a state.

Nation: (1) A fully sovereign state, or (2) a collection of people readily identifiable by each other and by outsiders, many of whom would like to form a fully sovereign state.

Law: A rule enforceable by government, which may be a statute, regulation, ordinance, precedential judicial opinion, etc.

Capacity: Ability to carry out a task or function, as measured by objective characteristics such as intelligence or physical capability. For example, one must be able to see and demonstrate knowledge of traffic law to drive an automobile.

Competence: Satisfaction of legal requirements to carry out a task or function, such as exceeding a certain age and passing a driving test to drive an automobile.

Table 1.1 Why be a parent

Benefit the world	Benefit oneself
Change the future for everyone[a]	To leave a legacy[b]
Invest in the human race[a]	"New life brings new responsibilities, new growth in yourself."[d]
Repay what I owe my parents[c]	Make oneself a better person[a]
Spiritual call to action[c]	Add to a greater sense of life's purpose
Fit in and meet society's expectations[b]	Feel the love of a child[c]
	Feel the love a parent has for a child[b]
Benefit the family	Personal growth[e]
To enrich our family[c]	New experience[c]
Grow and share familial love[a]	Kids are fun to hang out with and talk to[c]
Cultivate a strong lifelong bonds[c]	
	Other
Benefit the child	Give in to a biological urge[c]
Influence another person in how to live well[b]	It just happened
Re-create childhood joys[e]	
Be a better parent than I had[c]	

[a] Berry (2018)
[b] Dhel (2020), Mahon (2018)
[c] Allan (2017)
[d] Jensen (2018)
[e] Mitchell (2018)

1.1 The Problem

The subject of this book is the prerogatives, claims, powers, and immunities (see Chap. 2) of the stakeholders in parental decisions affecting a child's health. Stakeholders include parents, other family members, members of the child's local and cultural communities. They include the families and communities as discrete entities apart from their members. The health care team also has a stake, through their financial interest, their satisfaction at seeing children's health enhanced, and their moral distress when children suffer even though the suffering can be alleviated. Still other stakeholders include society as a whole, its members, and its government. The child, of course, usually is the primary stakeholder, while the state is the most powerful. Its power is limited only by its perceived legitimacy, by its practical ability to impose its will, and by constitutional guarantees that its citizens widely accept.

State interests inevitably come into conflict with parental interests with regard to decisions affecting children. Over two millennia ago, Euripides described the dilemma of King Agamemnon in his play, *Iphigenia at Aulis*. Agamemnon cannot sail with his Greek army to Troy because the goddess Artemis has sent unfavorable winds. Artemis will relent only if Agamemnon sacrifices his daughter, Iphigenia, who is in her teens. Agamemnon is under pressure from his army to slaughter his daughter. He must choose between his child and the good of the state.

Agamemnon faces two bad choices. So does every liberal state when confronted by the presence within them of groups with illiberal ideals, that govern themselves illiberally (Kymlicka andCohen-Almagor 2000). Examples of such authoritarian communities include company-owned mining towns, monasteries, and Old Amish settlements. The state, facing a *paradox of illiberalism*, has two bad choices. First, it can tolerate such groups. Schweder (2009) and Galston (2002) call it *liberal pluralism*. Such tolerance respects the citizens' prerogative of choice, but denies members of illiberal groups the presumed benefits of living in a liberal milieu. Second, the state can compel all citizens to abide by prevalent liberal norms. This view, called liberal imperialism (Shweder 2009), or liberal monism (Ye 2016), was famously championed by Okin (1998). A deficiency of this approach is that by forcing a liberal life on people who do not want it, the state is, itself, acting illiberally. A liberal state, then, must either act illiberally, tolerate illiberal enclaves, or find a balance between the two. One focus of this dilemma is how intrusively the state interferes with child raising practices.

The mirror image of Agamemnon's dilemma is Isaiah Berlin's *value pluralism*. The point of this doctrine is that there are too many good choices, and selection of the best choice cannot be done in a principled way that satisfies all (Berlin 1994). Desirable values and goods can conflict with each other. Thus, liberty and equality, justice and mercy, or knowledge and happiness may be incompatible. There often is no rational way to balance desirable values in tension with one another. Berlin's solution was tolerant compromise.

Consider the question of how to prioritize vaccination against COVID-19, when vaccines were first released and were scarce. People could be allowed to bid for the vaccine, if we believe that wealth roughly indicates a person's value to society and willingness to pay is a measure of the value of the vaccine to individuals. At the other extreme, the vaccine could be distributed by lottery, which removes all social distinctions as considerations. Third, people could be prioritized by risk of contracting COVID-19. A fourth way would be to prioritize distribution according to risk of death. A fifth allocation scheme would assign vaccine to those whose occupation or lifestyle made it most likely for them to spread the virus, with the goal of minimizing contagion. Sixth, healthcare workers could receive the vaccine preferentially, to induce them to stay on the job. Seventh, government could favor demographic groups on political grounds, such as compensation for prior injustice. Each of these rationales for distribution is based on a principle that might be a *pro tanto*[2] good. Each is in conflict with other distribution criteria motivated by other *pro tanto* justifications. No scheme is unequivocally ethically superior to the others.

Liberalism is a protean concept. Its political formulations range from libertarianism to the social democracy prevalent in Northern Europe. I characterize liberal democracy as majoritarianism constrained by the important negative liberties that characterize liberalism, such as freedom of expression and a fair criminal justice system. All current liberal democracy will provide a range of positive liberties, such as food and shelter. The extent of the welfare state differs from place to place. Liberalism is in conflict with equality (Kymlicka 1989) and with majoritarianism (Samet and Schmeidler 2003).

There need to be limitations on parental power. Almost everyone would protect children against grievous parental harm. There is little enthusiasm for repealing laws that criminalize child neglect and abuse. Illiberal groups must be subject to some state regulation. They must permit members to exit (Galston 2002), and must not use violence to undermine the state. Beyond such obvious examples, resolution of conflicts between parents and states regarding power over children must be based on a politically-determined *modus vivendi*. I prefer to minimize restrictions on citizens, and to maximize deference to parents. At the same time, society should guarantee that children's needs are met, irrespective of parental desire or ability to supply them.[3]

Practices of cultural and religious minorities are an ingredient of many conflicts with states, though others may be based on idiosyncratic parental beliefs. Governments may attempt to suppress minority practices that are in conflict with majority values, as with criminalization of corporal punishment. Alternatively, the state may force its own practices on minority children, as when mixed-sex physical education conflicts with traditional notions of modesty in Islam or Judaism. Governmental actions can reflect bias against parental status or beliefs. Recently, the German government removed four children from the care of parents who were home-schooling them instead of sending them to a government-approved school (*Wunderlich v. Germany*. Application #18925/15, European Court of Human Rights, 006 [2019]).

1.2 My Approach

I have been a child, a parent, a practicing physician, a medical administrator, and a lawyer. I have written about bioethics issues involving clashes between individual and state prerogatives. I am a member of a religious minority that has often been

---

[2] '*Pro tanto*,' literally, 'as far as it goes,' means that the item or argument at hand presents evidence toward justifying a point, but does not do so definitively.

[3] Although I mostly address liberal democracies, authoritarian states and illiberal democracies can also adopt my prescriptions. Empires such as the Mongols the Ottomans have tolerated extensive autonomy for linguistic and religious minorities. Israel and India, two democracies with strong established religious traditions, allow organized minority religions substantial authority over matters of personal status such as marriage and divorce.

subjected to persecution by governments and by private agents. My approach can be stated as follows:

1. This book does not ask what is right or wrong. Rather, my objective is to ask *whether states can use coercive means to right perceived wrongs.*
2. I assume that the family is the basic unit of social organization. However, families are fallible, and states should address serious flaws in family action. On the other hand, states are also fallible, and the scope of their power must be limited.
3. The work applies to liberal, Western societies, but can inform any society in which families are primary units of social organization.
4. The book seeks to develop a test to apply to parental actions, to evaluate whether the state may properly intervene. I call this test the State Intervention Test.
5. This requires excursions into political theory, as well as ethics and law. State exercise of power has its own intrinsic problems. We must balance tolerance of ills against the evils caused by governmental abuse of its power.
6. I consider the viewpoint of all stakeholders in these disputes, but I tend to be partial to the often-neglected parental perspective.
7. I value the findings of empirical investigators over speculation. Viewpoints based on false empirical premises are untenable, while those based on poorly demonstrated empirical affirmations are weak and unstable. Empirical studies in social and biological science are invoked in my discussion as relevant.

Any approach to resolving conflicts over child welfare should satisfy at least four elements. First, it must be compatible with the constitutional order and ethical values of the state. Second, the approach should be capable of generating both law- and ethics-based rules. Clinical ethics is toothless unless enacted into law. On the other hand, the law should reflect ethical values. Third, the approach must be able to address both general issues and individual disputes. Finally, the approach must be based on a clear and coherent account of the nature of the parent–child relationship.

I will attempt to develop a coherent, expedient approach to resolving parent/state conflicts over matters that affect child health. I first will discuss the relevant theoretical issues. I then will reify my approach as a test that I call the *State Intervention Test*. Finally, I will apply the test to important concrete examples.

I now propose a typology to classify theories of parent–child relationships. I identify four such types of relationships. These are stewardship, fidelity, ownership, and sovereignty, which may be democratic or paternalistic. I characterize Western families as being partially sovereign, with democratic and paternalistic elements.

1.3 Prioritization of Parental and Child Interests

Stewardship regards parents as being agents of the state in rearing children. Parenthood is a legally-defined status, which the state can assign, regulate, and revoke (Dwyer 2014). The rationale for the stewardship doctrine is twofold. First is concern regarding parental fitness (Dwyer 2014). The other is the desire to ensure that children are indoctrinated with appropriate values (Gutmann 1987). Supporters of the stewardship model tend to view citizenship as the most important connection among individuals. Rawls (2003), for example, considers the two goals of educating children, including education that occurs in the home, to be development of correct civic virtues, and producing self-supporting adults. A steward is the agent of a 'boss.' She looks after the boss's interests. The parent-steward is accountable to the state, which is the representative of the moral community (Dwyer 1994).

Those who see ties to the state as primary often are suspicious of intermediate groups besides the family. They frequently look at religion with a jaundiced eye. Some would forbid parents from indoctrinating children into their own religions (Shulman 2012). Brighouse and Swift (2014) are more moderate. They accept education in liberal religions such as Anglicanism, but not upbringing in fundamentalist denominations. They do not want parents to transmit bigotry to children (Sinclair et al. 2005).[4] Some would restrain parental rights if parents espouse intolerant ideas such as homophobia (Brennan and MacLeod 2017). It seems then, that a number of authors interested in restraining parental powers have political agendas.

The second model of the parent–child relationship is that parents are *fiduciaries* for their children (Fleishman et al. 1998). Parents do not fit the model of fiduciaries. Fiduciary relationships have five characteristics. The first is a limited, well-defined scope, such as lawyer or trustee. Second, fiduciaries typically receive compensation for their service, in consideration for the efforts and fiduciary restraints. The final three elements of a fiduciary relationship are the three fiduciary duties—care, loyalty, and abstention from self-dealing (*Cinerama v. Technicolor, Inc.*, 663 A. 2d 1156, Delaware Supreme Court, 1995). The duty of care requires that the fiduciary be attentive and somewhat competent (*Smith v. Van Gorkom*, 488 A. 2d 858, 873, Delaware Supreme Court, 1985). The fiduciary must act in the honest belief that her actions are in the beneficiary's best interest. Delaware Supreme Court). The duty of loyalty precludes conflicting duties to different fiduciary beneficiaries. Finally, abstention from self-dealing requires that fiduciaries subordinate their own interests to those of their beneficiaries.

The parental relationship does not meet any of these five criteria! It is not limited in scope. Parents are custodians, guides, protectors, etc. This exceeds the scope of a fiduciary relationship. Parents do not receive compensation for their services to their children. Rather, they must provide their children's material support. Finally, parents cannot avoid self-dealing or conflict of interest. Family life is a constant balancing of the interests of all family members.

The third model, the *ownership* model, holds that children are, in essence, parents' property until they reach legal majority. Apart from a few libertarians (Narveson 1988), the ownership model persists now only as a straw man proposed as the only alternative to state-empowering models.

---

[4] Other factors, such as peer interaction, may be at least as important in acquisition of bias (Zembylas et al. 2010).

The fourth model is *family sovereignty*. This can be *paternalistic*, *democratic*, or mixed. Family sovereignty corresponds most closely to the actual range of family structures across Western societies. A sovereign entity is a group that makes rules and decisions for itself. Sovereignty need not be complete. A group may be able to make decisions in some areas, but not in others. Also, the group's decisions may be subject to review by a higher sovereignty. Thus, state or provincial decisions may be subject to national law, and the state can review family decisions.

Aristotle (1999, Book 1, Part 12) advanced a *paternalistic sovereignty* model of the family; the father governed the family. But family sovereignty was partial, as families and their members were responsible to the state. Confucius and his successors elaborated another model of paternalistic sovereignty. The Confucian parent–child relationship is characterized by simultaneous hierarchy and mutuality (Tsai 2005). Although not based on equality, the superior should treat the dependent with beneficence and the dependent should treat the superior with respect. This reciprocal relationship, stripped of some of its sexist elements, is said to characterize the typical contemporary Chinese family (Qi 2015).

Democratic sovereignty seeks the contribution and assent of all members of a family. Parents might, for example, consult even a young child regarding what he wants to eat or wear. Decisions are not made by a single leader, but are negotiated within the family.

Actual family governance is intermediate between patriarchal and democratic. In optimal situations, parents give the child adequate care, and, in turn, receive the child's love (though not necessarily obedience!). Families may move from patriarchal toward democratic governance as children grow older, develop preferences and have greater capacity to form judgments and argue for them. State rules and norms constrain family decisions.

At this point it may be useful to describe in more detail the views of one of the most articulate advocates of the stewardship model (Dwyer 2021) (Table 1.2). James Dwyer believes that the only relevant issue is the best interests of the child, literally interpreted, with relevant interests and their importance defined by the state. The state should designate the best candidate for parenthood, based on empirically verifiable facts. Choice of biological parent is only a *ceteris paribus*[5] presumption. The state determines on an ongoing basis whether the parent it designates remains the best person to continue in the parental role, stability of the relationship being only one factor present in the consideration. Though Dwyer refers to the guardian as a fiduciary, his description of the parental role is closer to stewardship, a characterization he has used in the past (Dwyer 2014). In Dwyer's view the state determines the interests of the child, determines the parental role, and assesses the performance of the parents. Dwyer might be likely to disfavor religion and parents who espouse religion (Dwyer 1994). It is easy to see how this arrangement invites political abuse.

Dwyer's justifications are based on appeals to his conception of children's rights. His view is that the goal of child-rearing is to maximize the autonomy of the child and of the future adult—both controversial and vague propositions. The explicit and

[5] All other things being equal.

Table 1.2 Dwyer's assumptions versus more accurate assumptions (Dwyer2021)

Parameter	Dwyer's view (explicit or tacit)	Alternative to Dwyer's view
Primacy	Family ties are a creation of the state	Families are primary
Allegiance of the child	Primarily a citizen	Primarily friends and family
Nature of the state	Beneficent	Often indifferent, corrupt, or cruel
Role of the state	Plenary	Limited to prevent abuse of state power
Comparison with other vulnerable people	State-appointed guardians look out for their interests, which are clear-cut and limited	Children need to be taught morals, manners, survival skills, etc. There are many approaches, and solutions are controversial
What must be protected	Maximization of child's interest fulfillment	Needs
Determination of interests and needs	Can be done by government officials, aided by experts	Nature and priority of needs are controversial. Bias of experts disadvantages many citizens
Status of parent	Utterly subordinate to interests of children	Parenting is generally considered a great good—an interest tantamount to a need. And children grow up to be adults with this need
Parental motivation	Unclear	Love, perpetuation of identity, experience of participating in and watching development of child
Love	Does not appear in Dwyer's essay	A key part of parent–child bonding, and a good in itself
Biological relationship	Significance minimized	Important motivator per se. Also, similarities between children and parents are motivating and give pleasure to parents
"Daddy Warbucks" problem	Welcomed	Source of horror and disgust

implicit errors I believe Dwyer makes are outlined in Table 1.2. The table is self-explanatory except for the last line—the 'Daddy Warbucks' problem, named for the guardian of the comic strip character Orphan Annie. Imagine that the Warbucks, a wealthy, respectable couple, are universally regarded as excellent parents of their daughter, Wilma. When Wilma dies of leukemia at age 7, the Warbucks decide they want to adopt Annie, the winsome 5-year-old daughter of an unmarried meter maid. Annie spends much of her time in child care, because her mother has to work 60 h a week to support the family. A court awards parental rights to the Warbucks, deeming that although Annie's current mother is adequate, the Warbucks will make better parents.

There are potential negative externalities attached to a system such as Dwyer contemplates. For example, it exposes parents to denunciations by neighbors, and to hostile actions by government agencies, potentially creating a climate of suspicion and fear. It may invite children to denounce parents, as has been the case in China, Nazi Germany, the USSR, and even the United States (Watts 1987; *In re Grand Jury Proceedings, Unemancipated Minor Child.* 949 F. Supp. 1487, US District Court, E.D. Washington, 1996).

This book assumes that the family is a basic unit of society, and not a government creation. It is organized under a mixed, partial sovereignty model. States must meet a high burden of proof to interfere in family matters, let alone to break up a family.

1.4 What Parents Owe Children

Determining the adequacy of decisions regarding children relies on three components, which Buchanan and Brock (1989) call principles. First is the *guidance* principle—how parents should treat children under ideal circumstances. Second, there must be an *intervention* principle that provides clear standards for determining when parental care deviates so far from the ideal as to invite coercive state action. Finally, there must be recognition of a legitimate *authority* for formulating guidance and intervention standards, monitoring compliance with them, and intervening as needed. Any doctrinal approach to determine when states may intervene to change parental decisions must specify these principles.

The guidance principal I propose is that parents should promote children's *flourishing*. If this is the case, we must know what it is to flourish. The factors that contribute to flourishing must be fleshed out empirically. Armchair determination of what leads to flourishing are insufficient, though they may offer a framework for study. Theories of flourishing may be *subjective* or *objective* (Haybron 2016). *Subjective* approaches look to each individual to decide what makes her flourish, and whether she is flourishing. Theories asserting that flourishing consists of realization of one's desires are called *hedonic*. However, people make bad choices; they ride motorcycles and enter abusive relationships. The ability of individuals to align their desires with their overall goals is limited by the hurried nature of 'fast system' decisions, and by the distortion of 'slow system' decision from noise, bias, and heuristics (Kahneman 2011). It is axiomatic that any theory of human good must be compatible with human physiological and psychological capacities. This leads to interest in objective theories.

Objective theories either attribute the same needs to all people, or seek ways for outside observers to measure aspects of flourishing in any person. They fall into two categories: *eudaimonic* (or 'nature fulfillment'), or *list theories* (Haybron 2016).

Eudaimonic accounts are those that equate well-being with fulfilling one's role as a human, aligned with human nature (Haybron 2007, 2008). *List theories* such

Table 1.3 Proposed human capabilities (after Nussbaum 2007)

1. Life. Being able to live a life of normal length and decent quality
2. Adequate health, food, and housing
3. Bodily Integrity. Absence of domestic and outside violence, freedom of movement, sexual satisfaction, and reproductive choice
4. Senses, Imagination, and Thought. Education sufficient to use the senses, imagine, and reason. Experience and produce imaginative works of one's own choice. Political, artistic, and religious freedom. Avoid non-beneficial pain
5. Emotions. Being able to have attachments to things and people. Capacity for love, grief, anger, and other emotions. This requires forms of association necessary for emotional development
6. Practical Reason. Being able to form a conception of the good and to make life plans. This requires typical liberal negative rights
7. Affiliation A. Ability to live with others, empathize, have social interaction. This requires typical liberal negative rights B. Expectation of treatment as a dignified person whose moral worth is not subject to status considerations. This implies absence of inequality based on race, sex, sexual orientation, ethnicity, religion, etc
8. Non-human life. Being able to live with animals, plants, and the world of nature
9. Play. Recreation and enjoyment
10. Environment A. Political. Being able to participate effectively in political dialog and in politics B. Material. Being able to hold property. Equal basis for seeking and obtaining employment. Personal privacy

as Nussbaum's capability theory (Nussbaum 1997) and the functionality theory of Powers and Faden (2006) have been quite influential because they easily link to political programs. But the lists often are derived from speculation rather than from empiric validation. Table 1.3 details one list of capabilities or interests said to be important to children (Nussbaum 2007).

The large volume of empirical research on well-being has had an impact on the credibility of such lists. This impact undoubtedly will increase as psychological research deepens our understanding of flourishing. Subjective well-being has been linked to positive affective states, minimal experience of negative emotions, and global life satisfaction (Adler and Seligman 2016). Multiple factors contribute to flourishing, and are fairly consistent across societies. Seligman (2011) summarizes these factors using the acronym PERMA (pleasure, engagement, relationships, meaning, and accomplishment). 'Meaning,' to Seligman, is identifying and connecting with something larger than oneself. 'Accomplishment' is objective mastery or success in a field of endeavor. This may mean, for example, writing a book or mastering a language. It may also mean success in some form of competition. The other three items are self-explanatory.

Table 1.4 lists the factors that representative investigators have found to be most important for flourishing. Empiric findings such as these may serve as a basis for policy recommendations. People who tell investigators what is important to them

Table 1.4 Factors contributing to subjective well-being according to selected empirical studies

Author	Factors contributing to subjective well-being	
Kahneman and Deaton (2010)	Life evaluation Emotional health Physical health	Healthy behaviors Work environment Access to basic needs
Organization for Economic Cooperation and Development (Durand 2015)	Housing Income and wealth Jobs and earnings Social connections Education and skills Environmental quality	Civil engagement and governance Health status Life satisfaction Personal security Work-life balance
Ryff and Keyes (1995)	Self-acceptance Positive relationships with others Autonomy	Environmental mastery Purpose in life Personal growth
Seligman (2011)	Positive emotion Engagement Positive relationships	Meaning or purpose Achievement
VanderWeele (2017)	Family Work Religious community Happiness and life satisfaction	Physical and mental health Meaning and purpose Character and virtue Close social relationships
Węziak-Białowolska et al. (2018)	Happiness and life satisfaction Mental and physical health Meaning and purpose	Character and virtue Close social relationships Financial and material stability

consider health to be important, but autonomy less so. This relative lack of interest in autonomy stands in contrast to the emphasis on autonomy in philosophical writings. Most people prioritize relationships, meaning, physical security, and external validation. This should have major implications for the applied ethics of child-rearing.

1.5 Capabilities and Functioning

Sen (2011) explains capability in an intuitive and elegant way. At the individual level, Leah and Rachel (the names are of my choosing), each want to see a movie tomorrow. Leah can choose between seeing the movie and doing something else. Rachel will be compelled to go to the movie. Though both want to see the movie, Leah's capabilities are greater because she has a choice while Rachel does not. At the state level, compare Edom and Moab, which have comparable *overall* utility and wealth. In Edom, many people are malnourished, have cold dwellings in winter, and frequently die of preventable diseases. Married Edomite women are not allowed to leave their homes. Moabites enjoy greater gender equality and sufficient distribution of wealth that nobody starves or freezes. Sen would fault Edom for failing to provide all its citizens with fundamental capabilities.

Nussbaum (2007) has generated a list of capabilities she considers necessary to achieve a full human life (Table 1.3). She seems to have compiled the list without recourse to empiric social science literature. Nussbaum's capabilities are not fungible, so that a surplus of one capability does not compensate for a dearth of another. Upon reading the list, one wonders whether Nussbaum requires too much. Are humor and recreation really required for full humanity? Is a child with a serious permanent disability or a limited life span leading less than a fully human life? What about a sociopathic person with blunted emotional capacity? Malek (2009) created a widely cited inventory of 14 interests (Table 1.5) that closely resemble Nussbaum's capabilities. Powers and Faden (2006) emphasize the goal of not just having capabilities, but realization of these capabilities (which they call functioning) They propose that everyone is entitled as a matter of right to a sufficient level of well-being in each of six dimensions. These dimensions are health, personal security, reasoning (including the ability to formulate one's own way of life and life plan), respect from others, attachment, and self-determination. While most items on these lists are desirable, some are clearly more critical than others. The roster of capabilities is also highly aspirational. Few can achieve a full range of the things that these authors desire for

Table 1.5 Interests of children (after Malek 2009)

1. Life: To live and to anticipate a life of normal human length
2. Health and healthcare: To have good health and protection from pain, injury, and illness. To have access to medical care
3. Basic needs: To have an adequate standard of living, especially to be adequately nourished and sheltered
4. Protection from neglect and abuse: To be protected from physical or mental abuse, neglect, exploitation, and exposure to dangerous environments. To be secure that they will be safe and cared for
5. Emotional development: To experience emotion and have appropriate emotional development
6. Play and pleasure: To play, rest, and enjoy recreational activities. To have pleasurable experiences
7. Education and cognitive development: To have an education that includes information from diverse sources. To have the ability to learn, think, imagine, and reason
8. Expression and communication: To have the ability to express themselves and to communicate thoughts and feelings
9. Interaction: To interact with and care for others and the world around them. To have secure, empathetic, intimate, and consistent relationships with others
10. Parental relationship: To know and interact with their parents
11. Identity: To have an identity and connection to their culture. To be protected from discrimination
12. Sense of self: To have a sense of self, self-worth, and self-respect
13. Autonomy: To have the ability to influence the course of their lives. To act intentionally and with self-discipline. To reflect on the direction and meaning of their lives

everyone. Powers and Faden are more realistic than some authors in that they take a sufficientarian approach.

These lists seem informed primarily by feminist and egalitarian values. Evolutionary psychology might designate as an important capability a general capacity to compete (Buss and Schmitt 2019; Henrich 2016, 2020). Flourishing requires some ability to compete for mates, status, and resources. Buss and Henrich also would deem the ability to engage in goal directed social cooperation to be a necessary capability. Another important capability is the ability to make contributions that others value. Nussbaum cites the ability to work, but her concern is with equal rights and on the quality of the work experience. I am concerned with the capacity to produce output that is valued sufficiently by other people that it evokes a *quid pro quo*. This need not be an economic exchange; a stay-at-home parent is performing a valuable service, as, perhaps, is a member of a religious order. A final capability is resilience to stress.

Nussbaum may have been remiss in not discussing how to rank the value of her capabilities against each other, or to decide how much of each is necessary. And the central question of this book is deciding when things are so bad that the state should step in.[6]

I will expand on the key importance of being able to compete. Human existence is characterized by competition both among individuals and among groups of individuals. One basic field of competition is mating (Buss and Schmitt 2019). The ability to present oneself as an attractive mate is an important capability. There is differential desirability among potential mates whether mate choice is left to individuals themselves or determined by third parties (as with arranged marriages). Few would advocate overriding standards of mate desirability, as by forcibly assigning random mates. Humans also engage in interpersonal competition for resources important for well-being and for status, which is important for satisfaction as well as for reproductive success (Shenk et al. 2016). The ability to compete, and development of the emotional and cognitive habits that support this ability, are universally important capabilities.

The ability to engage in goal-directed social cooperation also is an important human capability. Whether involving hunting, war, or peaceful pursuits, it is vital for human success that individual people work together towards important goals. (Cosmides et al. 2018). Indeed, Curry (2016) calls cooperation the basis of all morality.

I would wish to see children equipped with these capabilities. Adequate health is important to achieve all of them. Since health is a prerequisite for attaining most capabilities in most catalogues of capabilities, it is important to *actually attain* health, and not just *to be able to attain* health (Tengland 2019). Ironically, some capabilities

[6] Security against physical violence may be important, for example, but if someone shoves me aside to take a seat on a subway car, I am not leading a significantly emptier human life. A *de minimis* dignitary violation is found in Jewish public worship, in which descendants of ancient priests (*Cohanim*) have certain liturgical privileges. Some congregations have eliminated this practice on egalitarian grounds. I doubt that either of these denials of Nussbaum's capabilities is worth much attention from the state.

are enhanced by activities that are detrimental to health. Quasi-competitive drinking behavior and some sports are examples of unhealthy behaviors that train for both competition and cooperation. Physical alteration, such as tattoos and circumcision, may be vital for belonging, status, and mating. The prevalence of these customs suggests they may confer a competitive advantage that outweighs their disadvantages to health. The capabilities approach is becoming increasingly influential in health care evaluation (Mitchell et al. 2017).

Paradoxically, conversion of capability into functioning is likely to reduce the scope of potential capabilities (Tengland 2016). I am born with the ability to learn any language. But as I learn to speak one or a few languages, I forego the ability to speak most of the thousands of languages that exist. As I make commitments with regard to occupation, belief, and spouse, I surrender myriad alternate, competing commitments. Parents inevitably direct their children's preferences and interests. They must find a mean between raising children to be narrow and bigoted, versus not providing a basic view of the world that provides a conceptual and spiritual anchor.[7] Parents have to make other choices in which children face opposing capabilities, one of which is health. Should parents, for instance, allow their children to play contact sports? Use sweets as a reward for desirable behavior? Too little personal security may lead to psychological unease and chronic fear. Too much may not allow the child to develop habits of resilience when challenged with a real threat.

The state should assure that the physical needs of children are met, and certainly provide sufficient health care. I will suggest a sufficientarian approach to this, arguing that the state should set a floor below which children cannot fall; it should not seek redistribution above that level. When possible, government should either defer to parents or use non-coercive means of influencing parental behavior.

1.6 Non-liberal Approaches

I will briefly summarize some important positions that would undermine either families or liberalism. These positions identify important problems. However, they do not make a plausible case for believing that their program would actually benefit children. Nor do they question whether states can be trusted to advance children's interests without restraint from non-governmental elements of civil society, including the family.

[7] Children do not necessarily follow their parents' lead. Some children may rebel against an authoritarian upbringing. Others, raised in a permissive home, may adopt views repugnant to their parents, be depressed because of lack of a lodestar of meaning in their lives, or fall in with a charismatic cult leader because the parent has failed to ground them in a thick set of values. A child whose temperament needs structure will seek structure, and one who wishes to be free of parental influence may well rebel against parental ideals and values.

1.6.1 Vulnerability

Vulnerability theory, expressed by Martha Fineman and Robert Goodin, demands vigorous state action and radical reorganization of the family. Vulnerability is susceptibility to harm. It may be *embodied*—intrinsic to human nature (Fineman 2015). Everyone is susceptible to pain, and we all eventually die. It may be *embedded*—caused by outside influences such as the possibility of violence or humiliation (Fineman 2008). The complexity and mutual dependence inherent in modern society enhances our vulnerability. An example of this is the shortage of medical equipment and supplies experienced during the early stages of the Covid-19 pandemic. Fineman (2019) emphasizes that our vulnerability shows that we are not the autonomous, independent beings that some writers assume we are. However, she proposes that, because women bear the brunt of caretaking, the family be radically reorganized. Furthermore, Goodin (1986) asserts an individual and joint responsibility for protecting the vulnerable. This joint responsibility falls, at least as a last resort, to the state.

The remedy for vulnerability is resilience, the ability to adapt successfully in the face of stress and adversity, when these threaten function, survival, or future development (Masten and Barnes 2018). Stressors are external to the individual, but resilience arises from factors that are both external and internal. Prenatal stressors include poor fetal weight gain, maternal drug use, and congenital defects. Children may be subject to neglect, malnutrition, physical or emotional abuse, absence or death of a parent, and grave illness or injury. Racial discrimination, and minority status per se, may be stressors. Severe stress produces adverse effects (Masten and Barnes 2018), but low-level stress may bolster resilience.

Innate differences in resilience are recognized (Richardson 2002), but have not been studied as much as external factors. Parent–child relationships are crucial to resilience in children (Traub and Boynton-Jarrett 2017). Small families with mature parents in a stable, intimate, relationship appear to promote resilience in children. Poverty is a significant stressor, as is lack of physical safety (Masten and Barnes 2018). It should not be surprising that the factors that contribute to flourishing also contribute to resilience. Resilience seems to be something like flourishing under adverse circumstances, as many of the same qualities and characteristics further both flourishing and resilience.

1.6.2 Critical Theory

Some scholars and activists believe that the primary focus should not be on individual needs. Rather, they would treat individuals as representative members of groups, subject to group vulnerabilities and group interests. Some of these views are profoundly anti-liberal, and certainly anti-pluralist. One such approach, critical social justice, has come to dominate academic discussion in many fields. I cannot discuss critical theory in detail, as it is not directly relevant to health. It is not incompatible with my prescriptions. Liberalism is not necessary to toleration, nor does democracy guarantee it.

Social justice and health equity have been widely adopted in American academic medical circles. The meanings of 'justice' and 'equity' are not traditional when used in these contexts. In common usage, social justice now usually refers to state programs designed to correct inequalities in Western liberal capitalist societies. This entails a focus on group differences. These approaches have some diagnostic validity. Group beliefs and practices can affect both health and the interaction between individuals and the health care system. Some members of minority cultural groups may, for example, refuse treatment by doctors on the basis of the doctors' gender or religion (Padela and del Pozo 2011). This exposes a conflict between liberal anti-discriminatory norms and the norm of respecting the perspective of the member of the less powerful group. Physicians, as well as patients, can be biased. Such bias can be based on class, race, or gender. This does not indicate that society is inexorably racist, despite the centrality of this concept in critical race theory (Brown and Jackson 2013).

Some critical social justice academicians maintain that oppression is inherent in the very notion of objectivity and clinical distance that are intrinsic to a traditional approach to medical professionalism (Thesen 2005). I am not as pessimistic. I believe that cultural groups can coexist under conditions of toleration and equality, if not necessarily amity. Physicians can take cultural differences into account, and provide the same level of care to all their patients. Many disputes involving parental decisions involve parental cultural practices which health professionals should tolerate. Patients in general, and those from subordinate groups, in particular, can be victimized by epistemic injustice (Kidd and Carel 2017).[8] At present, poor people and racial minorities may be given short shrift by physicians, consciously or not. Upper class Christian Scientist parents may have more leeway for withholding medical care from a child than lower class Jehovah's Witnesses parents. Furthermore, minority parents may be more likely to come under suspicion of child neglect or abuse (Lane et al. 2002).

Those treating children should be sensitive to the concerns and needs of children in marginalized groups, and should try to be sensitive to the parents' point of view, acceding to parents unless there is behavior that they would characterize as neglect or abuse in mainstream families.[9]

Critical social justice theories are antithetical to the liberal pluralism that I espouse. Many adherents advocate suppression of opposing points of view from academic and public life. At best, they emphasize groups over individuals, and tend to see competition for society's resources as a zero-sum game. I have devoted a space to

---

[8] Epistemic injustice consists of *hermeneutic injustice*, which is limitation in the ability of subordinate group members to present its knowledge, and *testimonial injustice* which is the diminished credibility of a person in a subordinate position (Fricker 2007).

[9] Or unless the child's assent is appropriate, or if the child is competent to make a medical decision without parental consent.

this movement because of its increasing predominance in professional life (American Medical Association 2021). While I agree with many of the goals of many critical social justice activists, I find their approach to be antithetical to a liberal democracy committed to the widest possible acceptance of all persons.

1.7 Procedural Fairness

Assurance that the process is perceived as legitimate and fair requires that the rules be *coherent*. Rules should be enforced consistently. Analogous cases should lead to similar outcomes. There will be borderline cases or new problems that prevent complete elimination of indeterminacy. Second, rules governing decision-making should be *transparent*. Third, there should be *societal consensus* as to the applicability of the standard. Intuitively, an approach that will be successful in Western societies will give greatest weight to the needs and interests of the child, while also addressing those of other interested parties. Fourth, child welfare should not be used as a pretext for attacks against minorities. Finally, the harms that comes from punishing or averting parental malfeasance should not exceed the harms of the malfeasance itself.

Conversely, the process for adjudicating parent/state conflicts should avoid indeterminacy and conclusory terms. *Indeterminacy* is a situation in which a rule as generally understood does not predict the outcome of a conflict described in a specific fact set. A *conclusory term* or *rule* is one in which the decision defines the term or the rule, rather than the reverse. Conclusory decisions occur when the meaning of indeterminate terms is influenced by different understandings and values of different deciders (Bazelon 1982). Birchley (2016) describes an excellent example of this. In London, two different judges in the same district at the same time came to opposite conclusions in cases with almost identical facts. The two mothers who were respondents in these cases went to a developing nation, were told they were pregnant, had a 'cesarean section,' and returned to London with babies that actually were not biologically theirs. Their care for the infants was excellent. The standard for whether the babies should be removed from the home was whether the child "is suffering, or is likely to suffer, *significant harm*" (UK *Children Act*, 1989, cl. 31(2), Eng, Wales, emphasis supplied). Judge Coleridge allowed the first mother to keep the child. Judge Ryder, though, terminated parental rights of the other mother, because being raised under false pretenses was a significant harm. A different couple was allowed to adopt the infant. "Significant harm" proved to be a conclusory term that meant what the sitting judge said it meant.

Considerations of fairness and justice are best served if rules minimize indeterminacy. Vague rules allow decisions involving children to be influenced by bias. It is difficult to completely avoid standards from being applied unfairly against unattractive individuals or marginalized groups, even when the standards appear clear and determinate. A British statute (UK *Female Genital Mutilation Act*, 2003, Eng., Wales) prohibits non-medical labial reduction (labioplasty) in women of any age. UK authorities consider cosmetic labioplasty, but not ritual labioplasty, as being medically appropriate. No society is perfectly liberal. But any approach to the problem of resolving parent-state conflict should attempt to secure both substantive and procedural fairness.

1.8 The Book's Project

I will propose a way to adjudicate parent/state conflicts involving children's health and safety. It will be based on a liberal pluralist perspective. It will respect individual and culturally-inspired choices up to the point where children's health and safety is seriously threatened, or there is unreasonable burden to society at large. A model for adjudicating parent-state disputes in a democracy must be consequentialist. First, liberal pluralism is incompatible with principled consensus, as there is no principled way to rank the importance of contradictory goals. Second, in a democracy, elections, legislation, and negotiated compromises are likely to center on substantive issues rather than on theoretical ones. This is because voters are likely to be swayed by concrete issues—both economic (Franzese 2002) and others. As well as self-perceived overall satisfaction (Liberini et al. 2017). My consequentialist, liberal pluralistic approach with constraints to protect unpopular ideas and practices will be reified as a two-step decision process which I call the State Intervention Test.

The State Intervention Test will accommodate the tension between the interests of children and those of other members of the family, including other children. Also, I will place greater stress on broad societal interests than has generally been seen in the ethics literature, which often views parents and children as an isolated dyad. The objective needs of the broader society should receive more attention from scholars in this area. Thus, my approach considers the interests of all significant stakeholders. I seek to guard against inappropriate bias against minority perspectives, whether idiosyncratic or culturally-based. I do this by proposing constraints against otherwise appropriate government action which disadvantages unpopular practices and groups.

1.9 Outline of the Book

The first several chapters set forth the theoretical basis for the State Intervention Test. This section of this book considers the interests and needs of the child, of the family, the culture or religion in which the family is embedded, and the broader society and its members. I desire extensive political liberty and safeguards for procedural fairness by the state. I thus reject approaches based both on liberal monism and illiberal theories such as Critical Race Theory and its analogs.

Chapter 2, ***The Primrose Path: Rights and Autonomy***, discusses putative rights of the child. It addresses both the concept of rights and specific rights, focusing especially on widely posited rights to autonomy. Rights may be legal or ethical.

Legal rights need no justification, but are enforceable. Rights proposed on ethical grounds are backed by attempts at intellectual justification, but are unenforceable. Rights may conflict, in which case there may or may not be guidelines for prioritizing some rights over others.

I describe rights as Hohfeldian relationships. Rights either direct or limit the scope of action of other parties with regard to the rightsholder's freedom or goods. I begin to examine the relationship between parents and children, and express some skepticism regarding whether rights language is useful in describing familial relationships under normal circumstances. I then address issues of autonomy as applied to the child. Respect for autonomy is a key constraint in professional relationships, but is not as important in all human intercourse. As we have seen, the emphasis on autonomy in the ethical literature ignores the vast body of empiric evidence on human flourishing that has been generated over the last 30 years, which does not assign the same importance to autonomy as philosophers often do. Actual individuals turn out to prioritize material satisfaction and relationships. Individuals understand that they are embedded members of wider local groups, such as families and networks of friends. I suggest that human flourishing is a more reasonable target of ethical and political theory. We should seek flourishing of the child, rather than make autonomy the *summum bonum*.

Chapter 3, ***What Is Relevant: Interests, Needs, and Harms***, analyzes the interests and needs of the child. It discusses the best interests standard and the harm principle, and tries to find a more sophisticated standard for the guidance and intervention principles. To this end, the chapter divides the intervention principle into two phases. It argues that there must be an *identification phase* governed by a standard for unacceptability of parental behavior. There is then a second *resolution phase*, whose standard is based on maximizing the interests of all stakeholders, which include family and society.

The approaches discussed so far devote little attention to parties other than the child affected by a parental decision. However, it is necessary to broaden the population of relevant interested parties to include the family and each of its members. Chapter 4, ***What We Owe Parents and Family***, discusses family-centered theoretical approaches, such as that of Ross (1998). In balancing the needs and interests of various family members, parents' decisions often satisfy the harm principal, but fail to pass a strictly construed best interests standard. These decisions fall into an intermediate category between categorically acceptable and unacceptable behavior, which Gillam (2016) called the Zone of Parental Discretion. I divide the Zone of Parental discretion into two categories, that I call the zone of state attention and the zone of concern. Parental behavior in the zone of state attention merits educational action and provision of services. Behavior in the zone of concern may call for a more interventionist approach, such as nudging, or mandatory programs with opt-out. Coercive measures are limited to the zone of unacceptable parental behavior, and that is what the State Intervention Test addresses.

Chapter 5, ***What Society May Claim: Public Health***, expands the horizon of interest beyond the child and family, considering the needs of society as a whole, and its members. States have a compelling interest in public health and safety, protecting citizens from threats to their health by other individuals and groups. The chapter reviews concepts in public heath ethics, providing a background for the State Intervention Test's emphasis on protecting society. It then turns to a brief review of currently fashionable anti-liberal ideology, explaining them and showing their incompatibility with liberal pluralism.

Chapter 6, ***Political Considerations in a Liberal Pluralist State***, provides the theoretical basis for the State Intervention Test. It discusses the appropriate limits of political action in an actual world, in which citizens pursue their own interests, and leaders often are corrupt and narcissistic. The chapter applies realist political theory to propose a political system based on negotiated *modus vivendi* constrained by constitutional guarantees. The chapter argues that systems constrained by scarcity, such as health care systems and matters requiring government oversight, must be sufficientarian. The currency that governs children's needs, as provided by parents, is *prevention of parental malfeasance*. The state must prevent parental malfeasance to a sufficient degree. The sufficiency limit for this currency is whether patents meet the child's fundamental needs, as defined in the State Intervention Test.

Chapter 7, ***The State Intervention Test: When to Interfere with Parental Decisions***, is the heart of the book. The State Intervention Test explicitly considers the needs of the child and the needs of society. Its consideration of the needs of other family members is implicit, and parents are given wide discretion. The State Intervention Test is the latest iteration of a test I first proposed in 2013 (Jacobs 2013) and which I refined in collaboration with Kavita Shah Arora and Hillel Levin. The State Intervention Test has two components. First, it stipulates two *bases* for limiting parental practices. One is that a parental practice should not create an unreasonable burden for either society as a whole or for members of society outside a family or group that endorses the controversial practice. The second basis is that there is a substantial chance that the child in question will be exposed to major physiological dysfunction, death, or comparable severe disadvantage (such as malnutrition or major psychological morbidity).

The Test then proposes three *constraints* on the state in so limiting such practices. The first constraint on government action is that the harm underlying restriction on parental decisions must be actual and likely, rather than hypothetical or rare. The second constraint is that harms forming the basis for a restriction must be greater than harms typically tolerated for comparable mainstream practices. This prevents governments from selectively stopping harmful practices, using the harm as a rationale for persecuting minorities. This is what happened in the Florida statutory schema that was overturned in *Church of the Lukumi Babalu Aye, Inc. v. City of Hialeah*, 508 U.S. 520, Supreme Court, 1993. Finally, the overall benefits of the restriction should foreseeably exceed overall harms.

The remainder of the book describes specific applications of the State Intervention Test.

Chapter 8, ***Treatment of Disease***, addresses treatment issues in children young enough that their consent or assent is not a factor. Four paradigms are explored. First is the situation in which custodial parents disagree on treatment. Second is the parent who does not want to accede to a physician's recommendations. The third paradigm is the reverse of this—the parent makes demands that the physician believes are inappropriate. Finally, the chapter discusses situations in which a parent or physician inappropriately tries to undermine the other's authority. This chapter demonstrates how the State Intervention Test can determine when to justify interference with parental decisions in medical decision-making for children.

Chapter 9, ***Prevention and Screening***, applies of the Test to parental refusal to expose children to disease prevention programs, using vaccination requirements as a paradigm. Here, honoring parental preferences has consequences to society and its members. I then discuss other low-risk screening and diagnostic procedures. Here, the primary risk is to the child at issue.

Some procedures are performed not to alleviate or prevent disease, but to enhance desired traits that benefit the child. This is the subject of Chap. 10, ***Enhancement of Function***. There are two paradigms here. One is a child with an attribute that falls below levels that might result in an average degree of secular success. An example is a cleft lip that does not interfere with nutrition. The other paradigm is the use of medicine to take a child with ordinary attributes and elevate them to excellence. In the context of the State Intervention Test, I discuss parental power to alleviate low function or to boost function in the absence of disability.

I then discuss ***The Maturing Minor*** in Chap. 11. This chapter concerns the child who is capable of understanding alternative courses of treatment and of forming relatively mature judgments. Unfortunately, intellectual capacity develops far sooner than the ability to apply rational understanding in a mature manner to personal medical decisions. Adolescents are inclined to be unduly optimistic, to prioritize possibility of reward over possibility of risk, and to be strongly influenced by actual or perceived group pressure and by the need for group approval. Furthermore, they are dependent on their parents to satisfy their material needs, and so subject to possible undue parental influence. The chapter scrutinizes approaches to such minors with partially mature higher brain function.

The next two chapters concern issues of sexuality and reproduction. Chapter 12, ***Sexual and Reproductive Issues I: Education; Reproductive Choices***, addresses the education that minors should receive in sexuality for their own protection and optimal sexual development. It goes on to discuss the rationales for bypassing the usual parental responsibility for minors' health care decisions in situations involving sexuality and reproduction, such as contraception and abortion. Parents' ideology regarding these issues may differ from those of their children, and the consequences of pregnancy may be great. Furthermore, there is a strong public health interest in avoiding adolescent pregnancy. Chapter 13, ***Sexual and Reproductive Issues II: Departures from Binary Sexual and Gender Viewpoints***, address principally disorders of sexual differentiation and gender incongruity. These are controversial issues in which parents and physicians are likely to disagree. Without arriving at a definitive conclusion, I maintain that the criteria of the State Intervention Test should set the standard for evaluating approaches to these issues.

The next two chapters concern ritual procedures that modify children's genitalia. Chapter 14, ***Genital Rituals: Circumcision***, concerns circumcision, or removal of the penile foreskin. It largely discusses ethical issues. Chapter 15, ***Female Genital***

Alteration concerns ritual female genital modification. Such alteration encompasses a wide range of procedures ranging from a simple nick drawing a drop of blood, to excision of the external genitalia and partial closure of the vaginal outlet. These chapters explore the rationale and effects of the procedures in question. They interrogate the appropriateness of non-genital ritual rites of passage that can cause various degrees of harm, such as ritual tattooing, breast augmentation, and participation of minors in contact sports. I apply the State Intervention Test to these procedures, and conclude that those procedures that do not meet the criteria for government action proposed by the test should be tolerated. Scrutiny, furthermore, should be applied to determine that mainstream and minority procedures are subject to the same sorts of analytical criteria. This chapter, then, will highlight the importance of the Comparability of Effect Constraint.

Finally, I summarize my ***Conclusions*** in Chap. 16. The family, consisting of adults and children, is an institution whose nature and scope have political, religious, cultural, psychological, and ethical facets. The functionality of families varies greatly. I will argue for broad parental discretion, and for limits on state coercion. I propose the State Intervention Test as a test to guide health care workers and state officials in resolving problems with parents. I approach this question primarily from the standpoint of health decisions. The State Intervention Test extends beyond medical matters. It addresses ethical and legal matters as well. I hope to improve consistency and equality in academic discourse, clinical decisions, policy, and law.

1.10 Conclusion: What, then, Do We Owe Children?

Society has to balance competing demands for resources, ethical stances, and political ideals. Should all citizens have the same access to health care (equality), or should one should affluent or medically sophisitcated citizens be able to purchase some advantage, such as choice of doctor (equity in its traditional meaning; also, liberty)? Should health care policy maximize mean life expectancy (efficiency) or minimize the standard deviation in life expectancy (equality)? And how much of the health care budget should be used to detect and prosecute fraud, irrespective of the financial and other impact of fraud on health (justice)? Empiric studies show varying views of fairness in allocation of health care resources, even among fairly homogeneous test subjects (Ahlert and Schwettmann 2017). These considerations may underlie disagreements among the triad of state, parents, and health care professionals.

There are many conceptions of social justice besides the critical theory vision I have discussed. One is the libertarian or neo-liberal conception propounded by Friedman (2002) and Nozick (2013). Another is the concept of a meritocracy, oligarchy or aristocracy that tempers its view with religiously-based social concern to provide dignity for those not as successful or fortunate. Traditional Catholic social teaching, as typified by Luigi Taparelli, falls into this category. Third is the liberal individualism of Rawls (1971) and the many theorists who use his work as a jumping-off point. They regard some leveling of distribution of basic goods as essential to the realization of individual goals. Fourth is a modified multicultural system that allows minority group identification provided the groups respect liberal norms (Kymlicka 1995). A fifth conception is a multiculturalism that allows cultural minority groups extensive power to define their communal life (Kukathas 2002). Sixth are monistic viewpoints that equate justice with conformity to an ideology, such as religious law or the program of a secular party. This is not an exhaustive list. Absent a consensus, the solution to resource allocation must be achieved through political *modus vivendi*.

It does not seem debatable that parents, civil society, and the state should meet the needs of children, and rear them to flourish and to function as productive members of society. This requires that most children attain a sufficient level of health to be able to meet reasonable personal goals. Several modest and pragmatic reasons justify the proposition that a society that has the resources to raise children to be healthy, well-nourished, and productive citizens should attempt to do so.

First is the emotional element. We are altruistic, by virtue of our religion, ideology, or mental structure. We want others to be comfortable and satisfied. We also may be concerned that seriously disaffected individuals or populations may resent us and threaten us, and wish to defuse this. So, we wish to create a society in which everyone feels invested. This requires caring for the important interests of all children.

Second, we may support welfare programs, including those supporting children, as a form of insurance. Even if prosperous today, any of us may be needy tomorrow. The fortunes of any family or child may change, and each of us benefits from the insurance provided by a social safety net.

Third, there also are specific threats against which the state can protect us. Mandatory vaccination, for example, can be justified by nothing more than a selfish desire to protect ourselves and our children against communicable diseases.

Finally, public security and welfare considerations can justify assuring children's health. Public goals, such as defense and the need for economic productivity, require a healthy, educated, productive population to sustain the necessary economic production and military capability. Child welfare is a public good. Everyone benefits from the ability of healthy, well-educated children to provide resources for the nation's economic well-being, and to defend everyone against violence.

On the basis of the arguments in this and the last chapter I conclude that children have interests in health, personal safety, and in developing the emotional, cognitive, and relational skills to function in society. This does not address the question of what the state can or must do to promote these interests, especially if it has a different conception of these interests than the child's parents. Many liberal and progressive theorists envision an expansive role for a beneficent state governed (hopefully) by statesmen who share these theorists' ideals and views. They also tend to have a limited focus on the needs of society overall.

In the next chapter I will discuss parental roles, including prerogatives, duties, and powers.

1.11 Nomenclature and Style

I conclude with some notes about stylistic decisions I have made.

- Pronouns. I have used male pronouns for children, and female or dual ('he or she') pronouns for adults, except when this would sound strange (as in discussing fathers). This choice was made for clarity.
- I use "double inverted commas" for direct quotations, and 'single inverted commas' in other situations in which inverted commas are called for.
- A *parent* is a guardian (with decisional authority) of a minor.
- I refer to parental approval of a child's medical treatment as *consent. Permission* may be a more accurate descriptor, but 'consent' is more widely used in practice, at least in the United States.
- In subsequent chapters, United States federal institutions and agencies will not be labeled as such, but those of other nations and American political subdivisions will be specifically identified (e.g., Canadian premier, Illinois Supreme Court; but [unmodified, meaning United States] Congress).
- Law cases will be cited in full in the text, rather than in the references. Rather than using a standard legal citation format, I will employ a reference format that will permit scholars in all field to identify the case and its provenance.
- In applying verbs to cited authors, I try to use the present tense when I believe authors to be alive ('Obama writes') but the past tense when I am aware that the author is dead ('Plato wrote').
- Abbreviations used throughout the book include
  - US: United States
  - UK: United Kingdom
  - UN: United Nations
  - WHO: World Health Organization.

References

Adler, Alejandro, and Martin E.P. Seligman. 2016. Using Wellbeing for Public Policy: Theory, Measurement, and Recommendations. *International Journal of Wellbeing* 6 (1): 1–35.

Ahlert, Marlies, and Lars Schwettmann. 2017. Allocating Health Care Resources: A Questionnaire Experiment on the Predictive Success of Rules. *International Journal for Equity in Health* 16: Article #112. https://equityhealthj.biomedcentral.com/articles/10.1186/s12939-017-0611-1.

Allan, David G. 2017. Why Did You Become a Parent? The Answer Could Help You Be a Better One. *CNN Health*, 3 November 2017. https://www.cnn.com/2017/11/03/health/parenting-wisdom-project/index.html.

American Medical Association. 2021. Organizational Strategic Plan to Embed Racial Justice and Advance Health Equity. https://www.ama-assn.org/system/files/2021-05/ama-equity-strategic-plan.pdf.
Aristotle. 1999. *Politics,* trans. Jowett, Benjamin. Kitchener: Batoche Books.
Bazelon, David. 1982. Veils, Values, and Social Responsibility. *American Psychologist* 37 (2): 115–121.
Berry, Mike. 2018. 5 Reasons We Become Parents. 19 May 2018, *The Good Men Project*. https://goodmenproject.com/ethics-values/5-reasons-we-become-parents-fiff/.
Berlin, Isaiah. 1994. *A Message to the 21st Century*. Lecture, University of Toronto, 1994 Nov 25. http://www.nybooks.com/articles/archives/2014/oct/23/message-21st-century. Accessed 22 Nov 2017.
Birchley, Giles. 2016. Harm Is All You Need? Best Interests and Disputes About Parental Decision-Making. *Journal of Medical Ethics* 42 (2): 111–115.
Brennan, Samantha, and Colin MacLeod. 2017. Fundamentally Incompetent: Homophobia, Religion, and the Right to Parent. In *Procreation, Parenthood, and Educational Rights*, ed. Jaime Ahlberg and Michael Chobli, 230–245. New York: Routledge.
Brighouse, Harry, and Adam Swift. 2014. *Family Values: The Ethics of Parent-Child Relationships*. Princeton, New Jersey, USA: Princeton University Press.
Brown, Kevin, and Darrell D. Jackson. 2013. The History and Conceptual Elements of Critical Race Theory. In *Handbook of Critical Race Theory in Education*, ed. M. Lynn and A. Dixon, 9–22. New York: Routledge.
Buchanan, Allen E., and Dan W. Brock. 1989. *Deciding for Others: The Ethics of Surrogate Decision Making*. Cambridge: Cambridge University Press.
Buss, David M., and David P. Schmitt. 2019. Mate Preferences and Their Behavioral Manifestations. *Annual Review of Psychology* 70 (1): 77–110.
Cosmides, Leda, Ricardo Andres Guzman, and John Tooby. 2018. The Evolution of Moral Cognition. In *The Routledge Handbook of Moral Epistemology*, ed. Aaron Zimmerman, Karen Jones, and Mark Timmons, 174–228. London: Routledge.
Curry, Oliver Scott. 2016. Morality as cooperation: A problem-centred approach. In *The evolution of morality. Evolutionary psychology*, ed. Todd K. Shackelford and Ranald G. Hansen. Cham: Springer, Cham, 27-51. https://doi.org/10.1007/978-3-319-19671-8_2.
Dhel, Rham. 2020. 10 Reasons Why People Want Kids (and 10 Reasons They Don't). *We Have Kids* (blog). 1 October 2020. https://wehavekids.com/having-baby/Most-Common-Reasons-Why-People-Want-Children.
Durand, Martine. 2015. The OECD Better Life Initiative: How's Life? And the Measurement of Well-Being. *Review of Income and Wealth* 61 (1): 4–17.
Dwyer, James G. 1994. Parents' Religion and Children's Welfare: Debunking the Doctrine of Parents' Rights. *California Law Review* 82 (6): 1371–1447.
Dwyer, James G. 2014. Who Decides? In *The Nature of Children's Well-Being: Theory and Practice*, ed. Alexander Bagattini and Colin MacLeod, 157–175. Dordrecht: Springer. https://doi.org/10.1111/j.1468-5930.2010.00497.x.
Dwyer, James G. 2021. Deflating Parental Rights. *Law and Philosophy*. https://doi.org/10.1007/s10982-021-09406-w.
Fineman, Martha A. 2008. The Vulnerable Subject: Anchoring Equality in the Human Condition. *Yale Journal of Law and Feminism* 20 (1): 1–23.
Fineman, Martha Albertson. 2015. Equality and Difference—The Restrained State. *Alabama Law Review* 66 (3): 609-626.
Fineman, Martha A. 2019. Vulnerability and Social Justice. *Valparaiso University Law Review* 53 (2): 341–369.
Fleischman, Alan R., Frank A. Chervenak, and Laurence B. McCullough. 1998. The Physician's Moral Obligations to the Pregnant Woman, the Fetus, and the Child. *Seminars in Perinatology* 22 (3): 184–188.

Franzese, Robert J., Jr. 2002. Electoral and Partisan Cycles in Economic Policies and Outcomes. *Annual Review of Political Science* 5: 369–421. https://doi.org/10.1146/annurev.polisci.5.112801.080924.

Fricker, Miranda. 2007. *Epistemic Injustice: Power and the Ethics of Knowing*. Oxford: Oxford University Press.

Friedman, Milton. 2002. *Capitalism and Freedom*. Chicago: University of Chicago.

Galston, William A. 2002. *Liberal Pluralism: The Implications of Value Pluralism for Political Theory and Practice*. Cambridge: Cambridge University Press.

Gillam, Lynn. 2016. The Zone of Parental Discretion: An Ethical Tool for Dealing with Disagreement Between Parents and Doctors About Medical Treatment for a Child. *Clinical Ethics* 11 (1): 1–8.

Goodin, Robert E. 1986. *Protecting the Vulnerable: A Reanalysis of our Social Responsibilities*. Chicago: University of Chicago Press.

Gutmann, Amy. 1987. *Democratic Education*. Princeton: Princeton University Press.

Haybron, Daniel M. 2007. Well-Being and Virtue. *Journal of Ethics and Social Philosophy* 2 (2): 1–27.

Haybron, Daniel M. 2008. Happiness, the Self, and Human Flourishing. *Utilitas* 20 (1): 21–49.

Haybron, Daniel M. 2016. The Philosophical Basis of Eudaimonic Psychology. In *Handbook of Eudaimonic Well-Being*, ed. J. Vittersø, 27–53. International Handbooks of Quality-of-Life. Dordrecht: Springer.

Henrich, Joseph. 2016. *The Secret of Our Success*. Princeton: Princeton University Press.

Henrich, Joseph. 2020. *The WIERDest People in the World*. New York: Farrar, Giroux, Straus.

Jacobs, Allan J. 2013. The Ethics of Circumcision of Male Infants. *Israel Medical Association. Journal: IMAJ* 15 (1):60-64.

Jensen, Sharon E. 2018. *Why Do You Want to Be a Parent?* (Blog post) Quora, 21 April 2018. https://www.quora.com/Why-do-you-want-to-be-a-parent.

Kahneman, Daniel. 2011. *Thinking, Fast and Slow*. New York: Farrar, Straus & Giroux.

Kahneman, Daniel, and Angus Deaton. 2010. High Income Improves Evaluation of Life but Not Emotional Well-Being. *Proceedings of the National Academy of Sciences* 107 (3): 16489–16493.

Kidd, Ian James, and Havi Carel. 2017. Epistemic Injustice and Illness. *Journal of Applied Philosophy* 34 (2): 172–190.

Kukathas, Chandran. 2002. Multiculturalism as Fairness: Will Kymlicka's Multicultural Citizenship. *Journal of Political Philosophy* 5 (4): 406–427.

Kymlicka, Will. 1989. Liberal Individualism and Liberal Neutrality. *Ethics* 99 (4): 883–905.

Kymlicka, Will. 1995. *Multicultural Citizenship: A Liberal Theory of Minority Rights*. Oxford: Clarendon.

Kymlicka, Will, and Raphael Cohen-Almagor. 2000. Democracy and Multiculturalism. In *Challenges to Democracy: Essays in Honour and Memory of Isaiah Berlin*, ed. Raphael Cohen-Almagor, 89–118. London: Ashgate Publishing Ltd.

Lane, Wendy G., David M. Rubin, Ragin Monteith, and Cindy W. Christian. 2002. Racial Differences in the Evaluation of Pediatric Fractures for Physical Abuse. *JAMA* 288 (13): 1603–1609.

Liberini, F., Michela Redoano, and E. Proto. 2017. Happy Voters. *Journal of Public Economics* 146 (1): 41–57. https://doi.org/10.1016/j.jpubeco.2016.11.013.

Mahon, Katherine. 2018. Why Do You Want to Be a Parent? (Blog post) *Quora*, 4 July 2018. https://www.quora.com/Why-do-you-want-to-be-a-parent.

Malek, Janet. 2009. What Really Is in a Child's Best Interest? Toward a More Precise Picture of the Interests of Children. *Journal of Clinical Ethics* 20 (2): 175–182.

Masten, Ann S., and Andrew J. Barnes. 2018. Resilience in Children: Developmental Perspectives. *Children (basel)* 5 (7): 98–113. https://doi.org/10.3390/children5070098.

Mitchell, Heather. 2018. 15 Reasons Why You Should Consider Becoming a Parent. *Adoption.com.*, 24 July 2018. https://adoption.com/15-reasons-why-consider-becoming-parent

Mitchell, Paul Mark, Tracy E. Roberts, Pelham M. Barton, and Joanna Coast. 2017. Applications of the Capability Approach in the Health Field: A Literature Review. *Social Indicators Research* 133 (1): 345–371.
Narveson, Jan. 1988. *The Libertarian Idea*. Philadelphia: Temple University Press.
Nozick, Robert. 2013. *Anarchy, State, and Utopia*. New York: Basic Books.
Nussbaum Martha C. 1997. Capabilities and Human Rights. *Fordham Law Review* 66 (2): 273–300.
Nussbaum, Martha C. 2007. Human Rights and Human Capabilities. *Harvard Human Rights Journal* 20 (1): 1–24.
Okin, Susan M. 1998. Feminism and Multiculturalism: Some Tensions. *Ethics* 108 (4): 661–684.
Padela, Aasim I., and Pablo Rodriguez del Pozo. 2011. Muslim Patients and Cross-Gender Interactions in Medicine: An Islamic Bioethical Perspective. *Journal of Medical Ethics* 37 (1): 40–44. https://doi.org/10.1136/jme.2010.037614.
Powers, Madison, and Ruth Faden. 2006. *Social Justice: The Moral Foundation of Public Health and Health Policy*. Oxford: Oxford University Press.
Qi, Xiaoying. 2015. Filial Obligation in Contemporary China: Evolution of the Culture-System. *Journal for the Theory of Social Behaviour* 45 (1): 141–161.
Rawls, John. 2003. *Political Liberalism*. Expanded. New York: Columbia University Press.
Richardson, Glenn E. 2002. The Metatheory of Resilience and Resiliency. *Journal of Clinical Psychology* 58 (3): 307–321. https://doi.org/10.1002/jclp.10020.
Ross, Lainie Friedman. 1998. *Children, Families, and Health Care Decision-Making*. Oxford: Clarendon Press.
Rawls, John. 1971. *A Theory of Justice*. Cambridge, Massachusetts: Belknap Press.
Ryff, Carol D., and Keyes, Corey L.M. 1995. The Structure of Psychological Well-Being Revisited. *Journal of Personality and Social Psychology* 69 (5): 719–727.
Samet, Dov, and David Schmeidler. 2003. Between Liberalism and Democracy. *Journal of Economic Theory* 110 (2): 213–233.
Seligman, Martin E. P. 2011. *Flourish*. New York, NY: Simon & Schuster.
Sen, Amartya. 2011. *The Idea of Justice*. Cambridge, MA: Belknap Press.
Shenk, Mary K., Kaplan, Hillard S., and Hooper, Paul L. 2016. Status Competition, Inequality, and Fertility: Implications for the Demographic Transition. *Philosophical Transactions of the Royal Society B: Biological Sciences* 371: 20150150. https://doi.org/10.1098/rstb.2015.0150.
Shulman, Jeffrey. 2012. Who Owns the Soul of the Child? An Essay on Religious Parenting Rights and the Enfranchisement of the Child. *Charleston Law Review* 6(1): 101–163.
Shweder, Richard A. 2009. Shouting at the Hebrews: Imperial Liberalism v. Liberal Pluralism and the Practice of Male Circumcision. *Law, Culture and the Humanities* 59 (2): 247–265.
Sinclair, Stacey, Elizabeth Dunn, and Brian S. Lowery. 2005. The Relationship Between Parental Racial Attitudes and Children's Implicit Prejudice. *Journal of Experimental Social Psychology* 41 (3): 283–289. https://doi.org/10.1111/sipr.12054.
Tengland, Per-Anders. 2016. Venkatapuram's Capability Theory of Health: A Critical Discussion. *Bioethics* 30 (1): 8–18.
Tengland, Per-Anders. 2019. Health and Capabilities: A Conceptual Clarification. *Medicine, Health Care and Philosophy*. https://doi.org/10.1007/s11019-019-09902-w.
Thesen, Janecke. 2005. From Oppression towards Empowerment in Clinical Practice—Offering Doctors a Model for Reflection. *Scandinavian Journal of Public Health* 66 (Suppl): 47–52.
Traub, Flora, and Renée Boynton-Jarrett. 2017. Modifiable Resilience Factors to Childhood Adversity for Clinical Pediatric Practice. *Pediatrics* 139 (5): e20162569. https://doi.org/10.1542/peds.2016-2569.
Tsai, Daniel Fu-Chang. 2005. The Bioethical Principles and Confucius' Moral Philosophy. *Journal of Medical Ethics* 31 (3): 159–163.
VanderWeele, Tyler J. 2017. On the Promotion of Human Flourishing. *Proceedings of the National Academy of Sciences, U.S.A.* 114 (31): 8148–8156.
Watts, Wendy Meredith. 1987. The Parent-Child Privileges: Hardly a New or Revolutionary Concept. *William and Mary Law Review* 28 (4): 583–631.

Węziak-Białowolska, Dorota, Eileen McNeely, and Tyler J. VanderWeele. 2018. Flourish Index and Secure Flourish Index—Development and Validation. https://www.researchgate.net/profile/Dorota_Weziak-Bialowolska/publication/324242500_Flourish_Index_and_Secure_Flourish_Index_Development_and_Validation/links/5afde80e458515e9a55a62ad/Flourish-Index-and-Secure-Flourish-Index-Development-and-Validation.pdf.

Ye, Jinzhou. 2016. To Infer Liberalism from Value Pluralism. *Ethical Perspectives* 23 (4): 663–688.

Zembylas, Michalins. 2010. Children's Construction and Experience of Racism and Nationalism in Greek-Cypriot Primary Schools. *Childhood* 17 (3): 312–328.

Part I
Prior Approaches to State Intervention

Chapter 2
The Primrose Path: Rights and Autonomy

Abstract Rights are relationships in which the rightsholder is categorically entitled to be left alone (prerogative), to demand some kind of good or performance (claim), to be able to change the status of another (power), or to be exempt from others' powers (immunity). Looked at ethically, rights are difficult to ground. In the real world, assertions of right tend to be based on specifics of relationships and of the type of situation involved. The existence of an ethical right is often controversial, and is unenforceable in any event. The almost infinite panoply of putative ethical rights-relationships must be reduced to legal rights. Legal rights are limited, written, enforceable, and have no justification except the legitimacy of the government that imposes and seeks to enforce them. Ethically-derived rights cannot serve as a theoretical basis for child welfare. Legal approaches generally prioritize children's beneficent interests over their abstract rights. Among the putative rights that laws tend to deemphasize, at least in the US, is a presumed right to autonomy. Autonomy is a cluster concept that includes independence from others, choice, authenticity, etc. Empirical studies suggest that most people prioritize relationships, security, and (to a point) material well-being over autonomy. This is in contrast to much philosophical speculation. Furthermore, attention to child autonomy is often a pretext for supplanting parental values. Thus, I reject concern for autonomy as a prominent feature in settling parent-state disputes.

2.1 Rights and Interests

This chapter will define rights, will distinguish them from interests, and will examine claimed entitlements to autonomy. I include this abstract, but short chapter to explain why I give rights and autonomy short shrift as an intellectual basis for my State Intervention Test (the Test). Even if we reject rights as an important concept in applied ethics, 'rights' is a vital legal concept. Ethical discussions need to be translated into legal terms to form the basis for action. The distinction between ethical and legal rights is important. If a dispute is litigated, the decision is based on the legal rights of the parties. If an issue is addressed through legislation, new legal rights or obligations

A. J. Jacobs, *Assigning Responsibility for Children's Health When Parents and Authorities Disagree: Whose Child?*, The International Library of Bioethics 90,
https://doi.org/10.1007/978-3-030-87698-2_2

are created. But legal rights are positive. That is to say, they need no justification except that they have been promulgated by a body with the capacity to enforce them (Hart 1961). Actual legal rights focus on children's needs and interests as the basis for custody, removing a child from parental care, etc. What is important, then, is meeting the needs and interests of children, and a rights model does not serve this purpose well.

Rights are not *interests*. An interest is anything that promotes one's well-being or prevents harm. We do not have a right to fulfill all of our interests. Scarcity creates interests without rights. Only three people can win the Nobel prize in physics each year. Winning this honor is in every physicist's interest, but is not a right. Matters beyond human control can lead to interests, but not rights. There is no right to have sun on the day of your picnic. Conversely, there may be rights that are not in people's interest, such as a right to smoke cigarettes.

Rights, unlike interests, inherently constrain parties other than the rightsholder. A child has a clear interest in eating. But only if a child has a right is someone forced to be fed to feed him. A right, then, is *a relationship in which a party can impose constraints upon another person or other entity*. Ethical justifications of rights are based on intellectual arguments. They may be accepted by the rightsholder or the burdened party because they are persuaded that the right exists, but an ethical right is not enforceable. Conversely, legal rights need no justification, because the state can enforce whatever relationships between people it wishes to. Someone obligated by the right must honor the terms of the right, however.

2.2 Rights as Hohfeldian Relationships

To the extent that rights exist, they can be classified. Wesley Hohfeld provided a cogent classification of rights, modified by Wenar (2005). I will describe the four kinds of rights, termed *Hohfeldian relationships*, using the example of a rightsholder named Rhonda, and her child, Burford, whom Rhonda's rights burden. Rhonda can prepare meals for herself and Burford with a time and menu of her choosing. A rightsholder who can act without interference holds a *prerogative*. This right *burdens* Burford, who can only eat when Rhonda feeds him. Burford, however, has a *claim* on Rhonda to be fed a nutritious diet. Rhonda has a corresponding *duty* to feed Burford a nutritious diet. A claim is the ability to make someone else act on one's behalf.

Rhonda may move to another city and has the *power* to take Burford with her. A power is the right to change someone else's status. Rhonda and Burford live in a city in which a parent is exempt from public transit fares when accompanied by a young child. This is an *immunity*. Immunities are exceptions from what would otherwise be burdens under prerogatives, claims, or powers.

Rights can be compound rights composed of more than one Hohfeldian relationship. Sita boards a bus, pays her fare, and sits in a vacant seat. She now has the prerogative of remaining in the seat and the power to deny others the opportunity to sit in the same seat. And she has a claim against a standee physically removing

Table 2.1 Corresponding rights and duties in the modified Hohfeldian scheme

Right	Duty
Prerogative	Absence of right
Claim	Duty
Power	Liability
Immunity	Disability

her from the seat; the standee has the duty to leave her where she is seated. In each type of Hohfeldian relationship, there is a burden corresponding to each right; these are named in Table 2.1. The terms outlined in Table 2.1 will be used throughout the book.

Individuals, groups, or organizations can be parties to a Hohfeldian relationships. Rights often can be delegated. Rights imply choice. If the state compels Rhonda to grow rhubarb on her land, then her growing rhubarb does not exercise a prerogative. Those without capacity cannot directly exercise rights, but designated surrogates can exercise as proxies for incompetent people.

Rights, if they exist, seldom apply to all people at all times. Rather, they depend on relationships (Ross 1930) and situations (Curry et al. 2020). Furthermore, assertions of rights may conflict, and then must be prioritized. In the context of the clinical encounter, familiar to all healthcare workers, the patient has a claim on physicians to do good, avoid harm, and respect the patient's right to choose. These claims do not exist in an encounter between a policeman and a lawbreaker, or a car salesperson and a customer. Each of these relationships is bound by different rights. And when there is more than one right, then each right is *prima facie*. That is, it is binding unless superseded by a stronger Hohfeldian right.[1]

If David Ross related morality to the uniqueness of relationships, Curry (2016) conceives of morality as solutions to the regular problems of cooperation common to human societies. He begins with the presumption that humans are social creature (Henrich 2016). Curry identifies seven types of cooperation: family values, group loyalty, reciprocity, heroism, deference, fairness and property rights. These give rise to the corresponding moral values of family values, group loyalty, reciprocity, heroism, deference, fairness and property rights. Curry et al. (2020) believe that these values are products of human evolution. They regard the values as a combinatorial system in which simple elements can combine to form many complex ones. Some combinatorial systems that readers will recognize include words/language, musical notes/melodies, and atoms/molecules. Curry et al. hold that the seven moral elements[2] function as elements of a combinatorial system. Examples of second order moral values include friendship (reciprocity and sharing group interests) or queuing

[1] Medical principlism was initially based on David Ross's concept, based on special relationships. Ultimately, though, Beauchamp and Childress (2013) have based principlism on a presumed consensus of a presumed common morality. The problems with the notion of a common morality are beyond the scope of this discussion.

[2] As this idea gains traction, more moral elements may develop. For example, raising a warning or an alarm may occur in ways that do not fit into Curry's seven modes of cooperation, even though

(dividing disputed resources and respecting first possession). Each principal has a negative counterpart (neglect, betrayal, cheating, cowardice, disrespect, unfairness, theft), so that group loyalty plus disrespect for authority is mutiny (considered immoral).

Goods and values can be arranged in different lexical orders. Ross showed that the different kinds of relationships carry different mutual Hohfeldian relationships. Different modes of cooperation are governed by different moral standards, per Curry et al. If each of these three parameters is a combinatorial system, then there are an almost infinite number of possibilities for moral choice that do not lead to an immoral result. However, states must establish rules based on a finite amount of text. This entails creation of a limited number of legal relationships. These rules cannot deal with the actual moral complexity that exists in even the simplest society. Legal rules are too blunt an instrument to finely regulate human relationships. Fitting parent–child relations into a legal framework introduces problems familiar to all who work with children. It follows that each family has its own set of moral standards. These depend on the needs and values of family members.

International organizations have issued declarations and conventions that stipulate purported rights. Posner (2014) documents over 300 enumerated rights stated in UN declarations and conventions. These range from fundamental (freedom of expression) to trivial (right to leisure) to impossible (the right to health). UN documents are cast as positive law. But the UN is not a sovereign, so these rights are not law unless adopted as legislation by sovereign states. The UN has not attempted serious ethical justification of the purported rights. Invoking these rights in argument is thus unconvincing. These rights statements serve neither as ethical arguments nor as positive law.

The Hohfeldian classification of rights is descriptive rather than normative. It merely tells us what rights would be if they exist. I regard it as axiomatic that *positive legal rights must, directly or indirectly, further the welfare of citizens. In other words, they must promote human flourishing*.

2.3 Dignity

I will briefly discuss 'dignity,' mostly to clarify the term and to dispose of it as a basis for justifying government action. Dignity has been invoked as the basis for morality (Cohen-Almagor 2017) and for claims of rights (Heselhaus and Hemsley 2019) as manifestations of universal dignity. There are two problems with reliance on dignity. First there are at least three bases for dignity, and we must decide which of these is appropriate in each circumstance. Second, we must to explain how dignity is derived.

---

they constitute positive social interaction. Regardless of how many elements there are, the main point that moral values or principles may form a combinatorial system has great appeal.

One of the bases for dignity is said to be one's status as a human, and is known as *human,* or *universal, dignity* (Schachter 1983). But there are other kinds of dignity that not everyone possesses to the same degree. *Status dignity* (Sulmasy 2013) attaches respect, privilege, and honor to individuals on the basis of positions they hold within society. Thus, as a physician, I am called "Dr. Jacobs" instead of "Mr. Jacobs," and I am allowed to cut into live human bodies. These are prerogatives based on my status as a physician. Dignity of station implies some inequality or power imbalance, but even in most hierarchical organizations both superiors and inferiors have status dignity. When an enlisted soldier salutes an officer, the officer must return the salute. Both parents and children have recognized status that carries status dignity. The Confucian parent is expected to show benevolence, and the child to show deference and obedience. In the West, the parent/child relationship is more egalitarian and less well-defined. Nevertheless, kinship remains an important determinant of dignity. This may be formally recognized, as in the power to bequeath property. Kinship dignity, a form of status dignity, may be extralegal, as in the phenomenon of Americans repeatedly electing presidents related to previous presidents.[3] *Dignity as recognition* is based on membership in identity groups (Rao 2011) such as national, religious, or gender identification. Rights emanating from recognition dignity depend on the culture. In Europe, dignity as a woman protects females from female genital alteration, while in other societies that status entitles (according to their lights) females to receive ritual genital procedures (Chiu 2007).

A fourth basis of dignity claims is dignity based on personal characteristics such as intelligence or strength. Rao (2011) calls this *substantive dignity*. It is the dignity of behaving in an appropriate or laudatory manner. A wise, reliable person with gravitas carries more dignity than an unstable clown.

If we accept the concept of dignity, we have to explain the derivation of dignity. We cannot use the circular argument of defining dignity and rights as the basis for each other. The Judeo-Christian Biblical dictum that God created humans in His image (Genesis 1: 26–27) will not be acceptable to secular scholars. It is no more comprehensible in secular terms than *grace, salvation,* or *satori.*

Invocation of dignity is a powerful rhetorical device, though; who could possibly oppose dignity? However, dignity is a conclusory term that can mean what the user wants it to mean. A famous legal case, *Miranda v. Arizona*, 384 U.S. 436, Supreme Court, 1966, limited the power of police to question detainees. Both the majority and the dissent invoked dignity. The majority supported the dignity of the prisoner, while the dissent lamented the loss of dignity that the decision would inflict on victims. It is not useful to view dignity as a formal or as an efficient cause of rights. Children can have rights claims based on their humanity, on their status as children, on their academic achievement, etc.

---

[3] Two Adamses, two Harrisons, two Roosevelts, and two Bushes.

2.4 A Rights-Based Philosophical Approach to Child-Rearing

I invite the reader to consider this hypothetical job posting:

> The successful candidate will assume full responsibility for the care of a child for 18-26 years, serving as steward of the child on behalf of the state. Commitment to the position is not categorical, but resignation involves major public shame. Responsibilities to the ward are deemed fiduciary. The ward will live in your home. For the first several years, responsibilities involve providing comprehensive physical care. You will have to feed your ward frequently, and keep him clean, as he will be incontinent of stool and urine. You will be sleep deprived. Eventually, your ward will be able to care for his physical needs, but you will still devote several hours a day to his care. You must meet his emotional needs as well as his physical needs. He will have a mercurial temper, and often will try to do dangerous or self-destructive things. He regularly will resist your attempts to guide him until he attains capacity. You must teach him appropriate modes of behavior necessary to relate to others in society. However, you are not allowed to try to influence him to adopt your values and beliefs. This function is assigned to state schools (which the ward must attend), his peer group, and mass culture. You will not be paid for this position. Rather, you are expected to bear most of the costs of your ward's care. At age 18 the ward attains legal maturity and the relationship is terminated, except to the extent you and the ward agree to maintain it.

Who would take this job?

As the concepts of political rights evolved in the eighteenth century, the Anglo-American view was that the state would always be in conflict with individuals over individual rights. The French, in contrast, saw positive law as a way to uphold rights. Thus, the Preamble to the US Constitution defines the state as the instrument of the people,[4] while the French Declaration of the Rights of Man and the Citizen states that "the principle of all sovereignty resides essentially in the nation" (Article 3). The American Bill of Rights restricts state power. In contrast, the French Constitution of 1848 provided that

> Education is free. [But t]he liberty of teaching is to be exercised according to the capacity and morality determined by conditions of the laws, and under the supervision of the State. (Article 9)

The French conception of a benevolent, powerful state enforcing both negative and positive legal rights was adopted in the UN Universal Declaration of Human Rights and other UN rights documents. It now at least tacitly accepted by many Anglo-American scholars, such as Brighouse and Swift (2014). I will relate and critique some of their ideas.

Brighouse and Swift believe it is best for children to be raised in a nuclear family, with one (or a few) adults who provide physical and material care, education in life skills, socialization, and morals education in a loving environment (p. 71). They view the priority of the child as categorical, however (p. 59). They assign parents the duty to raise children to attain extensive capabilities of the sort proposed by Nussbaum

[4] "*We the People of the United States*... do ordain and establish this Constitution for the United States of America. (Emphasis supplied.).

(2000). To this end, children have physical, educational, emotional, and moral claims. Parents must also promote the autonomy of their children. One facet of this is that children should be able to break from parental values at minimal cost.

But many parents attach great importance to their values and ways of life. Political views, religious practices, preferred recreational activities, or the way to handle household finances may be extremely salient to parents. Political, social, and religious views of potential mates are highly important in mate selection (Alford et al. 2011). The intrinsic importance of these subjects and the importance of family relationships would seem to make generational continuity of values an important good. This is especially true because of the evidence to be presented that autonomy seems to be of secondary important to personal flourishing.

The recommendations by Brighouse and Swift may not have much traction with actual parents. Reading the job description at the beginning of this section, which is based on Brighouse and Swift's conception of the family, one asks why anyone would want to be a parent. Brighouse and Swift would deny parents much of the satisfaction that made them want to be parents (Table 1.1). Also, their concerns with excess parental influence implies a degree of government intrusiveness that I will show is inappropriate in a liberal state.

Parents who belong to a minority culture may have strong feelings about raising their children in ways that differ from mainstream norms. If they are Jewish or Muslim, this entails circumcising their boys and refraining from pork consumption. Christian Science parents may be leery of what the medical profession has to offer to their sick children. A parent may refuse to let her son play American football because of the risk of head injury. Her neighbor may press her son to play football because of its social status. A deontic rights approach does not determine which parental choices are sufficiently bad for a child to invite government coercion. Nor is it clear that confronting parents by telling them that they are violating their child's rights is an effective way to influence them.

2.5 Summary of General Rights Discussion

This book looks at the narrow topic of what should happen when parents and state actors such as physicians disagree on medical care or other interventions with health implications for a child. Many rights claims proclaim universality of a catalog of rights. This is a bold statement, especially when applied to particular cases. Consider, first, that not all states are liberal states, or democratic, or committed to equality and solidarity. According to Sen (2004), the universality of human rights must be established by a general world consensus based on free discussion. This implies need for a wide cross-cultural consensus. Beyond Europe and North America, such a consensus would include China and India (each with 20% of the world's population) as well as African and Islamic nations. United Nations rights statements do not reflect a universal consensus (Mutua 1996). Attempts to assert their global applicability have at least a whiff of imperialism, and is arrogant at best. And, do Westerners want us to subject our own societies to the moral consensus of the rest of the world?

Any society, liberal or not, should make reasonable efforts to ensure that parents meet some basic physical and psychological needs of the child. They should try to ensure that their children are healthy, flourish, have sufficient economic resources, and are able to make a positive contribution to society. A strong, healthy, satisfied, and well-educated population benefits the nation as a whole as well as constituting conditions of flourishing for the individuals involved. Children also have a claim to a reasonable protection against physical harm.[5] The basis for this does not lie in rights narratives, but revolves around interests and needs. The child's interests must be balanced against those of other members of the family, and of people outside the family. This is best done without attempting to use rights claims as trump cards to stop discussion.

Before moving on to interests, I need to discuss assertions of the child's right to autonomy. The emphasis on autonomy by many ethicists impacts on some of the more controversial topics in the second half of this book. Space limitations require a discussion that will be too superficial to please philosophers, but I need to outline why I do not accept the primacy of autonomy.

2.6 Autonomy and Balance of Power

Arguments based on children's autonomy are, to a great extent, calls for restricting parental authority. Furthermore, they amount to an assertion of power by the leaders of society. It is the state, via media, schools, and organized activities, that will supply the formative influences on children in the absence of parental influence. I will try to rebut the idea that autonomy is of primary importance to human flourishing, and as a goal of child-rearing. I relate this to health care.

2.7 Consent as the Portal into Autonomy

The primary importance of autonomy in *clinical relationships* contrasts with overemphasis on its *general* importance. Clinical ethics is a special case of human interaction. Physicians and other healthcare providers are expert in health, but not in other topics that relate to a patient's interests and values. The decision to undertake medical care, however, requires consideration of more than the patient's health interests. There are very few occupations in which the customer pays the proprietor to do potentially

[5] This is not a simple matter. First, it isn't clear what pain is reasonable. Pain is not necessarily harmful, and controlled pain may be either part or a byproduct of a program designed to instill fortitude, as with contact sports. Rites of passage may involve painful or dangerous experiences (Johnson 2011).

dangerous things to her body. This, plus the power differential between patients and physicians, requires emphasis on patient consent, as classically stated by Judge Benjamin Cardozo:

> Every human being of adult years and sound mind has a right to determine what shall be done with his own body; and a surgeon who performs an operation without his patient's consent, commits an assault. (*Schloendorff v. Society of New York Hospital*, 105 N.E. 92, New York Court of Appeals, 1914, 94).[6]

Judge Spottswood Robinson, in *Canterbury v. Spence* (464 F.2d 772, US Court of Appeals D.C. Circuit, 1973), expanded the legal principle of consent to require *informed* consent as a valid legal claim by patients *against physicians*. In bioethical (as opposed to legal) discourse the need to respect patient autonomy originally was considered a prima facie claim based on David Ross's work (1930). The medical relationship is unique in at least two salient ways. First, physicians alter the patient's body with drugs, surgery, etc., in potentially dangerous ways. Second, patients may have considerations that are not health-related, but which they prioritize over health. Physicians' health-related recommendations must be reconciled with patients' other interests, and patients themselves are in the best position to perform this reconciliation. A clinical relationship is neither an arm's length commercial relationship nor a typical fiduciary bond; it is *sui generis*.

The consensus of empiric studies outside the context of clinical relationships, however, shows that autonomy is generally not a prominent component of flourishing. Parents serve as surrogates for their children with regard to consent, making decisions on their behalf that adults would make on their own. Legally, these decisions for minors without decisional capacity must be based on children's interests. Children have never been capable of formulating autonomous decisions, so we cannot rely on their prior legally competent wishes. Pure autonomy is impossible, and parental decisions must therefore be based on considerations of beneficence and nonmaleficence.

2.8 Autonomy and Choice

Bioethicists have used the concept of autonomy to justify their positions on matters outside the scope of clinical relationships. Some have applied it to parent–child relationships.

Autonomy is a cluster concept. Cluster concepts (Pigliucci 2003) are terms that occupy several different meanings which are close enough to be related but not

[6] Ironically, this quote was *obiter dictum*, that is, a passage in a judicial opinion that did not apply to the issue that the court was considering. The court actually unanimously excused the hospital! This opinion is widely cited because of Cardozo's reputation and fine writing style, but the opinion technically has never been precedent for consent requirements. In fact, consent requirements had been established in American common law at least 9 years before *Schloendorff* by the less quotable cases of *Mohr v. Williams*, 104 N.W. 12, Minnesota Supreme Court, 1905, and *Pratt v. Davis*, 79 NE 562, Illinois Supreme Court, 1905!

close enough to lend themselves to a precise definition. Dworkin (2015) notes that autonomy has been equated with liberty, self-rule, freedom of the will, individuality, integrity, responsibility, and self-knowledge. It applies to actions, beliefs, and relationships. John Stuart Mill wrote that "the only purpose for which power can be rightfully exercised over any member of a civilised community, against his will, is to prevent harm to others." (Mill 1859, Chapter I. *Introductory*). In context, this pronouncement means less than it seems to. Mill was speaking only of state action. Indeed, Mill explicitly recognized that children are subject to paternalistic intervention (Idem. Chapter IV: *Of the Limits to the Authority of Society over the Individual*). One cannot infer that Mill regarded autonomy as an important consideration in child-raising.

Kant, unlike Mill, argued that that moral principles were derived independently of empirical considerations or of imposed authority, and that morality of an action is divorced from the action's tangible effects. Autonomy meant that individuals were to use their innate moral sense to generate universally applicable maxims (Kant 1785). His sense was that if people were attentive to their a priori moral sense, they would often come to similar conclusions about moral matters. In his little-read *On Education*, Kant (1803) favored parental discipline to guide children toward autonomous life. Although parents had great power to teach their children moral precepts, their only prerogatives stemmed from their duty to rear their children. That duty involves physical care, training a child to function in society, and moral education (Kant 1803). In practice, though, parents care mostly that children can make their way in the world, so Kant would send children to schools to learn to be moral people.

Kant (1785) believed that actions or maxims determined by custom or religion, or directed to instrumental ends, do not comport with autonomy; rather, they were *heteronomous*. It is likely that he would have required parents to prioritize their children's health over dictates of religion or custom. This would require that parents obtain effective medical care for their children. Furthermore, Kant likely would have prioritized the scientific bases and benevolent motivations of physicians over the heteronomous and unreasoned opinions of parents. Regardless of where Kant's conclusions would fall, his outlook is incompatible with liberal pluralism. Furthermore, Kant tended to equate his categorical imperative—that universally applicable maxims spring a priori from the mind—with contemporaneous notions of morality. An example of this is his condemnation of masturbation. (Kant 1803).

Contemporary accounts of autonomy are likely to resemble those of Gerald Dworkin (1988). Dworkin speaks of autonomy as being able to critically reflect on one's first order preferences, and to use these reflections—second order preferences—to modify initial choices as needed. The difference between first- and second-order preferences might best be illustrated by example. Leonid eats a package of cupcakes. He understands that his health requires that he lose weight, and wishes to stop eating cupcakes. Eating the cupcakes expresses a first-order preference. His desire to lose weight reflects a second-order preference. His choice of eating or not eating cupcakes is autonomous. Autonomy as so conceived has three elements: reflection, exercise of will, and freedom from undue external constraint. Those immersed in a cult may not be able to reflect critically. Addicts (or anyone with a well-established habit) may not have the will to act on second-order preferences. Undue influence is a more difficult concept. It is important, though, to note that autonomy is *not* the same thing as wide availability of choice (Dworkin 1982).

While autonomy as so defined is desirable, it is not an overarching goal either of life or of child rearing. Autonomy may be important in realizing one's second-order preferences (which are more important than first order preferences), but autonomy does not shape these second-order preferences. Bernard Madoff and Robert Mugabe undoubtedly enjoyed great autonomy, viewed in Dworkin's terms.

2.9 Undue Influence and Coercion

Parents may be subject to undue influence as surrogates. They may also attempt to exercise undue influence over an older child. Consider the following vignette. Aquila Adler, the richest person in the world, will soon die if she does not receive a liver transplant. Eight-year-old Prometheus Kazbek is a perfect immunological match. Aquila asks Prometheus' mother, Clymene, to have Prometheus donate half his liver to her. The postoperative course will be difficult, but most donors survive. In return, Aquila will establish an irrevocable trust whose income will pay for Prometheus's education and allow him to enjoy an upper-middle class style for his entire life. Clymene is a single parent with limited income, and sees this as an opportunity that will benefit Prometheus. She accepts Aquila's offer.

It is important to distinguish among three concepts. *Paternalism* is restriction of the freedom of another for that person's own good.*Coercion* is the imposition of the will of a stronger party upon a weaker party through the threat of harm. *Undue influence* is an offer to provide a benefit that results in the recipient's bad judgment (Largent and Fernandez 2017). For the minor child, parentalism is what parents appropriately do. Parental direction of children is necessary for the child's safety, growth, development, and flourishing. Coercion is a necessary tool used by both parents and state. It is sometimes appropriate and sometimes not. The reason for the coercion, the appropriateness of coercion in a particular circumstance, and the proportionality of the coercive measure, all contribute to the morality of coercion in any specific instance. In my community, a parent would generally not be criticized for withholding screen time until a child finishes his homework, but would be considered too strict for using loss of screen time as a punishment for dressing too slowly. As for the state, it seems reasonable for the state to remove a child from a home in which he is sexually abused, but removal from the home is not an appropriate remedy for a parent occasionally missing a routine medical appointment. Finally, undue influence is, by definition, never appropriate. It also is a conclusory term, meaning that we first decide what is inappropriate and then call it undue influence, rather than use fixed standards (see Chap. 1).

In the Prometheus example, it would be within Clymene's discretion to paternalistically allow Prometheus to donate his liver to Aquila, provided the transaction were reasonable. Whether the deal is reasonable is open to discussion, though the circumstances leave a bad taste in the mouth. This is because Aquila clearly subjected Clymene to undue influence. This book does not discuss the influence of undue influence and coercion on the state's appropriate power to interfere with parental decisions that are reasonable, but elicited under conditions of coercion or undue influence. My intuition is that the only party that should be subject to punishment in such cases is the person who exerted the undue influence. The decision itself should be subject to state review, with a court assuming authority in the matter. Space considerations prevent me from exploring the implications of coercion and undue influence in detail.

Those involved in health care decisions will frequently hear the terms 'paternalism' and coercion misused, or used in a derogatory manner. This purpose of this discussion is to clarify the terms, and to establish the point that adults have to make many important decisions for children who lack the judgment to make those decisions themselves. Readers will note that situations involving coercion are ubiquitous in this book. The book has been written to suggest when states may coerce parental behavior. In addition, physicians and parents may try to use coercive tactics against each other. As for children, they rarely have a say in their medical treatment until adolescence. Even then, they are at implicitly or explicitly subject to coercion or inappropriate incentives. The possibility of coercion underlies all hierarchical relationships. Indeed, the possibility of using coercion is necessary to realize our legal prerogatives, duties, powers, and immunities. Undue influence is not as important to the topics discussed in this book, except as regarding adolescents responding to peers.

2.10 Autonomy and Relationships

Autonomy considerations have potential impact on decisions regarding children's health. There are at least three specific areas in which this is important in ethical analysis. First, to what extent should maximization of autonomy or choice—and these are not the same thing—be a factor in exposing children to experiences with anatomical, physiological, or psychological consequences? The second issue is what the appropriate balance of power between parents and health care workers in health-related treatment should be. The third question is when it is appropriate for the state to determine when to allow a physical procedure on a child for non-medical reasons. Decisions regarding children generally should not detract from their flourishing. Value pluralism provides the insight that it can be impossible to determine whether a given intervention promotes or is detrimental to flourishing. This is because flourishing includes physical, psychological, relational, and spiritual elements, as well fostering autonomy. From the standpoint of the state, parental responsibility is to provide adequate care, and not perfect care.

Goals in raising children must be based on appreciation of psychological needs and capabilities. Ethical dictates cannot be based on impossible or erroneous behavioral expectations, such as John Rawls' three 'Laws of Moral Psychology' (Rawls

1971, §75), which do not conform to empirical understanding and were not based on experimental data.[7] Nor did Rawls (1971) empirically ground his minimization of the importance of envy (§81), competition (Idem.), or hedonism (§84) He did not discuss greed at all. His notion that children's positive relationships are based on his perception of the just behavior of others is not borne out by Piaget (Ginsburg and Opper 1988), attachment theory (Mikulincer et al. 2003), or evolutionary psychology (Henrich 2016). Indeed, the consensus derived from empiric research is that children acquire moral judgment largely by learning from individuals close to them, and they can acquire immoral modes of behavior as well as moral ones. This was established in classic studies by Bandura (1969), which were well known when Rawls (1971) published his book. Furthermore, a great deal of the social behavioral repertoire is innate and group-directed (Henrich 2016). Indeed, learning is a two-way street in which infants elicit a psychological and physiological maternal response and vice versa (Nagy and Molnar 2004).

A number of authors have proposed alternatives to ethical and political individualism based on concepts compatible with the insights of evolutionary psychology. Hazony (2018) posits that social organization is a pyramid of associations uniting individuals for mutual protection against adversity, and based on affinity and loyalty. The family is primary. Families unite to form more complex organizations, consisting of extended families, then clans, tribes, and, finally, nations. The basis for society is not individual consent or social contract, but evolution, economics and safety. Hazony regards the ultimate purpose of these complex associations—including society—as protection of primary relationships and the people involved in them. Henrich (2020) cites compelling evidence that kinship structures form the basis of most societies, and that this was universally true in ancient times, His data support Hazony's speculation. Outside of what Henrich (2020) calls WEIRD (Western, educated, industrialized, rich, and democratic) societies, kinship bonds and the supreme importance of relationships predominate in most societies.

Stable relationships are of utmost importance for children. Relationships, not autonomy, are key in child development, and to flourishing in general (Hinde and Stevenson-Hinde 1987; Lally and Mangione 2017). The widespread preference for security over freedom is eloquently expressed in iconic religious (1 Samuel 8:4–20) and literary (Dostoyevsky 1879; the Grand Inquisitor parable) passages. Both of these texts, incidentally, disapprove of this preference.

Even if usually a positive feature, there is little reason to believe that freedom from constraint is equally beneficial to all. Both autonomy and choice are likely to be less important to a person who seeks to belong to a monastery than to a philosophy professor. Furthermore, it is doubtful that, for most people, either maximizing choice (Dworkin 1982) or maximizing autonomy does much to enhance either hedonic or eudaimonic flourishing. Much flourishing is dependent on voluntary limitation of one's choices. Marrying one of many potential spouses, pursuing one of many potential professions, and choosing one of many potential dwellings all limit choice,

[7] Rawls wrote his treatise in 1971. I am not implying that Rawls intended to mislead, but only that he proposed unsubstantiated views on factual matters.

but forming commitments is part of flourishing. Being a chattel slave certainly is not compatible with flourishing (or with any conception of dignity), but using an extreme case like this is to present a straw man argument. At the other extreme, frequent reevaluation of one's commitments and choices in order to preserve one's autonomy from unthinking habits is also likely to detract from flourishing.

Parents seek close relationships with their children as well as the converse. They seldom hope to cut parental ties when their children leave home. Reproducing oneself is part of the pleasure of parenthood. We flourish when we see our children experience the same milestones and problems that we did. If we have biological children, we are apt to discuss our children's physical and character similarities to others. Such similarities ('Lars looks like his mother;' 'Yoko is a picky eater like her grandfather') foster closeness. Such identification may include, among other things, physical similarities, other resemblances to family, common experiences, shared interests, and shared values. We love our children regardless, but the to the extent that there is mutual identification the relationship is apt to be closer.[8]

Children, of course, will absorb values from parents as well as from other people they know, regardless of parental intent. Thus, our relational environment necessarily shapes our choices and frames our beliefs and values. Had I been switched at birth with Princess Marijka of the Netherlands, who was born the same day as I was, each of us would have grown up with a different set of interests and beliefs. Restraints on autonomy inevitably occur as a result of personal and environmental influences during childhood, and by societal pressure to conform. A child that grows up in Manhattan, for example, is likely to speak English as a primary language, wear a shirt, and be politcally liberal. It is highly unlikely that a graduate of an elite American or British secondary school would consider a career as a plumber, or marry and have a child immediately after graduation. Few become military officers or priests, though these are prestigious occupations with important responsibilities. Some of these influences are caused by unshared environment, which is the differences in experiences of children in the same family (Plomin and Daniels 1987). SStudies have implicated unshared environment as a factor leading to youth criminal behavior (Wallace 2017). Other studies have documented an important role of unshared environmental factors in genesis of eating disorders (Yao et al. 2019), optimism (Mavioğlu et al. 2015), and educational achievement.

Thus, relationships are of primary importance both in shaping people's preferences and their behavior. Much of what we think we do by choice is actually strongly shpaed by influences of other people.

---

[8] This is not to say that adopted children and their parents cannot form wonderful, loving relationships, but only that parent–child relationships are enhanced by perceived similarities.

2.11 Autonomy, the State, Health, and Education

Moving from ethics to law, American constitutional norms are more protective of parents than are European norms. In the United States, "marriage, procreation, contraception, family relationships, child rearing, and education" are considered central to defining one's identity (*Lawrence v. Texas*, 539 U.S. 558, Supreme Court, 2003, 574). As such, there is a strong presumption against state interference in these matters. American constitutional law reflects a perception that family autonomy is necessary for human flourishing. Two Supreme Court cases decided almost a century ago, *Meyer v. Nebraska* (262 US 390, 1923), and *Pierce v. Society of Sisters*, (268 U.S. 510, 1925, and subsequent derivative cases, are the basis of this understanding.

European constitutional law is more deferential to state intervention in family matters. It tends to focus on the child in question:

> Spouses shall enjoy equality of rights and responsibilities of a private law character between them, and in their relations with their children ... *This Article shall not prevent States from taking such measures as are necessary in the interestsof the children.* (*European Convention on Human Rights*, Protocol 7, Article 5, emphasis supplied).

States have important reasons to be concerned with children's health and education. First is a concern for physical and social reproduction. Perceived overpopulation has led to coercive population control measures in heavily populated nations such as China and India (Sollinger and Nakachi 2016). Some European nations with low fecundity have taken the opposite tack, and have incentivized parents to have more children. All states legislate some coercive sexual and reproductive measures, such as a minimum age for sexual consent. This is consistent with a traditional legal view that certain behavior should not be allowed before age has given individuals sufficient maturity and perspective to allow them to make wise decisions.

A second government interest is the necessity for a healthy and educated workforce to compete with other societies and deal with environmental challenges. Children must be raised to participate in the economic, military, and social life of the nation. The state has an interest in children's health to the extent that this contributes to children's being able to mature into adults that can perform the tasks needed to maintain and advance society. They can stop parents, then, from making choices that foreseeably and unnecessarily lead to their children's major disabilities. Furthermore, the state has an interest in controlling activities that jeopardize public health. State interest in its citizens' health has been recognized for well over two centuries (Frank 1976). Third, children can be vectors for communicable diseases. Individual and group criminal activities harm individuals and society as a whole. These societal interests make states stakeholders in decisions affecting children's health.

I now briefly consider a clever, but invalid, argument that parents are responsible for enhancing the adult choice opportunities for their currently minor children. The open future doctrine will arise in discussion of several substantive issues in the second half of this book.

2.12 Choice and Its Preservation: Open Future

Children's prerogatives and claims merge with an expansive view of autonomy in Feinberg's (1980) assertion of a child's claim to an open future. This attack on parental powers was written as criticism of a Supreme Court decision, *Wisconsin v. Yoder* (406 U.S. 205, 1972). The court had ruled that Old Order Amish parents could withdraw their children from school after 8th grade notwithstanding a state law requiring education through 10th grade. The open future doctrine has gained much traction since Feinberg proposed it.

The argument asserts a breathtakingly broad compound right for children. As a general principle, minor children are said have certain claims on their parents to preserve future claims and prerogatives that the children cannot exercise until they are adults. Feinberg called such claims 'rights-in-trust.' He asserted that one such right-in-trust was that parents must preserve for the child the broadest possible range of adult choices. He termed a child's claim to be raised in a manner that allows him to maximize access to a wide panoply of future claims and prerogatives later to be a right-in-trust a known as a *right to an open future*.

The open future doctrine has proven to be influential—in my opinion, unfortunately so. It has been used to argue that certain decisions should be deferred to legal maturity regardless of parental wishes, to allow children who otherwise would be the subject of the decisions to be able when adult to decide for themselves whether he wanted it. One example is the use by Davis (1997) of the open future principle to argue against testing children for late-onset genetic diseases.

To the extent that it is desirable, open future considerations clash with other rights and interests. For example, the open future doctrine has been used to justify mandatory maternal drug testing (Kanaris 2016), since in uteroharm from drugs narrows the options of the fetus-turned-human. This conclusion conflicts with the American consensus in law and medical ethics that mothers have the right to refuse such testing (American College of Obstetricians and Gynecologists 2016; *Ferguson v. City of Charleston*, 532 U.S. 67, Supreme Court, 2001).

Observing that rights function as moral trump cards, Garrett er al. (2019) suggest that protecting future choice should be considered an interest, rather than a right. In this way an open future can be balanced against other interests of the child and against the interests of others. This seems correct to me.

2.13 Conclusion

Rights, as conceived positively (legally) lack justification. Rights, as conceived ethically, conflict with one another, without a way to resolve the conflict. The priorities commonly established by ethicists in ranking the salience of rights is not the same as the ranking suggested by people who evaluate what is important for their own flourishing. Neither does it reflects the mode of interaction with children that psychologists believe is key to optimum child development. Thus, if autonomy is seen as maximization of choice, its priority in child-rearing is limited. Even if it is seen as second order reflection on one's primary choices, combined with the ability to act on one's choices, autonomy is not a *summum bonum*.

Parents' duty is to prepare children to cope with the challenges of adulthood. First, parents should educate children to be economically or socially productive.[9] Second, the child must be able to successfully navigate the environment in which he likely will live. This may be different for a farmer than for an urban lawyer. Third, education should teach children to deal with the sorts of competition the child will experience, including competition for resources, status, and mates. Finally, parents must provide moral education, as well as must provide physical care and psychological security. They are in a better position to understand how to do this than the state, though the state must serve as a last resort in rescuing children whose parents are unable to meet their needs.

Most parental duties are better explained through a model of interests, rather than through a model of rights. It is to interests, then, that I now turn.

References

Alford, John R., Peter K. Hatemi, John R. Hibbing, Nicholas G. Martin, and Lindon J. Eaves. 2011. The Politics of Mate Choice. *Journal of Politics* 73 (2): 362–379. https://doi.org/10.1017/S0022381611000016.

American College of Obstetricians and Gynecologists. 2016. American College of Obstetricians and Gynecologists, Committee on Ethics. *Committee Opinion 664: Refusal of Medically Recommended Treatment During Pregnancy*. https://www.acog.org/Clinical-Guidance-and-Publications/Committee-Opinions/Committee-on-Ethics/Refusal-of-Medically-Recommended-Treatment-During-Pregnancy?IsMobileSet=false.

Bandura, Albert. 1969. Social-Learning Theory of Identificatory Processes. In *Handbook of Socialization Theory and Research, Chicago*, ed. David Goslin, 213–262. Chicago: Rand McNally.

Beauchamp, Tom, and James F. Childress. 2013. *Principles of Biomedical Ethics*, 7th ed. New York: Oxford University Press.

Brighouse, Harry, and Adam Swift. 2014. *Family Values: The Ethics of Parent-Child Relationships*. Princeton: Princeton University Press.

Chiu, Elaine M. 2007. The Culture Differential in Parental Autonomy. *University of California, Davis Law Review* 41 (6): 1773–1828.

Cohen-Almagor, Raphael. 2017. On the Philosophical Foundations of Medical Ethics: Aristotle, Kant, JS Mill and Rawls. *Ethics, Medicine and Public Health* 3 (4): 436–444.

[9] There are many valuable and praiseworthy adult vocations that provide no remuneration.

Curry, Oliver S. 2016. Morality as Cooperation: A Problem-Centred Approach. In *The Evolution of Morality. Evolutionary Psychology*, ed. T. Shackelford and R. Hansen, 27–51. Cham: Springer. https://doi.org/10.1007/978-3-319-19671-8_2.

Curry, Oliver S., Mark Alfano, Mark J. Brandt, and Christine Pelican. 2020. Moral Molecules: Morality as a Combinatorial System. OSF Preprints. June 9. https://doi.org/10.31219/osf.io/xnstk.

Davis, Dena S. 1997. The Child's Right to an Open Future: Yoder and Beyond. *Capital University Law Review* 26 (1): 93–105.

Dostoyevsky, Fyodor. 1879. *The Brothers Karamazov*, 258–262. Translated by Richard Pevear and Larissa Volokhonsky. London: Vintage Books.

Dworkin, Gerald. 1982. Is More Choice Better than Less? In *Midwest Studies in Philosophy, volume* 7, ed. Peter French, 47–61.

Dworkin, Gerald. 1988. *The Theory and Practice of Autonomy*. Cambridge: Cambridge University Press.

Dworkin, Gerald. 2015. The Nature of Autonomy. *Nordic Journal of Studies in Educational Policy* 2: 28479. https://doi.org/10.3402/nstep.v1.28479.

Feinberg, Joel. 1980. The Child's Right to an Open Future. In *Whose Child? Children's Rights, Parental Authority, and State*, ed. William Aiken and Hugh LaFollette, 124–153. Totowa, NJ: Rowman & Littlefield.

Frank, Johann Peter. 1976. *A System of Complete Medical Police: Selections*. Translated by E. Velum. Edited by Erna Lesly. Baltimore: Johns Hopkins University Press.

French Constitution. 1848. *French Constitution of 1848*. https://en.wikisource.org/wiki/French_Constitution_of_1848.

Garrett, Jeremy R., John D. Lantos, Leslie G. Biesecker, Janet E. Childerhose, Wendy K. Chung, Ingrid A. Holm, Barbara A. Koenig, Jean E. McEwen, Benjamin S. Wilfond, MD, & Kyle Brothers, Clinical Sequencing Exploratory Research (CSER) Consortium Pediatrics Working Group. 2019. Rethinking the "Open Future" Argument Against Predictive Genetic Testing of Children. *Genetic Medicine* 21 (10): 2190–2198. https://doi.org/10.1038/s41436-019-0483-4.

Ginsburg, Herbert P., and Sylvia Opper. 1988. *Piaget's Theory of Intellectual Development*, 3rd ed. Englewood Cliffs, NJ: Prentice Hall.

Hart, H.L.A. 1961. *The Concept of Law*. Oxford: Clarendon Law Series.

Hazony, Yoram. 2018. *The Virtues of Nationalism*. New York: Basic Books.

Henrich, Joseph. 2016. *The Secret of Our Success*. Princeton, New Jersey: Princeton University Press.

Henrich, Joseph. 2020. *The WIERDest People in the World*. New York: Farrar, Straus and Giroux.

Heselhaus, Sebastian, and Ralph Hemsley. 2019. Human Dignity and the European Convention on Human Rights. In *Handbook of Human Dignity in Europe*, ed. Paolo Becchi and Klaus Mathis, 969–992. Cham: Springer.

Hinde, Robert A., and Joan Stevenson-Hinde. 1987. Interpersonal Relationships and Child Development. *Developmental Review* 7 (1): 1–21. https://doi.org/10.1016/0273-2297(87)90002-5.

Johnson, Jay. 2011. Across the Threshold: A Comparative Analysis of Communitas and Rites of Passage in Sport Hazing and Initiations. *Canadian Journal of Sociology* 3 (3): 199–227.

Kanaris, Constantinos. 2016. *The Concept of Prenatal Screening as an Enforceable Parental Duty*. Ph.D. Dissertation, University of Manchester. https://www.research.manchester.ac.uk/portal/files/54589339/FULL_TEXT.PDF. Accessed 15 Jan 2019.

Kant, Immanuel. 1785. *Groundwork to the Metaphysics of Morals*, translated by Allen E Wood. New Haven, CT, USA: Yale University Press.

Kant, Immanuel. 1803. *On Education (Ueber Pädagogik)* [inconsistency of umlaut use in original]. Translated by Annette Churton. Boston: D. C. Heath. http://files.libertyfund.org/files/356/0235_Bk.pdf.

Lally, J. Ronald., and Peter L. Mangione. 2017. Caring Relationships: The Heart of Early Brain Development. *Young Children* 72 (2): 17–24.

Largent, Emily A., and Holly Fernandez Lynch. 2017. Paying Research Participants: The Outsized Influence of Undue Influence. *IRB* 39 (4): 1–9.
Mavioğlu, Rezan Nehir, Dorret I. Boomsma, and Meike Bartels. 2015. Causes of individual differences in adolescent optimism: a study in Dutch twins and their siblings. *European Child and Adolescent Psychiatry* 24 (11): 1381–1388. https://doi.org/10.1007/s00787-015-0680-x.
Mikulincer, Mario, Phillip R. Shaver, and Dana Pereg. 2003. Attachment Theory and Affect Regulation: The Dynamics, Development, and Cognitive Consequences of Attachment-Related Strategies. *Motivation and Emotion* 27 (2): 77–102.
Mill, John Stuart. 1859. *On Liberty*. New York: Bartleby.com. https://www.bartleby.com/130/1.html.
Mutua, Makau wa. 1996. The Ideology of Human Rights. *Virginia Journal of International Law* 36 (3): 589–657.
Nagy, Emese, and Peter Molnar. 2004. *Homo Imitans* or *Homo Provocans*? Human Imprinting Model of Neonatal Imitation. *Infant Behavior & Development* 27 (1): 54–63.
Nussbaum, M. 2000. *Women and Human Development: The Capabilities Approach*. New York: Cambridge University Press.
Pigliucci, Massimo. 2003. Species as Family Resemblance Concepts. *BioEssays* 25 (4): 596–602.
Plomin, Robert, and Denise Daniels. 1987. Why Are Children in the Same Family So Different from One Another? *Behavioral and Brain Sciences* 10 (1): 1–60.
Posner, Eric A. 2014. *The Twilight of Human Rights Law*. Oxford: Oxford University Press.
Rao, Neomi. 2011. Three Concepts of Dignity in Constitutional Law. *Notre Dame Law Review* 86 (1): 183–272.
Rawls, John. 1971. *A Theory of Justice*. Cambridge, Massachusetts: Belknap Press.
Ross, W. David. 1930. *The Right and the Good*. Oxford: Oxford University Press.
Schachter, Oscar. 1983. Human Dignity as a Normative Concept. *American Journal of International Law* 77 (6): 848–854.
Sen, Amartya. 2004. Elements of a Theory of Human Rights. *Philosophy and Public Affairs* 32 (4): 315–356.
Sollinger, Rickie, and Mie Nakachi. 2016. *Reproductive States: Global Perspectives on the Invention and Implementation of Population Policy*. New York: Oxford University Press.
Sulmasy, Daniel P. 2013. The Varieties of Human Dignity: A Logical and Conceptual Analysis. *Medicine, Health Care and Philosophy* 16 (4): 937–944. https://doi.org/10.1007/s11019-012-9400-1.
United Nations. 1948. United Nations General Assembly *Universal Declaration of Human Rights*.
United Nations. 1969. United Nations General Assembly *Declaration on Social Progress and Development*. Resolution 2542 (XXIV), 11 December 1969, Article 4.
United Nations. 1989. United Nations General Assembly. 1989. *Convention on the Rights of the Child*.
Wallace, Lacey N. 2017. Siblings and Adolescent Weapon Carrying: Contributions of Genetics, Shared Environment, and Unshared Environment. *Youth Violence and Juvenile Justice* 15 (3): 264–280. https://doi.org/10.1177/1541204016639354.
Wenar, Leif. 2005. The Nature of Rights. *Philosophy and Public Affairs* 33 (3): 223–253.
Yao, Shuyang, Henrik Larsson, Claes Norring, Andreas Birgegård, Paul Lichtenstein, Brian M. D'Onofrio, Catarina Almqvist, Laura M. Thornton, Cynthia M. Bulik, and Ralf Kuja-Halkola. 2019. Genetic and Environmental Contributions to Diagnostic Fluctuation in Anorexia Nervosa and Bulimia Nervosa. *Psychological Medicine* 1–8. https://doi.org/10.1017/S0033291719002976.

Chapter 3
What is Relevant: Interests, Needs, and Harms

Abstract A right is a relationship that allows one person or entity to alter the behavior of another. An interest, on the other hand, is something that benefits a person or entity. At an auction, I may have an interest in acquiring an object, but I do not have a right to win the auction. There is a reciprocal relationship between interests and harms. It is against one's interests to be harmed, while frustration of one's interest is a harm. Legal consideration of children's welfare has been based on interests, often expressed as the "best interests standard." The term "best interests" has multiple conflicting meanings. First intended as a legal term of art, the term unfortunately has often been construed literally by bioethicists and by others who should know better. This undiluted focus on the child has led to a salutary attempt to replace the best interests standard as a state intervention principle with a "harm principle" that is closer to legal intent and much legal practice. Reasonable discussion will be difficult unless nomenclature changes. I propose that the intervention principle should be divided into (1) an identification principle for determining when the state may coercively intervene; and (2) a resolution principle for determining how the state should act. Identification of grounds for intervention should be based on failure to meet children's needs; a need is an especially important kind of interest. Resolution should maximize fulfillment of the interests and needs of all stakeholders. It should not necessarily privilege the child in question, nor should health concerns necessarily be prioritized. Parents are to be accepted as the default deciders, and the state has the burden of showing that parents are failing to meet children's needs.

I have argued that stakeholders' rights do not provide a good foundation for resolving conflicts regarding children's health. Indeed, most writers in this area have focused on *interests*, and especially children's interests. Some have emphasized *fulfilling interests* of children, while others have focused on *minimizing harm*. But reduction of harm is an interest. This chapter will focus on the relation between interests and harms, and will define a subset of interests that I call *needs*. I will emphasize that there are non-coercive forms of government intervention, and I will titrate parents' departure from ideal care to appropriate government response.

A. J. Jacobs, *Assigning Responsibility for Children's Health When Parents and Authorities Disagree: Whose Child?*, The International Library of Bioethics 90,
https://doi.org/10.1007/978-3-030-87698-2_3

Interests are something that one person possesses to her benefit. A right is a relationship between at least two people: the rightsholder and those who must accommodate the right. Whenever there are at least two alternative outcomes that can make a person better or worse off it is an interest of that person to achieve the best outcome. Every candidate for political office in a contested election has an interest in winning the position, but none has a right to it. Whether or not Oliver Twist had a right to more porridge, he had an interest in receiving it. The scope of interests is vast. Some interests rise to le level of needs. I hold that it is needs, rather than interests as a whole, that the state may coercively protect.

Two areas of confusion make it difficult to use interests as an intervention principle, which is a basis for coercive state intervention in a family relationship. First is the indeterminacy of interests—it is not clear what they are, or how to prioritize them when they conflict. The second is that the word 'interest' has all but been cemented into the concept of the '*best interests standard*.' This standard has several different meanings with important differences that are not always carefully distinguished. This has led some ethicists to advocate harm avoidance as an alternative to pursuit of best interests.

3.1 Natural History of the Parent-State Conflict

Consider a paradigm for consent to treatment. A decision to actively treat is analogous to the unlocking a safe deposit box. The physician and the patient each must turn a different key for a treatment to proceed. The physician uses the 'key' of professional judgment (beneficence and nonmaleficence) to agree to *perform* the intervention. The patient's key is her informed consent to *receive* the intervention. Dialog between the physician and patient (or surrogate) optimally results in a situation in which the patient receives the treatment that is compatible with the physician's knowledge and the patient's needs and values. This is called *shared decision making* (Elwyn et al. 2012). Procedures require informed consent. Though the ideal of informed consent is not often fully realized it usually is sufficiently approximated to allow care decisions to be implemented without gross injustice. When a patient cannot make a rational decision, a surrogate must make the decision on behalf of the patient (Beauchamp and Childress 2013). The child's parent ordinarily fills this role. Since the child can never have made a legally competent judgment, the child's parent cannot exercise the standards of *pure autonomy* or of *substituted judgment*, which apply to surrogates for adults who become legally incompetent. The appropriate legal decisional standard for children is the *best interests standard*. (Beauchamp & Childress 2013). Some have construed this literally, to mean achieving the highest possible net benefit to the child (Beauchamp and Childress 2013). I will term this construction of the best interests standard the *ideal best interests* standard. It seeks to maximize the child's interest irrespective of other considerations, including the interests of others. It is neither desirable nor possible to use the ideal best interests standard.

When the state alters a parental decision, it is, in effect, limiting parental custody. All parents are imperfect in supporting their children's best interests, sometimes in major respects and sometimes in trivial respects. Not all deficiencies of parental care should be subject to legal intervention. All parents lose their temper, postpone their children's medical appointments, or commit similar venial offences. The trigger for state intervention needs to involve more serious deficits than imperfect parenting. Rather, it seems intuitive that state intervention should be reserved for seriously inadequate care.

American law (Meyer v. Nebraska, 262 US 390, Supreme Court, 1923; *Pierce v. Society of Sisters*, 268 U.S. 510, Supreme Court, 1925) and European law (Charter of Fundamental Rights, 2009, Arts. 7, 9, 33) hold the family to be a fundamental unit of society and the natural environment for the flourishing of children. This entitles the family to a high degree of deference in connection with childrearing. Beyond the shelter of positive law, there are at least eight reasons why parents should be the default surrogate decision-makers for their children:

1. Parents know their children and their needs better than others (Buchanan and Brock 1989).
2. Parents bear many of the consequences of choices made for their children (Buchanan and Brock 1989)
3. The family itself is a valuable social institution (Buchanan and Brock, 1989)
4. The opportunity to perpetuate one's values and concerns is a prime motivation for having children, and reproduction is a fundamental need of society. Conversely, a social system that regards parents as stewards of children on behalf of the state will discourage people from having children (Jacobs and Arora 2018).
5. The vast number of decisions parents make cannot be supervised by the state or others without undue intrusion (Iltis, 2010).
6. The state cannot raise children by itself (Schneider 1995); furthermore, state officials lack expertise and insight sufficient to overrule parental judgment in most cases.
7. Parents need to be able to balance children's interests against those of other members of the family, including their own (Schneider 1995).
8. There is an important state interest in maintaining pluralism. Allowing members of minority communities to live in families that express their values makes pluralism meaningful (Schneider 1995).

Parental prerogatives are not absolute, and there are occasions in which state intervention is justified. The state has the power, and perhaps the responsibility, to protect the vulnerable from harm—even from their legitimate guardians. This power is known in Anglo-American law as the *parens patriae* doctrine (*Prince v. Massachusetts*. 321 U.S. 158, Supreme Court, 1944. *Parenspatriae* has been applied to cases involving disputes over medical care (*Van Winkle v. Nichols*, No. 1:15-cv-01082-JMS-MJD, Southern District, Indiana, 2017; *In re Piland*, No. 340754 Michigan Court of Appeals, 2018). States also have a power to act on behalf of the health, safety, and welfare of their citizens; in the United States this is called *police power* (*Home Building & Loan Association v. Blaisdell*, 290 U.S. 398, 437, Supreme Court, 1934). Finally, the state has a general interest in a healthy, strong, well-educated citizenry for its own reasonable purposes.

Government action against parents entails two phases (Kopelman 2018). First is the decision that a parent's actions are so deficient that the state should step in to reverse the decision or punish the parent. I term this the *identification* phase. Second, the state must determine a remedy for this situation. The state may either refrain from action, or may act to change the parental decision. This is the *resolution* phase of the process. Identification of a serious deficiency and its resolution on behalf of a burdened child require separate intellectual underpinning, much like conviction and sentencing in the criminal justice system. Identification is focused on the child. Just resolution, however, must balance the interests of the child and other stakeholders, including parents and society.

3.2 The Guidance Principle

The guidance principle sets the standard for optimal parenting (Buchanan and Brock 1989). It stipulates the best thing to do, but violation of a guidance principle does not necessarily merit state action. Thus, Kopelman (1997) distinguishes among three senses of the best interests standard. She sees these three different meanings as bases for, respectively, the guidance principal, the identification step in state intervention, and the resolution step. The ideal best interests standard serves as a guidance principle, but encompasses flaws too trivial to justify coercive intervention. Government coercion involving family affairs should be applied mainly to assure that needs are met.

Let us distinguish between interests and needs. If we can identify and set a value to each of a child's interests, then maximization of a child's interests is a prima facie parental duty. Satisfying any single interest is a relatively weak duty, as it is overridden by meeting more compelling interests held by the child and others, including the other members of the family. Suppose that Dr. Baudelaire, a cosmetic surgeon, has promised to take her son Sunny to a museum, but her other son, Klaus, has a medical emergency. Baudelaire clearly is justified in breaking her promise to Sunny, even if this violates Sunny's ideal interests. But Dr. Baudelaire might be morally obliged to cancel a scheduled elective rhinoplasty ('nose job') to attend a school play in which Sunny is acting. Since conflicting interests must be prioritized, and since there is disagreement regarding the importance identity of children's interests, I prefer to call the prima facie duty to maximize a child's interest the *child's interest principle*, which I propose as the guidance principle. I will distinguish this from the *needs principle*, which I use as the identification principle.

3.3 Using the Needs Principle to Govern the Identification Phase of State Intervention

Kopelman's next sense of the best interests standard is as a minimum standard for parental behavior. She calls this the threshold for identification and judgment, (Kopelman 1997) and it is the basis for the identification phase. I will call this the *minimalist best interestsstandard* for the time being. Kopelman believes that this minimalist standard requires a showing of harm. She wants states to intervene based on rules that strike a balance between too much and too little intervention. We do not want to remove a child from a home just because it is untidy.[1] To Kopelman (1997), an overly intrusive state is not acting in a child's best interest. But a child may be removed from a home so dirty as to be dangerous—for example if it is overrun with rats, or if there are feces on the floors. It seems to me that rhetorical clarity requires using different language to distinguish ideal behavior and non-dangerous behavior. Use of the term 'best interests' to characterize both will confuse those who deal with children but are not accustomed to making subtle verbal distinctions or to using terms of art in the course of work.

Identifying the threshold for sanctions generates controversy. Most would agree with overruling parents to allow children to receive lifesaving blood transfusions (*State v. Perricone*, 181 A.2d 751, New Jersey Supreme Court, 1962. Compelling parents to take their children for prophylactic dental exams would be less popular. The line between permitted and impermissible parental departure from the child interest standard lies somewhere in between. American courts have required demonstration of actual or pending harm due to parental unfitness as a condition of restricting custody.[2] Parental deficiency now must be proven by clear and convincing evidence (*Matter of NJ*, 8 P. 3d 126, Nevada Supreme Court, 2000)[3]—meaning that the adjudicator has "an abiding conviction that the truth of its factual contentions are [sic] highly probable." (*Colorado v. New Mexico*, 467 U.S. 310, Supreme Court, 1984, 467).

European jurisdictions place greater limits on parental authority. The European constitutional rights regime recognizes children's claims against parents that American law does not allow. It also grants broader prerogatives and immunities than exist in the United States (Council of Europe 2015). Thus, in contrast to the United States, any spanking, even by parents, is illegal in most European countries. The margin of appreciation doctrine allows differences in the deference that individual states give to parents. Thus, although home schooling is legal in many European countries,

---

[1] This is my example, not Kopelman's.

[2] The Heinemann case (*Heinemann's Appeal*, 96 Pa. 112, Pennsylvania Supreme Court, 1880) may be the first American case to restrict parental rights based on a parent's decision regarding health care. Though the court mentioned the children's interests the case is better construed as relying on imminent parental harm. A father was treating his five children's diphtheria using unproven, nonmedical methods. After three children died the court removed the remaining two from the father's custody. The opinion was based on a child neglect statute, and the father is noted several times in the opinion to have treated the children in a neglectful manner.

[3] To appreciate how the court decided this case, see *Matter of NJ*, 129–130. The mechanism of determination is fairly typical in the US.

Germany terminated parental care of children the parents insisted on home-schooling (*Wunderlich v. Germany*. Application #18,925/15, European Court of Human Rights, 006 (2019).

Using interests as a basis for government action maximizes the flourishing of the child. Different situations, personality, and skill sets of different children may result in different interests. Music lessons may be a more important interest for a child who is interested and gifted in music than for a child who doesn't care about music. But a need is a matter of fundamental importance, and music lessons are not a need. Needs, such as adequate nutrition and protection from violence, are more similar from child to child than are many interests.

3.4 Harm and the Harm Principle

Interests and harm are two sides of the same coin. It is in one's interest not to be harmed. And it is harmful not to have one's interests realized. But neither interests nor harms can be precisely defined, let alone be assigned relative values. There can be tradeoffs between harms and interests. Perhaps Helen Keller led a happier, more fulfilled, and even more independent life than would have been the case had she not been rendered blind and deaf in early childhood. Furthermore, current and future harms and interests may be inversely related. A child's illness (a harm) may contribute to his subsequence resilience. It may make him more empathic toward ill people. It may inspire him to go into a health profession.

A *need* is a kind of interest that must be satisfied in order to avoid a high probability of tangible serious harm. We do not remove children from their homes for their parents' failure to meet the ideal best interest standard. We remove children only for parental deficiencies that may result in grievous harm. To put it another way, the state intervenes when a parent is not meeting, or is likely not to meet in the future, a child's needs. We expect parents to satisfy their children's needs. Parental failure to meet a need is unacceptable if the need can be addressed. Fulfilling interests that do not rise to the level of needs does not carry the same moral weight as meeting needs. We demand that the state and parents provide children with literacy and with vaccination against serious communicable diseases, but not that they provide chess lessons and cosmetic orthodontia. Thus, I will call this principle governing the identification phase of intervention the *needs principle.*

One reason to distinguish among interests and needs is to define state authority and limit state abuses. The government-perceived interests of children from aboriginal groups formed the rationale for forced adoption into ethnically European families in Australia (Cuthbert and Quartly 2012) and Canada (Sinclair 2007), and for forced relocation to residential schools in Canada (Bombay et al. 2009) and the United States (Trennert 1983). Without clearly defined rules, parental care can be terminated when the parents do not value the sort of education that the government values. This potentially endangers the integrity of minority families whose cultures do not sufficiently value secular education. This might include aboriginal children, Amish children, Chasidic Jewish children, etc. The state may say that it is not in the child's *interest* to be raised in a communist home, a homophobic home, or one that is not 'anti-racist' (choose your unpopular political belief). Use of the needs principle may make abuses of interest principles less likely.

I now address the relationship between needs and harms. My needs principle encompasses somewhat more parental deviation than Douglas Diekema's respected *harm principle* (Diekema 2004). Diekema modifies John Stuart Mill's harm principle, which states that the only justification a government has for action against an individual is to prevent harm to other individuals. He and his colleagues then use harm to a child as an identification principle (Hester et al. 2018). The harm principle is better identification principle than is best interests, an imprecise and indeterminate term with maximalist implications in the eyes of some of its prominent proponents. Diekema (2004) modifies Mill's harm principle to demand that the threat of harm be imminent, and that the intervention is one that most parents would believe is reasonable (Diekema 2004). Diekema believes that his application of the harm principle is similar to that used by contemporary in making determinations of child abuse or neglect, and that it accommodates the needs of children.

I prefer the needs principle to the harm principle for the following reasons. First, though Diekema (2004) acknowledged public health rationales for intervention, he explicitly declined to discuss them. Also, Diekema defines harm allowing intervention as being immediate and serious. I consider this to be too narrow. Consider a child with severe obesity whose parents continue to feed him a high calorie, high carbohydrate diet. This may cause complications that gradually lead to disability and death. End stage obesity complications include insulin-dependent Type 2 diabetes, obstructive airway disease leading to heart failure, and fatty hepatitis and cirrhosis (Varness et al. 2009). These harms, including death, even occur in some children. Thus, some would remove a child from a home if there is high likelihood of serious harm, removal is likely to result in effective weight loss, and other interventions with the family have been exhausted. The needs principle might sanction removal of an obese child with systemic health problems from parental care sooner than would a version of the harm principle that required imminent serious harm.[4]

Also, consider a society in which literacy were important for full participation, and in which ample resources were available for medical care. Myron, age 7, is not learning to read. A screen by the school nurse shows that Myron is severely myopic. Myron's parents, for idiosyncratic reasons, refuse to allow Myron to receive optometric evaluation or to wear glasses. The needs principle might require parents to cooperate with use of visual prostheses or risk state intervention. As I read Diekema's harm principle, the parents would be allowed to refuse treatment for Myron, even if he never learns to read.

---

[4] Of course, if poor parenting is not to blame for a child's obesity (Merry and Voight 2014) then it would be unjust to remove the child from his home.

3.5 An Ideal Best Interests Standard is Incompatible with Liberal Pluralism

I have suggested that the best interests standard could be abused. The ideal best interests principle, if used as an identification principle, gives cover undermining parental relationships in favor of state policy. Shah (2013) distinguishes an ideal best interests legal standard, which she calls a "*paramount*" or absolute standard, from a "*primary*" standard which allows courts to weigh considerations besides a child's interests.

An ideal, absolute, or paramount standard has three problems, First, it allows courts to interfere deeply in family affairs. Consider the custody of Orpheus, whose parents recently died, and whose two uncles each want to adopt him. Orpheus's upbringing will be identical in the two homes except for the recreational interests that the uncles will try to cultivate. Uncle Basil will play baseball with Orpheus, while Uncle Chester will play chess. The judge awards custody to Chester, ruling (within her appropriate discretion) that chess is a more valuable pastime than baseball. It transpires after a year that Chester is not playing chess with Orpheus. Though Orpheus is happy and thriving, and loves Chester. Basil sues for custody. Basil claims that even if chess is more valuable than baseball, baseball is more valuable than no pastime. Judge Hans finds that the deciding factor is the stability of the relationship, and that the difference in recreation is less important. Chester retains custody. Basil appeals, and Judge Hestia awards custody to Basil, using the paramount standard. Hestia accepts Basil's argument that a shared recreational activity is more in Orpheus's interest than no shared recreation, and that the ideal objective situation must be sought.

Those who agree with Judge Hestia may now consider the next case on the judge's docket. It shows that an ideal best interests standard can be used to break up families, even if parental care is adequate. Bruce Wayne,a rich bachelor (known not to be a pedophile) encountered 9-year-old Dewey Ostavil at a settlement house.[5] Dewey and his three siblings live with their mother, Eudora, who works 80 h a week to support the family. She is a loving, caring parent who is fit by usual standards. Dewey performs above grade level at an inner-city school. The family is poor, though. Bruce files a request to adopt Dewey. Bruce can provide Dewey with a more fashionable name (Robin), private tutors, and a thrilling life as a vigilante. After Bruce dies, Dewey/Robin, as his heir, will be a billionaire. Hestia awards custody to Bruce.

This illustrates another problem. The best interests standard elevates tangible over relational needs. If one accepts the intuitive conclusion that a stranger should not be allowed to break up a family that is taking satisfactory care of a child no matter how much more this alternative adult has to offer the child, then one must abandon the ideal best interests principle. There are several ways to do this. One is to postulate that the family is a foundational element of society that can only be dismembered for inadequate parental care. Another is to balance the interests of other interested parties. Eudora and her other four children have an interest in family continuity.

---

[5] I have taken. extensive liberties with the back story of the Batman comics and films.

Indeed, all members of all families have an interest in preventing raids by rich and powerful people who take a fancy to our children. A third approach is to single out relational interests as relatively inviolable.

A third problem is that if majority values are accepted as the basis for identifying and determining the priority of interests, minorities are disadvantaged. Consider a state, Denisovia, with an implacably hostile cultural minority, the Neandertals. The Neandertals remain impoverished and unhealthy because of their cultural norms. Denisovia decides to solve the problem by removing all newborn Neandertals from their homes and adopting them into Denisovian families. The Neandertal-born children live comfortably. Neandertal parents are otherwise left undisturbed as long as they obey the laws. Denisovia becomes a more pleasant and prosperous place as the Neandertal culture fades. (Similar polices have actually been adopted in enlightened Anglophone democracies.) Application of the paramount principle as an identification principle can rationalize massive injustice, and even cultural genocide.

In conclusion, the needs principle should be used as an identification principle. It will be reified to this end in the State Intervention Test.

3.5.1 The Resolution Step

Let us assume the needs standard is the identification principle, and look at how to resolve parental violations of the needs principle. Kopelman's (1997) third and last construction of the best interests standard is as a standard of *reasonableness*. Kopelman identifies this construction of best interests—the best interests under the circumstances—with the standard legal use of best interests standard as used in settling custody disputes. The best interests standard originated as a legal concept for determination of child custody in the English case in chancery of *de Manneville v. de Manneville*, 32 Eng. Rep. 762 (Ch. 1804) (Abramowicz 2009). This case is the root of American law of custody, which considers the child's situation as well as the parents' (Dolgin 1996).[6] Paternal custody gave way to less gender-specific doctrines still based on parental status, such as the Tender Years doctrine, which rebuttably presumed maternal custody for young children. Subsequent rules included the less gender-specific Primary Caretaker and Psychological Parent doctrines. The best interests standard ultimately prevailed because it was based on the child's welfare, rather than on the status of the parental litigants (Mason 2011).

Used in the context of parental custody, 'best' in best interests standard never meant 'the very best possible.' Rather, it means 'best choice among legally possible options.' Pope (2011) asserts that the body of jurisprudence provides an adequate

[6] In one early case custody was awarded to the mother because of the father's incapacity to care for the children. (*Commonwealth v. Addicks*, 5 Binn. 520, Pennsylvania Supreme Court, 1813). Two years later, the father regained custody because the adulterous mother was found to be a bad moral influence (*Commonwealth v. Addicks & Lee*, 2 Serg. & Rawle 174, Pennsylvania Supreme Court, 1815) In each case, the court considered the effects on the child, albeit with differing outcomes.

guide using best interests standard as a reasonably precise legal term of art in this way, as applied to the narrow context of custody. I call this the *best choice best interest standard* to distinguish it from the ideal and minimalist best interest standards.

Empirical findings contradict Pope's hope that courts will apply the best choice version of the best interest standard rather than the ideal version (paramount principle, in Shah's terms). Shah (2013) reviewed actual court resolutions of health care disputes. In the 56 cases that met her criteria for analysis, 44 courts applied the paramount principle to the child in question, using only health considerations. Proposed organ or bone marrow donations to a sibling were disfavored even though there might be psychological benefits to the donor and there were great benefits to the recipient sibling. Shah believes that the best interests standard is a 'legal fiction'—a false or unproven supposition that provides cover for a legal rule (Smith 2007). Use of legal fictions is conclusory (see next section) and creates lack of transparency and predictability. The ideal best interests standard serves as a fig leaf for whatever a judge wants to decide. Saying that we are using the ideal best interests standard for any determination regarding a child (ignoring, now, for the sake of argument, the interests of other individuals) does not say what interests to consider, or what weight to assign different interests. These two determinations are hampered by the multitude of interests, the controversiality of some of them, and the varying degree of their importance when these interests conflict. (This problem applies not only to interests, but to harms.)

This book is primarily about resolutions of parent-state conflicts that coerce parents. There are other kinds of resolutions, and the interests of all stakeholders must be considered in the resolution process. The subject will be addressed in detail in the next chapter.

3.5.2 Delineation of Interests and Harms is Conclusory

A conclusory principle is one that pretends a deductive approach to solve problems, while it actually uses an inductive approach. A typical judgment based on a legal principle is deductivist; it can be phrased as a syllogism. Consider a law that defines a mother as parent by birth or adoption. Eve brings Cain to a pediatric clinic, and a female wolf named Louve brings Romulus. The major premise determines the conclusion, even if it is counterintuitive (as in the second syllogism):

Someone who gives birth to a child is that child's mother. (Legal principle)

Eve gave birth to Cain. (Fact)

Eve is Cain's mother. (Law is correctly applied to fact)

A parent by adoption is the child's mother. (Legal principle)

Louve, a female adult wolf, has formally adopted Romulus. (Fact)

Louve is the mother of Romulus. (Law is correctly applied to fact).

Clearly, legislative drafting should have been more careful in defining mothers, but a court has an easy time deciding that Eve and Louve are mothers. But try to define privacy. This is a conclusory term (Gavison 1980). Privacy has something to do with being let alone. But it seems not to cover, for example, imprisonment for crimes, disclosure of sensitive information to obtain occupational licenses, or a requirement that people carry identification on their persons in public. These invasions are not considered invasions of privacy in democratic nations in which they are in effect. Privacy is what a government says it is. Rather than the term defining the immunity (privacy implies immunity from government action), the government decides when it wants to interfere with people, and calls other areas private. But, unlike the case with the motherhood law described above, there is no bright line that says when a decision on privacy is deductive or is inductive and conclusory.

Best interests analysis is highly conclusory. An example is Connecticut General Statutes 46b–56(c),[7] a law concerning custody. This law appears to tell the judge what to do, but it provides so much wiggle room that a judge can decide pretty much as she pleases. This statute, though it supposedly provides a detailed framework for analysis of best interests, is conclusory in practice. The legal fiction of best interests is actually a cover for judges' subjective views.

Mnookin (1975) used the indeterminacy of best interests standard to launch a devastating criticism. A rational decision-maker can use a rule to specify possible alternative resolutions. She then can apply rules to specify which of these outcomes she prefers. He notes that the best interests standard neither allows formulation of specific rules nor provides metrics to rank possible solutions. Another problem with

---

[7] In making or modifying any order as provided in subsections (a) and (b) of this section, *the court shall consider the best interestsof the child, and in doing so may consider, but shall not be limited to, one or more of the following factors*: (1) The temperament and developmental needs of the child; (2) the capacity and the disposition of the parents to understand and meet the needs of the child; (3) any relevant and material information obtained from the child, including the informed preferences of the child; (4) the wishes of the child's parents as to custody; (5) the past and current interaction and relationship of the child with each parent, the child's siblings and any other person who may significantly affect the best interests of the child; (6) the willingness and ability of each parent to facilitate and encourage such continuing parent–child relationship between the child and the other parent as is appropriate, including compliance with any court orders; (7) any manipulation by or coercive behavior of the parents in an effort to involve the child in the parents' dispute; (8) the ability of each parent to be actively involved in the life of the child; (9) the child's adjustment to his or her home, school and community environments; (10) the length of time that the child has lived in a stable and satisfactory environment and the desirability of maintaining continuity in such environment, provided the court may consider favorably a parent who voluntarily leaves the child's family home pendente lite in order to alleviate stress in the household; (11) the stability of the child's existing or proposed residences, or both; (12) the mental and physical health of all individuals involved, except that a disability of a proposed custodial parent or other party, in and of itself, shall not be determinative of custody unless the proposed custodial arrangement is not in the best interests of the child; (13) the child's cultural background; (14) the effect on the child of the actions of an abuser, if any domestic violence has occurred between the parents or between a parent and another individual or the child; (15) whether the child or a sibling of the child has been abused or neglected… and (16) whether the party satisfactorily completed participation in a parenting education program … *The court is not required to assign any weight to any of the factors that it considers, but shall articulate the basis for its decision.* (Emphasis supplied.).

best interests standard is that in order to determine what is best, one must be able to predict the future (Mnookin 1975). In order to determine whether best interests dictate teaching my child French or Japanese I need to know which will serve his interests in the future, which is related to (1) the future geopolitical importance of these two nations; and (2) whether people in these countries are willing to communicate in English. Neither this nor many other future events that determine what is in the best interests of children can be determined accurately. Regarding health, medical diagnoses may be incorrect, or may be based on imprecise criteria defining a disease. Also, and more important, there may be no objective way to determine the values that should inform the resolution of conflicts between parents and a medical team or other public agency. For the child lacking legal competence, there are many possible things for decision-makers to consider. These include, for example, the child's happiness, his career prospects, and his religious training. How does one balance commitment to interpersonal relations, disciplined, self-abnegating pursuit of personal goals, and intellectual life? Judges seeking to determine cases involving children must consider such factors, and many others.

Some interests of children are present interests, and others are future interests. There may be trade-offs between present and future interests, and these must be balanced (Salter 2012). Current discomfort may improve future prospects, and vice versa. What may seem to be harmful in the short run may be beneficial in the long run. Considerations may include objective physical benefits, such as comfort and prosperity. In addition, a child's putative direct interests may be psychological-emotional, cognitive-developmental, relational, or spiritual. Furthermore, interests may be either self-regarding or others-regarding (Salter 2012). Self-regarding interests provide a direct benefit. Others-regarding interests are those apropos to maintaining a relationship with others. An example of this is a child who donates an organ or bone marrow to a sibling. In cases such as this, imposing a narrow, self-regarding best interests standard precludes children from making altruistic decisions, requiring them to pursue 'self-seeking' values. *Curran v. Bosze*, 566 N.E.2d 1319, Illinois Supreme Court, 1990, for example refused a parental request for a bone marrow transplant from one 3-year-old twin to the other twin, despite the low risk of serious complications.

The health care team is apt to limit their consideration to children's health interests. All of us, including children, have many other interests, though. Setting aside cases in which parents' opposition to medical science barred clearly effective treatment, cases in which treatment is of limited effectiveness but has great impact on quality of life have led enlightened courts to weigh.

> [parents'] interest in making fundamental decisions regarding the care of their minor child, the state's interest in preserving human life, and the child's own welfare and best interests, in light of the severity of the child's illness, the likelihood as to whether the proposed treatment will be effective, the child's chances of survival with and without such treatment, and the invasiveness and *nature of the treatment with regard to its effect on the child* [i.e., quality of life considerations]. *M.N. v. Southern Baptist Hospital of Florida*, 648 So.2d 769, District Court of Appeal of Florida, First District, 1994, 771; emphasis supplied.

The harm principle is indeterminate as well, as evidenced by Birchley's (2016) example described in Chap. 1. Two mothers received babies under similar circumstances outside the UK which they mistakenly believed to be theirs. One mother's baby was taken away, while the other mother got to keep her baby. These decisions were made in the same judicial district, based on almost identical facts.

Lack of objective standards allow doctors and courts to render decisions reflecting their profession, class, and community. Physicians, of course, tend to prioritize their patient's health interests, perhaps at the expense of relational and psychological interests. Jehovah's Witnesses will not be allowed to deny their children essential transfusions (*State v. Perricone*, 181 A. 2d 751, New Jersey Supreme Court, 1962; a neglect standard was used to decide this case). But parents are free to refuse life-saving transfusions even if the consequence is to leave their children parentless (*Public HealthTrust v. Wons*, 541 So. 2d 96, Florida Supreme Court, 1989).The life of the patient in question is considered, but the effect of treatment on the lives of others is not.

3.6 Conflicts Between Health and Other Interests

I now consider conflict between children's health interests and their other interests. Rather than using extreme examples such as life-saving transfusions to justify best interests (when application of the harm principle would carry the load) I will use a less dramatic situation.

Extensive near work such as reading is associated with development of myopia in children (Ku et al. 2018). A great deal of near work is also a feature of challenging academic programs beginning in primary school. Myopia interferes with, or forecloses, performance at a high level in certain sports, and also precludes certain occupations, such as piloting planes commercially. How shall we regard parents who encourage or compel their children to spend long hours studying, knowing that their children are more likely to develop myopia—a physical disability that causes some occupational limitation? I think we should not act against them or discourage them. Conversely, we should not take action against parents who, in order to produce aviators, limit children's study time to preserve their eyesight, even at the risk of lower grades that interfere with academic success at a high level. Readers of this article are likely to have advanced degrees and to consider academic and professional achievement to be of high value. My readers (many of whom are myopic, as am I) may regard their child's interest in becoming a doctor, lawyer, or academician as greater than her interest in retaining visual acuity and becoming a pilot or a sniper. High school contact sports can impair cognition by causing brain trauma. American football is a prestigious pastime for young men, though. Many believe that it teaches group cooperation (Wistrom 2018), competition, and resilience. Some proponents and opponents of close work may consider the risks of football to be worth the benefits, but others will not. Ranking a child's interest in these examples is indeterminate, and children may not be mature enough to make those decisions in an autonomous manner. Parents' values play a part in how they prioritize the various aspects of their children's health. State intervention, either at a policy or individual level, is inappropriate.

Spiritual and relational interests are especially likely to lead to controversy. A religious belief is a concept that has a transcendental or numinous component that cannot be inferred from empirical observation (Jacobs and Arora 2018), A religion is an organization or community dedicated to affirming common religious beliefs and acting in a manner consonant with those beliefs. This includes performing rituals and activities the religion requires, and refraining from engaging in behavior the religion forbids. A religious person is likely to prioritize his religious beliefs and practices over other commitments. This is because either she wishes to align herself with the purpose of the cosmos or because she is concerned with the consequences of doing or not doing so (George 2008). Consequently, someone who takes her religious beliefs seriously cannot accept the plenary power of the state (Hauerwas and Baxter 1992).

On the other hand, monist liberal secular belief sees the state as a being a collective of free and equal citizens whose categorical power is limited only by a few basic constraints. Rawls (1997) held that the only justifications or arguments that are acceptable for public discussion are those which all citizens might reasonably accept. These exclude religious views, as everyone accepts inference from empirical data but not everyone recognizes the validity of testimonies based on faith (Audi 2011). But many people feel as though they have a personal relationship with God, and communicate with demiurges such as saints and angels. These same people may have limited exposure to inferential statistics. They may believe that being asked to accept the conclusions of climate scientists without having been presented with any of the reasoning behind the models was being asked to accept something on faith.[8] I am not arguing against the reality of climate change here. Rather, I am pointing out that understandings of what is reasonable are not culturally neutral. However, religious or spiritual claims that disadvantage children's health must be balanced against those health claims. The state should use the needs principle to determine whether parental behavior merits interference, bearing in mind that, as stated in the Convention on the Rights of the Child, Art. 30, "a child belonging to [a minority group] shall not be denied the right, in community with other members of his or her group, to enjoy his or her own culture, [or] to profess and practice his or her own religion."

Children have an important direct interest in stable, supportive, loving relationships (McLaughlin 2009). They consequently have an interest in the well-being of those they love. In addition, loss of a loved one often has deleterious social, economic, and psychological consequences.

Cunningham (2016) points out that mainstream bioethics is not value free, and tends to prioritize individual over relational considerations. That this prioritization does not necessarily resonate outside professional and academic circles was shown by the international attention given to Charlie Gard (Lantos 2017), an infant whose

[8] Indeed, how many humanities professors understand the science that supports the existence of climate change?

parents' request for futile treatment at no expense to the UK national health system was denied by British courts (*Great Ormond Street Hospital v Yates & Ors*, [2017] EWHC 972 (Fam) (England and Wales High Court [Family Division]) April 11, 2017.

In some instances, the likelihood, or certainty, of harm from parental decisions not to treat a child for illness is clear-cut (Offit 2015). At other times, physicians and medical facilities have initiated legal action culminating in long-distance police chases (Cohen and Bonifeld 2018)[9] or SWAT team invasion of homes (Adeel 2019) based on assessments of young patients' medical needs that may not have been well-founded. State intervention is more likely when parents are difficult to deal with (Cohen and Bonifeld 2018), doubt the efficacy of medical science (Adeel 2019), are uneducated and inarticulate (Cunningham 2016), belong to disfavored minority religious and cultures (Gray and Brunger 2018), or when a combination of these elements is present.

Bester would like to place identification and resolution on a normative footing (Bester 2018). I believe it is impossible to do this. There is inevitably some arbitrariness in these decisions. There are at least four reasons for this. One is Berlin's value pluralism. Another is the paradox of illiberalism in the liberal state. Third, most normative systems lead to at least some results that offend our intuitive sense of justice. Utilitarianism offers the vulnerable too little protection (note my earlier Bruce Wayne/Robin example), while Rawls's maximin justice principle of favoring the welfare of the worst-off may offer the vulnerable too much protection. The fourth reason is the difficulty of applying general concepts to specific situations, as whether late abortion is murder, or whether statutes criminalizing incest violate the right to establish families (Frick 2019). The putative interests that a society will accept as valid, and their relative importance, then, may be political matters—determined by societal preference. Some moral rules are universal, and are necessary for people to live together in societies (Haidt 2012; Henrich 2016; Curry 2021). Regulation of violence within society, honesty, and physical and social reproduction are some examples of such moral rules. Frick (2019) demonstrates that even among societies committed to the European rights regime there is great room for variation based on local conditions and mores; she calls this *relative universalism* (Frick 2019).

As I have noted, members of society, and society as a whole, have interests. Some of these that are politically relevant are succinctly summarized in the Preamble to the United States Constitution (1787):

> …establish Justice, insure domestic Tranquility, provide for the common defense, promote the general Welfare, and secure the Blessings of Liberty to ourselves and our Posterity…

If these political considerations are salient, then public health policy may, at times, supersede individual interests and opinions regarding children's health as well as general policy that affects children. Parents and other persons and groups with which a child is connected have interests as well. A child's interest is not absolute

[9] But see the response to the media story by the facility involved, at https://newsnetwork.mayoclinic.org/CNN-Letter-08-15-2018.pdf, accessed April 27, 2019.

(Shah 2013). The need to reconcile interests of children with those of others is one reason I recommend the needs principle over other identification standards more deferential to the child. I believe that the needs principle is similar to Shah's (2014) *secure child standard* for parental consent to medical research. This standard requires deference to parental decisions unless the child is exposed to an unjustified risk of significant harm. Other similar standards include Wilder's (2009) *substantial harm* standard proposed for custody cases, and Mutcherson's (2002) *actual or imminent harm* standard for superseding parental authority to authorize treatment of potentially fatal diseases.

Ideally, the resolution phase should be a *comprehensive utilitarianresolution* based on maximizing the interests of all concerned. Physicians' recommendations as their patients' health fiduciaries must, at times be subordinate to their patients' non-medical needs. Physicians may also have to accommodate to the interests, and especially needs, of other stakeholders, such as family members. Non-medical interests include psychological and direct relational interests, and may also include a child's spiritual interests, dignitary interests or even (in the case of an older child with well-formed ideas) ideological preferences, all balanced in accordance with the doctrine of value pluralism. We must ask not only about what we must provide to the child (Bester 2018), but also what we ought to provide to other interested parties.

3.7 Conclusion

I have advocated that parents be the default decision-makers for their children, with the state serving to correct gross parental malfeasance. I have tried to establish that neither considerations of rights nor protection of autonomy is an appropriate basis for state intervention. In this Chap. 1 began to formulate a doctrine to delineate when state intervention is justified and when it is not. Interests and needs are the currency of my approach. Taken literally, the best interests standard is useful only as a guidance standard. As a standard for identifying actionable parental malfeasance, we must look to needs, which are a subset of interests that command special respect. However, I believe that Diekema's iteration of the harm principle is too stringent. Furthermore, decisions must consider the interests of all stakeholders, and not just those of the child in question. Once a situation is identified as requiring state action, the resolution should take into consideration the interests of all parties involved, including those of society.

I now will examine the child as a member of the family and as a member of society.

References

Abramowitz, Sarah. 2009. Childhood and the limits of contract. *Yale Journal of Law and Humanities* 21 (1): 37–100.

Adeel, Hassan. 2019. *Officers Take Sick Toddler, Unvaccinated, from House.* New York Times, March 30, 2019. https://www.nytimes.com/2019/03/29/us/unvaccinated-children-home-raids.html

Beauchamp, Tom L., and James F. Childress. 2013. *Principles of Biomedical Ethics*, 7th edn. New York: Oxford University Press.

Bester, Johan Christiaan. 2018. The harm principle cannot replace the best interests standard: Problems with using the harm principle for medical decision-making for children. *American Journal of Bioethics* 18 (8): 9–19.

Birchley, Giles. 2016. Harm is all you need? Best interests and disputes about parental decision-making. *Journal of Medical Ethics* 42 (2): 111–115.

Bombay, Amy, Kim Matheson, and Hymie Anisman. 2009. Intergenerational trauma: Convergence of multiple processes among first nations peoples in Canada. *Journal of: Aboriginal Health* 5 (3): 6–47.

Buchanan, Allen E., and Dan W. Brock. 1989. *Deciding for Others: The Ethics of Surrogate Decision Making.* Cambridge: Cambridge University Press.

Cohen, Elizabeth, and John Bonifield. 2018. *Escape from the Mayo Clinic: Parents Break Teen Out of World-Famous Hospital.* CNN Health. August 17, 2018. https://www.cnn.com/2018/08/13/health/mayo-clinic-escape-2-eprise/index.html

Council of Europe. 2015. *European Union Agency for Fundamental Rights and Council of Europe. Handbook on European Law Relating to the Rights of the Child.* https://www.echr.coe.int/Documents/Handbook_rights_child_ENG.pdf

Cunningham, Thomas V. 2016. A life below the threshold? Examining conflict between ethical principles and parental values in neonatal treatment decision making. *Narrative Inquiry in Bioethics* 6 (1): 63–71.

Cuthbert, Denise M., and Marian Quartly. 2012. 'Forced adoption' in the Australian story of national story of national regret and apology. *Australian Journal of Politics and History* 58 (1): 82–96.

Diekema, Douglas S. 2004. Parental refusals of medical treatment: The harm principle as threshold for state intervention. *Theoretical Medicine* 25 (4): 241–264.

Dolgin, Janet L. 1996. Why has the best interest standard survived? The historic and social context. *Children's Legal Rights Journal* 16 (1): 2–10.

Elwyn, Glyn, Dominick Frosh, Richard Thompson, Natalie Joseph-Williams, Amy Lloyd, Paul Kinnersley, Emma Cording, et al. 2012. Shared Decision making: A model for clinical practice. *Journal of General Internal Medicine* 27 (10): 1361–1367. https://doi.org/10.1007/s11606-012-2077-6.

Frick, Marie-Luisa. 2019. *Human Rights and Relative Universalism.* Cham: Palgrave Macmillan.

Gavison, Ruth. 1980. Privacy and the limits of law. *Yale Law Journal* 89 (3): 421–471.

George, Robert P. 2008. Natural law. *Harvard Journal of Law and Public Policy* 31 (1): 171–196.

Gray, Ben, and Fern Brunger. 2018. (Mis)understandings and uses of 'Culture' in bioethics deliberations over parental refusal of treatment: Children with cancer. *Clinical Ethics* 13 (2): 55–66.

Haidt, Jonathan. 2012. *The Righteous Mind: Why Good People are Divided by Politics and Religion.* New York: Pantheon.

Hauerwas, Stanley, and Michael Baxter. 1992. The kingship of Christ: Why freedom of "Belief" is not enough. *De Paul Law Review* 42 (1): 107–127.

Henrich, Joseph. 2016. *The Secret of Our Success: How Culture is Driving Human Evolution, Domesticating Our Species, and Making Us Smarter*. Princeton: Princeton University Press.

Hester, D. Micah, Kellie R. Lang, Nanibaa' A. Garrison, and Douglas S. Diekema. 2018. Agreed: The harm principle cannot replace the best interest standard ... but the best interest standard cannot replace the harm principle either. *American Journal of Bioethics* 18 (8): 38–40.

Iltis, Ana S. 2010. Toward a coherent account of pediatric decision making. *Journal of Medicine and Philosophy* 35 (5): 526–552.

Jacobs, Allan J., and Kavita Shah Arora. 2018. When may government interfere with religious practices to protect the health and safety of children? *Ethics in Medicine and Public Health* 5 (1): 86–93.

Kopelman, Loretta M. 1997. The best-interests standard as threshold, ideal, and standard of reasonableness. *Journal of Medicine and Philosophy* 22 (3): 271–289.

Kopelman, Loretta M. 2018. Why the best interest standard is not self-defeating, too individualistic, unknowable, vague or subjective. *American Journal of Bioethics* 18 (8): 34–36.

Ku, Po-Wen, Andrew Steptoe, Yun-Ju Lai, Hsiao-Yun Hu, Dachen Chu, Yung-Feng Yen, Yung Liao, and Li-Jung Chen. 2018. The associations between near visual activity and incident myopia in children: A nationwide 4-year follow-up study. *Ophthalmology* 126 (2): 214–20

Lantos, John D. 2017. The tragic case of Charlie Gard. *JAMA Pediatrics* 171 (1): 935–936.

Mason, Mary Ann. 2011. The roller coaster of child custody law over the last half century. *Journal of the American Academy of Matrimonial Lawyers* 24 (2): 451–466.

McLaughlin, Julia Halloran. 2009. The fundamental truth about best interests. *Saint Louis University Law Journal* 54 (1): 116–165.

Merry, Michael S., and Kristin Voigt. 2014. Risk, harm and intervention: The case of child obesity. *Medical and Health Care Philosophy* 17 (2): 191–200.

Mnookin, Robert H. 1975. Child-custody adjudication: Judicial functions in the face of indeterminacy. *Law and Contemporary Problems* 39 (3): 226–293.

Mutcherson, Kimberly M. 2002. No way to treat a woman: Creating an appropriate standard for resolving medical treatment disputes involving HIV-positive children. *Harvard Women's Law Journal* 25 (2): 221–279.

Offit, Paul. 2015. *Bad Faith: When Religious Belief Undermines Modern Medicine*. New York: Basic Books.

Pope, Thaddeus M. 2011. The best interest standard: Both guide and limit to medical decision making on behalf of incapacitated patients. *Journal of Clinical Ethics* 22 (2): 134–140.

Salter, Erica K. 2012. Deciding for a child: A comprehensive analysis of the best interest standard. *Theoretical Medicine and Bioethics*. 33 (3): 179–198.

Schneider, Carl E. 1995. On the duties and rights of parents. *Virginia Law Review* 81 (8): 2477–2491.

Shah, Seema. 2013. Does Research with children violate the best interests standard? An empirical and conceptual analysis. *Northwestern Journal of Law and Social Policy* 8 (2): 121–173.

Sinclair, Raven. 2007. Identity lost and found: Lessons from the sixties scoop. *First Peoples Child and Family Review* 3 (1): 65–82.

Smith, Peter J. 2007. New legal fictions. *Georgetown Law Journal* 95 (5): 1435–1496.

Trennert, Robert A. 1983. From Carlisle to Phoenix: The rise and fall of the Indian outing system, 1878–1930. *Pacific Historical Review* 52 (3): 267–291.

Varness, Todd, David B. Allen, Aaron L. Carrel, and Norman Fost. 2009. Childhood obesity and medical neglect. *Pediatrics* 123 (1): 399–406.

Wilder, Joanne Ross. 2009. Resolving religious disputes in custody cases: It's really not about best interests. *Journal of the American Academy of Matrimonial Lawyers* 22: 411–423.

Wistrom, Grant. 2018. The Importance of Teamwork: What Football Can Teach Us About Finding Success as a Team. February 14, 2018. https://www.linkedin.com/pulse/importance-teamwork-what-football-can-teach-us-finding-grant-wistrom/

Chapter 4
What We Owe Parents and Family

Abstract The family is the basic unit of society, and the interests of family members and the family unit are always relevant. Despite much rhetoric, neither parents nor physicians (let alone the state!) have a true fiduciary relationship with children under their care. Parents are responsible for the physical care of their children, and for their education leading them to a status as productive adults. They are responsible for their children's flourishing. Neither their responsibility to an individual child nor their responsibility to the government is categorical. First, parents appropriately balance the interests of all family members (including their own), and the corporate interests of the family as a whole. Second, the state has non-coercive means of intervention at its disposal. This chapter reviews and expands on some prior approaches to parental authority and responsibility. The chapter classifies parental behavior into four categories, based on the maximum appropriate state response. Parental behavior within the Zone of Acceptability warrants no government attention. The next two zones represent divisions of Gillam's Zone of Parental Discretion. Parental action within the Zone of State Attention may elicit educational efforts and the provision of services. Parental behavior within the Zone of Concern invites nudges, mandatory programs with op-out possibilities, etc. Finally, parental behavior within the Zone of Unacceptability justifies coercive state action to reverse or punish potential or actual harm. Harm may not involve the child per se, but can involve third parties, as with parental vaccination refusal.

4.1 Introduction: What Are Family Interests?

I have argued that fulfilling interests, and especially that subset of interests called needs, should be the basis for judging parents' treatment of their children. The interests of all stakeholders must be considered. Families and their members usually are most directly and forcefully affected by these decisions. In this Chap. 1 will explore the family as stakeholders and as decision-makers for children.

Groll (2014) identifies four non-exclusive ways to conceive of family relationships involving sick children. First, the *sick child's interestsare primary*. The relevance of

A. J. Jacobs, *Assigning Responsibility for Children's Health When Parents and Authorities Disagree: Whose Child?*, The International Library of Bioethics 90,
https://doi.org/10.1007/978-3-030-87698-2_4

parents' interests is to optimize their ability to care for their children. Second, *the well-being of the child is also a parental interest*. Third, the *family may have corporate interests* beyond those of its members. Kinship identity, kinship cooperation, and competition among kindreds are basic to human psychology (Henrich 2016, 2020). From ancient times to the present (Asma 2013; Hazony 2018) many have regarded the family as being a fundamental basis for human organization, more basic than the state. Schoeman (1985) described the family as organic, enduring, and possessing goals and purposes. The family has interests apart from individual interests. Weakening it deprives its children of physical, and especially, social and psychological needs. (Lindemann 2014). The fourth and last consideration is the form of family relationship is the *individual interestsof all family members*, as these will be affected by decisions involving a single member.

Being ill does not automatically trump another interest of another family member. Consider the Talleyrand family, which lives in Paris, Texas, where Talia Talleyrand is a professor of diplomacy. She has an offer of a high government job in Vienna, Virginia. Her hemophiliac son, Alexis, would be best treated in St. Petersburg, Florida. Her other son, Plácido, has great musical talent, and would benefit from studying at a world-class opera school in Milan, Michigan. The children do not want to move. Talia can and should make the decision that is best overall for the family, provided that Alexis gets adequate care. She need not maximize his care at the expense of her career or Plácido's musical development.

4.2 Different Roles

Parents, physicians and the state have different roles and interests. Although parents and physicians have both been described as fiduciaries, each has a unique mission with regard to the child (Table 4.1).

4.2.1 Parents

Parental influence on children is greater than that of professionals. Parents, however, are not as highly trained in theoretical aspects of child development as are pediatricians or psychologists. Children live with their parents. Parents make scores of decisions on behalf of their children each day, some with long-term consequences. Parents decide when and how to feed, dress, and bathe their small children. They supervise children's access to media. Parents guide children in forming habits of time management, interaction with other people, and other interactive skills. They provide moral education. Parents have primary responsibility for their children's health and safety. Reasons for primary parental authority are summarized in Table 4.2.

It is inevitable that parents will make some suboptimal decisions. Many of these decisions are made under conditions of stress or fatigue. Some will lose their temper,

Table 4.1 Differences between fiduciaries, parents, and physicians

Parameter	Fiduciary	Parent	Physician
Scope	Limited	Comprehensive	Limited to health matters; controversial whether these are prioritized over other patient interests
Creation	Contract or trust	Procreation	Contract with parents
Payment	Beneficiary pays fee	Parents are financially responsible for children; reverse of fiduciary	Either fee to parent or public funding
Affect	Professional	Love	Professional or sympathy
Dependency of beneficiary	Limited	Extensive	Limited
Permanence	Potentially temporary	Throughout life	Potentially temporary
Contact	Occasional	Constant	Intermittently frequent (if child is ill)
Duty of care	Reasonable judgment	No neglect/abuse	Standard of medicine
Self-dealing[a]	Forbidden	Inevitable	Impermissible if self-employed[b]
Conflict of interest[a]	Forbidden	Inevitable if family has >2 members	Between patient and employer, if physician is not self-employed
Termination	Per terms of contract or trust	Child reaches age of maturity, or if parent is found unfit	By decision of parent or guardian

[a] *Self-dealing* means the legal right to profit from the relationship, other than a legal fee for services rendered. *Conflict of interest* means that duties to different parties with whom the person has a professional relationship are at odds

[b] There are exceptions. For example, academic physicians need to recruit research subjects, and to use patients in the course of medical education

be slow to change diapers, or establish unreasonable rules. A few parents put their children in harm's way through neglect, abuse, or even through reasonable decisions that take into account risks, benefits and alternatives.

Communitarians, traditionalists, conservatives, religious thinkers and liberal pluralists have seen the family as a fundamental cornerstone of society, although subject to some state oversight. Many feminists have accepted the centrality of the family, although with concerns about longstanding gender inequities in distribution of responsibilities. Few professionals who deal with children believe that parents should not be the primary caretakers of children (but see, Gheaus 2018).

Table 4.2 Reasons for parental authority

Parents best understand their children's interests, and are best positioned to make decisions that will enhance their children's welfare[a]
Since parents bear many of the consequences of choices made for their children, they should exert some control over these choices[a]
Parents have a prima facie right to raise children according to their own values[a]
The family is a valuable social institution, *per se*[a]
Parents can point out suboptimal aspects of their children's treatment, and advocate for their children[b]
Much treatment occurs at home, and parents are more likely to participate in treatment plans if they have bought into the plan[b]
Parental assertiveness sets an example for children to develop autonomous behavior as they mature[b]
The vast number of quotidian parental decisions cannot be supervised without undue intrusion[c]
Perpetuating one's fascinations, beliefs, and way of life is a prime motivation for having children, and reproduction is essential to society.
Parents are aware of environmental obstacles to treatment outside health care facilities[b]

[a]Buchanan and Brock (1989); [b]Navin and Wasserman (2017); [c]Iltis (2010)

4.2.2 Physicians and Other Professionals

Medical doctors usually devote themselves to school and professional training until they are about 30 years old. They say they enter medicine primarily because of an interest in people and in the subject of medicine (Goel et al. 2018). If they do not prioritize health as a value when they begin, they are apt to do so later, as it is the focus of their professional lives. They are successful students, and future oriented. Physicians[1] know more than most parents about health and its maintenance, disease and its treatment, and finding paths through complex medical systems. There is a power imbalance between physicians and patients. This power imbalance is partially contained and channeled to patients' benefit by physicians' professional ethics, by shared decision-making (Elwyn et al. 2012), and by the influence of bioethics.

4.2.3 Differences in Stance with Respect to the Child: Physician, Parent, and State

Parents and healthcare providers may clash over care. Lindemann (2014) suggests that healthcare workers are individualistic, and are concerned with the immediate patient, while the ethics of families is communal, relational, and balances the interests and views of its members. Focusing on medical treatment can forget, misunderstand,

[1] 'Physician' is used to refer to all health care professionals.

or disapprove of what family members choose. Parents and physicians each have their own special relationship with a child. Physicians' fiduciary obligations are confined to health and often focus on medical features of a case. They may give short shrift to the non-medical implications of a parental decision.

Parents, in their capacity as medical surrogates, have a legal responsibility to make decisions in the best interests of their children. As we have seen, this is a protean concept. Interests can be present-directed or future directed. They can be directed toward positive goods or avoidance of harm. They can be related to any and all facets of a person's life. They include physical security, education, relationships, psychological well-being, spiritual well-being, etc. Parents must balance the interests of all members of the family. This contrasts with the doctor, who is responsible only to her patient. She better understands a child's medical interests than most parents, but she does not live with the child and may not understand his personality, desires, and priorities.

Finally, there is the state. The state has some responsibility to protect children from harm. This is operationalized as the common law *parens patriae* doctrine in Anglophone nations (*Prince v. Massachusetts*, 321 U.S. 158, Supreme Court, 1944). The state also has a general power, known as *police power*, to act on behalf of its citizens' health, safety, and welfare (Abramowicz 1999). These doctrines provide justification for the state to intervene against parental malfeasance. Furthermore, the state requires physicians, teachers, and other designated professions to report suspected neglect or abuse of children to state enforcement authorities. Clinicians may feel uncomfortable when families disagree with their medical management proposals, though, even if no actual abuse or neglect is present.

4.3 Interests, Needs, and Everything in Between

4.3.1 Who are the Stakeholders?

Prevailing US legal and bioethics standards ask decisional surrogates for people incapable of consent to apply, in descending order of preference: the pure autonomy standard, the substituted judgment standard, and the best interests standard (Beauchamp and Childress 2013). In mainstream bioethics, and possibly in law, the interests of other family members have low priority. The law demands that parental decision be in the best interests of the child. But there may be good reasons to take the interests of others into account (Hardwig 1993). If long-term care is necessary, the child's family will deliver much of it. If the child is terminally ill, the family members the burden of grief, guilt, and possibly financial cost. Love and loyalty are emotions more powerful than duty. If a child's illness has morally relevant impact on family members, then it is wrong to place the sole focus of moral attention on the patient. Hardwig considers the interests of all persons involved by the decision to be important, and does not see why medical interests have priority over other interests.

The argument for prioritizing patient interests arises from patient vulnerability (Fineman 2010).[2] However, the patient whose care is at issue is not necessarily the most vulnerable person involved. Even in permanently unconscious children with no prospects for recovery, interests of children must be balanced against those of other family members (Weise et al. 2017). Parents may feel guilty about allowing such a child to die, or be unwilling to accede to cessation of active treatment. Alternatively, and the feelings are not incompatible, they may be physically and emotionally burdened by the sick child—not just the burden of care, but the burden of living with their child's suffering. They may feel that they are neglecting other children, or other family and friends.

Consider another situation—the prospect for a trans-sibling donation of a kidney or of bone marrow. Organ transplantation to a sibling is disfavored in Europe, but allowed in the US. At first glance, the value of a highly functioning life to the recipient seems more valuable than the low risk of renal donation and lower risk of bone marrow transplantation. However, the relationship is more complicated (Holm 2004). The family dynamics change. Recipients feel obligation and guilt. It is normative for a gift to be reciprocated, and an organ donation is a truly major gift. Donors often feel neglected despite their sacrifice, as focus is on the recovery and health of the recipient. Transfer of tissue may psychologically traduce the strong taboo against cannibalism (Holm 2004).

Parental surrogates are rarely explicitly informed of the criteria they are supposed to use when making decisions for a minor child. Parental scope of duty is broader than fidelity relationships encompass. Parents, unlike fiduciaries, must consider their own interests along with their children's. They have unresolvable conflicting obligations to their different children. These conflicting loyalties were illustrated earlier in the Talleyrand example. Physicians are not disinterested parties, either. They are not neutrals capable of providing oversight of biased parents. Make no mistake about it—physicians have the opportunity for self-dealing. Even if they are not paid fees for procedures, they are under pressure from employers to tailor their practice patterns to the employers' financial incentives.

Hardwig (Hardwig 1993) would allow surrogates to make decisions that benefit themselves as long as they are fair to the patient. He begins to develop a doctrine of family-based decision-making. First, he includes as stakeholders anyone with an important interest in the medical decision—whether or not actually related, and whether or not the patient and stakeholder are mutually fond or hostile. Second, he favors a resolution fair to all stakeholders. He decries bias in favor of any stakeholder, including the patient. However, Hardwig does not tackle the question of how to

---

[2] Hardwig convincingly shows that substituted judgment does not help, using a *reductio ad absurdum* argument that I here concretize. Imagine two comatose 16-year-old boys, Harry and Draco. Dr. Ridgeon can cure them with a new medicine, but there is only enough to treat one of them. Using the substituted judgment standard Ridgeon notes that Harry is altruistic, and has risked his life several times to help other people—even people he disliked. Draco, on the other hand, regularly boasted that he would drown his mother to achieve fame and fortune. Ridgeon appropriately concludes that Harry would offer the drug to Draco, who would take it. She cures Draco, and lets Harry die on the basis of substituted judgment.

ensure fairness of surrogates, and accepts that people who need an agent may be treated unfairly.

One approach to fairness is relational autonomy. It begins with the premise that our personality and values are inextricably linked with and flow from, our social matrix. We exist in relation to others (Baier 1985). Walter and Ross (2014) characterize relational autonomy as taking advantage of the social matrix in which we are embedded. Relational autonomy encourages decision-makers to consult with those close to them, rather than avoiding any contacts that might lead to others influencing their decisions. Relational autonomy expects clinicians to aid patients in helping make difficult choices, without coercing them. This entails shared decision-making rather than a non-directive approach, in which physicians merely offer a menu of options with advantages and disadvantages. Patients' emotions and preferences, as well as medical reasons, can appropriately influence a decision. Relational autonomy arose as a feminist concept, but has wider appeal in the context of the physician–patient relationship (Stoljar 2011; Sullivan and Niker 2018). A physician who is respectful and trusted, and who tries to accommodate the family's needs, can be part of the relational web.

A parent will be more invested in the child/patient than the physician will be. Physicians would best familiarize themselves with the non-clinical aspects of their patients' care. They also should accept justifications for decisions that consider both the child's interests and needs as part of a family, and the interests and needs of other members of the family as they relate to the child. Provided the minor's needs are met, it may be reasonable to overrule the child's expressed desire, in order to meet interests of family members. Walter and Ross (2014) describe a family that authorized Catholic last rites for their non-religious, comatose, dying adolescent child. The rationale was that the minor incurred no tangible harm, but the parents were distressed by the moral and religious implications of their child's not receiving the sacrament.

Iltis (2010) shows why a family-centered model is superior to a legalistic human rights model as applied to parental decisions regarding children. She notes that the United Nations Convention on the Rights of the Child (1990; CRC) identifies three principles. These are the best interests of children, autonomy of children, and family centrality to children's upbringing. These are mutually incompatible. CRC does not state how to reconcile these principles (Iltis 2010). Indeed, the best interests standard conflicts with itself if there is more than one child in a family.

When a dispute involves conflicting principles, a moral foundation is required to resolve the conflict (Iltis 2010). Beauchamp and Childress (2013) hold that such a foundation might be supplied by balancing defined ethical principles, which they say are based on a common morality that morally serious people share. But defining the universe of morally serious persons is conclusory, and even morally serious persons differ in their interpretation of principles. So ultimately, resolving conflicts among the principles is subjective, and going from the realm of ethics to the realm of action requires an authority whose determinations will be at least partially subjective and partly determined by the ability of the authority to exert its power. In actuality, then, the foundational question is the question of who is in authority (Iltis 2010). The question of 'how to use rights to resolve principled differences' over decisions regarding children, then, ultimately is reducible to a different question—'who is in charge?' If there is no true consensus, positive law governs.

4.4 The Extent and Limits of Family Authority

Even if interests or needs are used as an identification principle, the conundrum just described applies to converting principles to legal oversight. The fundamental question still is: who is to decide? Iltis concludes, for reasons similar to those I have elaborated earlier, that there should be a strong presumption in favor of parental authority, and that the state must hold parents to a more lenient standard than a rigid best interests standard. Defining the realms of parent and non-parental authority is a task of pediatric bioethics (Iltis 2010). Action in response to suboptimal parenting should be calibrated with factors such as the gravity of potential harm the parental decision might inflict, parental motivation, and the likelihood that the parents will correct their behavior.

This section will describe how various scholars addressed this problem of parental authority, exploring the region between harm and optimal care. To lay the groundwork for this discussion, I note that criminal offenses classically require both a criminal action and a criminal purpose. Only rarely is this rule breached (Manchester 1977). State interference with parental prerogatives, immunities, and powers is punishment analogous to punishment of a crime. When the state applies coercive measures against parents, the rules they write, the procedures they conduct, and the sanctions they impose are parallel criminal law. So, it is necessary to designate the *mens rea*, which is unacceptable parental motivation; and the *actus* reus, the minimally tolerable parental behavior.[3]

4.4.1 The Rational Parent

Imagine this scenario:

> Drs. Albert and Teresa Duguid have two young children, Fritz and Ernest. They establish a missionary hospital in Zeray, where malaria is endemic and where there are frequent deaths and injuries due to civil unrest and predatory reptiles. They will have to home-school their children, as educational facilities are absent. The Drs. Duguid are aware of the problem, but believe they have a calling from God to care for the people in Zeray. A crocodile bites off Fritz's leg. Their neighbors, Richard and Cosima Rheingold, also move with their young children, Jack and Franz, to Zeray, exposing the family to the same hazards, in order to try to become rich from mining precious metals. Franz contracts malaria, and dies. Both the Duguids and the Rheingolds are deported to their native European nation, where the

[3] Sometimes a *mens rea* is not necessary, as when a parent is physically unable to exercise parental functions.

government wishes to remove the surviving children from parental care on the grounds of child endangerment.

How important is the motivation of these parents in deciding whether to terminate parental rights for endangering their children?

Parham v JR, 442 U.S. 584, Supreme Court, 1979 gave parents wide discretion to determine their children's care. Unfortunately, this decision established best interests as a resolution standard, essentially creating a legal fiction. In cases such as Baby K (*Matter of Baby K*, 16 F.3d 590, US 4th Cir. Ct. of Appeals, 1994) and Charlie Gard (*Great Ormond Street Hospital v Yates & Ors*, [2017] EWHC 972 (Fam) (England and Wales High Court [Family Division]), courts bound by the best interests standard had to decide whether death, was better for the child than living with permanent unconsciousness and self-awareness (Annas 1994; Lantos 2017).[4] When parental decisions are based on religious grounds, judicial determination is even more difficult, as the benefits cannot be measured in reductionist terms. The value of a heavily burdened life is God's secret (Post 1995).

Schoeman (1985) would defer to rational parental decisions that a responsible person could justify. Cooper and Koch (1996) write of the rational parent. Such a rational parent should be granted decisional authority except in cases of child neglect or abuse. Rationality is determined by presence of a stable belief system (even if unusual), decisional consistency over time, and comprehension of the material facts (Cooper and Koch 1996). When there is a conflict between interests of different children, utilitarian considerations apply, with the parents determining the weight of the benefits and harms to the children involved.

Rhodes and Holzman (2004) elaborated on reasonableness. They distinguished among three types of judgments: those that reasonable people cannot reject, those that no reasonable person could accept, and an intermediate category that one can reject without being unreasonable. Medical situations can also be divided into four categories (I have modified their description slightly). First are *strongly indicated* treatments, where there is a likely good outcome with treatment, but a bad outcome without treatment. An example is surgery for a ruptured appendix. Second are situations in which a *bad outcome is expected*, such as ventilator care for an anencephalic infant. Third are situations in which treatment may be helpful, but not dramatically so. I will call this *mildly effective* treatment, and the use of diphenhydramine for motion sickness is an example. Fourth is treatment with *uncertain outcomes*, in which the outcome may be either good or bad. Treating cancer with a taxing regimen of drugs and radiation with an expectation of a 50% cure rate and a high probability of permanent sequelae of treatment would be an example of uncertain outcome. The interaction between the four kinds of clinical outcome and parental decisions is stated in Table 4.3:

Bester (2018) approaches reasonableness from a different perspective. He is committed to the best interest principle, but accepts that medical interests are not the

---

[4] The Charlie Gard litigation took place in the UK, where *Parham* was not precedential.

Table 4.3 Consequences of parental refusal of medical advice recommending intervention. Modified from recommendations of Rhodes and Holzman (2004)

Assessment of likely clinical outcome	Parental decision		
	Patently reasonable	Reasonable people can disagree	Patently unreasonable
Strongly indicated	Parent and physician will agree to treat	Parent and physician likely will agree to treat, but treatment is mandatory	Reject parental refusal
Mildly effective	Defer to parent	Defer to parent	Defer to parent[b]
Uncertain outcome	Defer to parent	Defer to parent	Defer to parent[b]
Likely bad outcome regardless of treatment	Parent and physician will agree that no treatment is warranted	Defer to patient[a] except as overall justice requires	May reject parental insistence on treatment if child is suffering from treatment[b]

[a]Considerations of justice may require overriding parental wishes if extensive or scarce resources are needed to comply with those wishes. This is my position, and not necessarily that of Rhodes and Holzman

[b]Regardless, if a surrogate is uninterested, seems hostile to the child's welfare, or globally lacks capacity, consideration of referral for legal action should be considered

only interest of sick children, and that the interests of other stakeholders are important. That being said (and as I understand his points), he sets a high bar for parents to challenge medical advice. If they mount a challenge, they should use factual premises and clear values, they should draw logical inferences from these. The conclusion, however, can consider all interests of all stakeholders, and not just medical interests of the child. It is not clear whether he appreciates that differences involving conscience may not be amenable to public reason (Andrew and Lindsay 2008). Both Cooper and Koch, and Rhodes and Holzman, accepted religious premises. If there is a disagreement, should it be settled by preponderance of evidence (i.e., by whose plan seems better).

I have three concerns with 'reasonable parent' approaches. First, 'reasonable' is a placeholder to smooth over a controversial issue. Someone who cannot make a decision, or who is frankly delusional, is unreasonable. But what about parents like the Rheingolds who go to an unhealthy, dangerous place in search of riches, and take young children with them? As for religion, some believe that it has no place in public discussion (Audi 2011), which presumably includes the courts. Indeed, Dawkins (2006), among others, regards religious beliefs as delusional, and teaching them to children as child abuse. Some prominent philosophers see religion as a pernicious and epistemically culpable false belief (Leiter 2014). It is easy to conceive of people labeling other motivators as unreasonable.

Second, the demand for a consistent, self-consciously held, defensible value system privileges intelligent, educated people who attack problems using a rational approach. It handicaps those with a more intuitive approach. Perhaps more seriously, it disfavors the less educated, less sophisticated, inarticulate parents (Cunningham 2016).

Finally, in contemplating effects on children, the consequences of the decision seem intuitively to be more important than the parents' motivation, or even the badness of the act (*actus reus*). Does the Duguids altruism give them more leeway to endanger their children than does the Rheingolds' greed? If a single parent became paralyzed and indigent, and was patently unable to care for her child through no fault of her own, would we not find alternatives to her parental care? The concept of strict liability (Epstein 1973)—basing legal action only upon the consequences of the action—may have a role in this area. We will now explore the space between ideal parenting and harm.

4.4.2 The Space Between Ideal Parenting and Harm

McDougall and Notini (2014) review efforts to define a middle ground between a literal reading of best interests and harm as an identification principle., and Diekema's (2004) use of harm criteria for intervention.

I will begin with the brilliant work of Lainie Friedman Ross (1998). Ross defines family structure in preparation for discussing how families treat their children. She is critical of the influential proclamation by Buchanan and Brock (1989, 133) that parental surrogate decisions must maximize the self-regarding interests of children. In fact, all of us, including children, live in a web of relationships in which we care about other people and in which almost all of us will sacrifice some of our immediate interests for those of others (Ross 1998). This is why so many are moved by The Gift of the Magi (Henry 1905) the story of a poor woman who sold her hair to buy a watch chain for her husband, who had meanwhile sold his watch to purchase ornamental combs for his wife's beautiful hair. It is not appropriate for physicians to consider only a patient's self-directed goals, even though the patient is a child whose opinions have no standing in law. There is a middle ground between overprotectiveness of a child's tangible, self-directed interests and acquiescing to the manipulation or coercion of a vulnerable child. The intimate family is a community with its own goals (Ross 1998). Parents will make decisions for minors in a family, but must show their children respect, which is tripartite. First, there is respect due to every human. Second, there is respect that flows from status as children, which, in Confucian terms, requires parental benevolence toward the child (Rosemont 2015). In the Confucian view, the ideal child is obedient, grateful, and loyal, while the ideal parent cares for and encourage the child. Finally, there is respect derived from the child's capabilities. To the extent that a child is cognitively and emotionally capable, he should have a voice in decisions made on his behalf.

Parents should consider the interests of all members of the family, including their own (Ross 1998). Parents are bound by constraints. First, parents may not neglect, abuse, or exploit their children. Second, parents must provide children with the education, behavioral skills, and opportunities that will allow them to function as adults. But they may otherwise direct their child's future in accordance with their own conception of the good. Ross calls this approach *constrained parental autonomy*.

When the probability of serious harm from a parental decision is low, the parent's wishes generally should be honored (Ross 1998). Physicians should seek state intervention when each of three conditions is met. First, proposed treatment is appropriate and non-experimental. Second, failure to treat is likely to seriously jeopardize the child's basic needs. Finally, the treatment must give the child a reasonable chance for a life worth living, as evaluated from the child's perspective. When parents demand care that is highly unlikely to be of benefit as seen by most people, Ross would still defer to the parents. An exception is care that is painful to the child, or otherwise causes extreme suffering, when neither the condition nor the suffering is likely to improve.

The constrained parental autonomy analysis seems to leave two loose ends. First is definition of basic needs. Second is the limit of parental autonomy. Ross does not want minors to be compelled to be indoctrinated through high school in views of good that parents do not share. Ross would have little problem with the child directed towards being an Amish farmer or a Talmudic scholar, provided the child were productive within the context of his society. But what about a parent who raises a child within a tightly insular cult, such as the Waco Branch Davidians, from which there was no effective exit? (Kerstetter 2004). (Assume that the rampant physical and sexual abuse did not exist.)

I will now turn to two approaches based on economic analysis. This approach makes some bioethicists uncomfortable, but is useful in comparing beneficial and detrimental consequences of alternative programs. I first discuss the microeconomic analysis of De Marco et al. (2011). In microeconomics, a price point is reached when the marginal benefit—the benefit produced by the next increment of production—equals the cost of that margin of benefit. If gold sells for $1,500/oz, a mine that produces the next day's output at a cost of $1,490/oz will extract gold. If it costs the mine $1,510/oz to produce gold, the mine will not operate.[5] If we treat cancer with chemotherapy, the notion of marginal cost and benefit will direct that we choose a regimen where the marginal toxicity of increasing the chemotherapy dose is slightly less than the marginal increase in antineoplastic effectiveness caused by that increase in dose. All physicians intuitively understand this concept as balancing harms and benefits, but microeconomic analysis tries to quantify this. De Marco et al. do more: they propose to consider *externalities*—i.e., the cost of treatment and non-treatment on *both* the pediatric patient *and* other people. De Marco, like Ross, wants to include the external costs and benefits on other individuals as part of the equation, and not discriminate for or against the sick child's interest in the analysis. This is a utilitarian analysis involving the family as the universe to which the sum of goods and harms applies. Although physicians may believe that they have a fiduciary duty to steer decision-making to exclusively address the self-interested medical needs of children,

[5] The FreeEconhelp (2020) blog provides a very simple explanation of marginal benefit and cost, with a helpful graph.

there is no good ethical reason why someone who does not have a fiduciary medical relationship with the pediatric patient should accede to this.

The problem with De Marco's approach is that the currency of interest is not fungible. We can apply microeconomic analysis to fungible commodities or interests such as time or money. When one compares length of life, cost of treatment, quality of life, and degree of love of one person for another, one is comparing apples with oranges. There is no common variable that one can place along the *y*-axis of the cost/benefit curve. So, cost/benefit with consideration of externalities is a useful way of framing the problem, and seems correct in principle, but it does not provide a useful tool for settling disputes.

A second approach is to try to achieve a Pareto optimization among family members to achieve a fair or just outcome. Pareto efficiency is a state that, considering all possible decision combinations, finds a point that is impossible to change without worsening the condition of at least one individual in the system being considered. The range of choices is constrained by resources and opportunities. Also, it is necessary to specify the scope of the community for which Pareto efficiency is evaluated. Here, it may include the child/patient and her siblings, or the nuclear family, or even a larger group, such as the state as a whole. Furthermore, the concept of Pareto efficiency can apply to overall satisfaction and not just to material economic efficiency (Frisch 1955).

This means that non-economic interests such as relational and psychological considerations are germane, as well as health and safety. Pareto optimization would take into account both present and future interests. It also would include both self-regarding interests and other-regarding interests—i.e., the stake each member of a family has in the well-being of other family members. I will assume that the group to which Pareto efficiency applies is the nuclear family, and call this Pareto-optimal state *comprehensive Pareto efficiency of the family* (CPEF).

CPEF will not solve problems of this kind. Let us return to the Talleyrands to demonstrate this. Let's assume that the interests are of comparable magnitude. The well-being for each Talleyrand, measured in hypothetical utility units,[6] is 25 units it the family remains in Paris. Talia teaches at a decent university; and there is a fair voice school for Plácido and fair hemophilia treatment for Alexis. Milan has world-class music training and decent hemophilia care, but no university, and Talia would have to teach high school. St. Petersburg has a prestigious university that would hire Talia. It has great medical care, but no music school. Finally, Talia would have a high government position in Vienna (a suburb of Washington), and Plácido could get excellent voice instruction, but there is no pediatric hematologist in the area. The utility of living in each city is shown in Table 4.4.

Several things are apparent. First, the Pareto-efficient solution is for the Talleyrands to remain where they are. Someone in the family is worse off with any move. Second, any move has more utility for the family than remaining. Paris has 75 total utility units, while any move would give the family 135 units. Finally,

[6] The interests of the three Talleyrands are not fungible, but I will compare them anyway to make a point about Pareto analysis.

Table 4.4 Relative utility of residence in four cities for each member of the Talleyrand family

	Opportunities to satisfy interests		
	Talia	Alexis	Plácido
Paris, TX (current residence)	25	25	25
Milan, MI	5	40	90
St. Petersburg, FL	40	90	5
Vienna, VA	90	5	40

any move would make two people better off and one person worse off. This tie means that there is no clear utilitarian solution either. Alexis's physician might demand the move to satisfy Alexis' best interests. However, if Talia is a superb diplomat, national interest might trump Alexis' illness and dictate a move to Vienna. One thing that is not immediately apparent when a Pareto analysis is proposed is that inertia is inherent in this model. This example is governed by a loser's veto.

We now go to Gillam's *Zone of Parental Discretion*, probably the most cogent analysis of the identification principle to date. Wilkinson (2013) observed (1) that there are medical treatments so effective against serious diseases that they ought to be mandatory, and (2) there are other situations in which the prognosis is so poor irrespective of treatment that physicians should be able to eschew or discontinue treatment without parental consent. There is a large zone in between. Rhodes and Holzman (2004) implicitly made this point as well.

Gillam (2016) uses the term *Zone of Parental Discretion* (ZPD) to denote the in-between zone—between optimal conditions for a child and conditions that are likely to cause serious harm to the child. If physicians are unhappy with a parental decision, they or a court must determine whether the child in question is in the ZPD or is in danger of harm. This is done by explicitly answering three questions as precisely as possible. First, what do the parents overall goals and specific thoughts regarding treatment plan? Second, what effects would the physician's proposed plan have on the child? The answer to this may be in terms of probabilities. Finally, is the likely effect of the parents' desires so detrimental as to present probable significant harm to the child? (Gillam 2016). If the proposed parental action does not threaten the child with significant harm, that decision falls within the ZPD, and must be tolerated.

If not, there are two additional necessary inquiries to determine whether it would cause the child more harm than good if the state proceeded against the parents for their proposed action. First, what would happen if the physician attempted to override a parental decision? Second, would overriding the parent's decision cause greater harm or good to the child than accepting that decision? (Gillam 2016). Parents frequently do not comply with court-ordered treatment, and may move the family out of a court's jurisdiction to avoid compelled treatment (Caruso Brown and Slutzsky 2017). On the other hand, parental disagreement with more powerful entities or with individuals with more education constitutes neither child abuse nor an assertion of ownership.

The Gillam approach provides clear procedural guidance for those caring for the child. It leaves undefined the limits of unacceptable harm. That is a goal that never can be reached in a world of value pluralism.

Most of this discussion has addressed coercive state intervention. I now will reclassify the three zones (Ideal behavior, ZPD, and zone of harm) into four zones to calibrate parental deviation from ideal judgment with the strength of the state response.

4.5 Four Zones of Parental Behavior

State response to parental decisions falls into four categories. First is *complete toleration* of parental action. Second is *expansion of parental choice*, through means such as education or provision of additional services. Third is *channeling parental choice*. This can be done by providing programs with possibility of opt-out, such as vision and hearing testing in schools. Another such measure might be cash rewards for participation in health activities. Nudges (Thaler and Sunstein 2008) as such as making healthier food easier to obtain in school dining facilities, provide another example. Fourth, and finally, there is *coercive action*, such as, compulsory vaccination, limitation of parental custody, and criminal punishment.

I propose four *zones* of parental behavior, ranked by their degree of departure from ideal behavior, and each linked to one of these four levels of state action. The behaviors encompassed within each zone must be defined in a conclusory manner. In other words, the Zones ultimately are defined by what the government thinks it should do about the behavior, rather than the reverse. An inductive approach that prospectively states rules for zone assignment would be preferable, with government action following from that placement. However, there is no uniformity regarding the seriousness of a parental departure from ideal, and liberal pluralism does not accommodate any sort of principled mechanism for assignment. Therefore, the examples I provide as types of parental behavior or decisions that fall into each zone are based on my own opinion.

I characterize each zone by its effect on the child, and not by the motives of the parent. Some parents with severe physical or economic limitations may fail to meet their children's needs, though there is no intent to harm. Though there is no *mens rea*, children cannot remain in a situation in which their needs are not met. Government action should be based on a child's welfare, rather than on a parent's intent.

The first zone is the *Zone of Acceptability* (ZA), which encompasses all behavior that should not trigger any state action. ZA encompasses optimal parental choices and also *de minimis* departures from the ideal. The state need not, for example, concern itself with parents who occasionally miss a medical or dental appointment, whose meals are not always highly nutritious, or who only brush their children's teeth once a day.

This next zone is the *Zone of State Attention* (ZSA). Parental behavior that falls within this zone allows government measures to influence parents by expanding their choices through education or provision of additional services. In this spirit, a comprehensive program to prevent and manage obesity through education and intervention through schools is said to have reduced the incidence of childhood obesity (Hoelscher et al. 2015). Biomedical interventions for enhancement may also fall into ZSA. Some parents treat their short sons with hGH to increase their final height, because stature may be correlated with psychological, social and economic success (Tyrrell et al. 2016). The relative safety of hGH treatment places it in ZSA. The state might opt to make the procedure readily available and maximally safe. The unusual circumstance of child-to-child renal transplant may fall into ZSA. The recipient has an other-directed interest in the health of the diseased sibling. Regardless, the parents must weigh the harms and benefits to which all their children may be exposed. Unless the risks or the threat to the quality of the donor's life are unconscionable, there seems to be no compelling reason for the state to limit parental discretion to permit or deny such a transplant. The principle of liberty compels respect for parental choice.

Finally, ZSA encompasses some parental decisions to allow children to participate in potentially harmful activities which may have compensating advantages not related to health, such as scholastic contact sports. The state can ensure that parents make informed choices, and that risks are minimized.

ZSA, then, includes those activities which warrant that governments provide education and improvements of the circumstances in which the activity is carried out. It seems that such government action is warranted in three sorts of situation. First is to avoid a high likelihood of mild harm. Second is to allow parents to obtain enhancements for their children despite mild to moderate risks that are commensurate with potential gains. Finally, parents may make choices that expose children to some danger, which the parents accept because they perceive that the activity generates a greater good that is not related to health.

The third category is the *Zone of Concern* (ZC). This consists of parental choices that the state considers important to alter, but which do not present the level of danger that merits coercive action. The state, therefore, can direct parental choices but not compel them. Mandatory vaccination programs with non-medical parental opt-out are in place in 46 American states (California, Mississippi, New York, and West Virginia are exceptions as I write this). Incentivization is another sort of behavior-directing option. Adults with children were given gifts in India in exchange for their accepting IUD insertion or vasectomy.

ZSA addresses parental choices of commission or omission that have a significant negative health impact but either fall short of the harm threshold or are sufficiently unpopular that political considerations preclude coercive measures. An example of the latter is a regulation adopted in 1970 (since repealed) as a result of lobbying by the Christian Science church, which precluded state prosecution of parents who eschewed medical treatment in favor of treatment by faith-healing practitioners (45 C.F.R. § 1340.1–2(b)(1) (1975). ZSA also could also encompass situations in which enforcement would be difficult or impossible, as with the practice of direct oral aspiration (*Metzitzah B'peh*) of blood from the penis at the time of circumcision (Davis 2013). This oral contact occasionally causes serious herpetic infections in circumcised infant newborns.

Finally, the *Zone of Unacceptability* (ZU) allows the state to take coercive action in response to parental decisions. Diekema (2004), and Hickey and Lyckholm (2004), simultaneously proposed that measures designed to avoid harm to children be the least possible commensurate with achieving the primary goal of the action (Hickey and Lyckholm 2004), and that deciders should minimize the negative effects of such measures. Sometimes this requires coercion. A state interest in the health of its children has also been cited in support of restrictive measures in these circumstances (Williams 2012). Frank (1976) propounded the existence of such a state interest over 200 years ago in a work that came to be considered foundational in the ethical justification of public health ethics (Semba 2008). Also, individuals have some rights to state protection against dangers threatened by others.

Taxes are an example of mild restriction in the of ZU. Consumption of sweetened beverages are associated with many health problems, including obesity, diabetes Type 2, and metabolic syndrome (Basu and Madsen). Taxation has reduced consumption of these beverages in many localities (Roache and Gostin 2017).

Court orders to compel treatment, which represent partial limitation of parental prerogative, are the classic scenario in discussions of government action. Since 1952, American courts have generally granted injunctions to administer life-saving blood transfusions to children against parental objection. This is parallel to international practice (Wooley 2005; Conti et al. 2018). Courts often order other necessary medical care for children over parental objection (Bross 1982). Parents also have been prosecuted for refusing to provide medical care, and have been convicted of charges as serious as homicide (*Walker v. Superior Court*, 763 P. 2d 852, California Supreme Court, 1988; *Statev. Neumann*, 832 NW 2d 560, Wisconsin Supreme Court, 2013).

ZU permits the most radical state action, and thus requires the strictest identification threshold. Threat of harm from a parental decision is required (Diekema 2004), but what kind of harm? Harms triggering restrictive measures may threaten either the child in question or others. The state ethically may protect unaffected individuals against communicable disease through public health programs. These programs burden the liberties of individuals who are forced to receive vaccines (Dawson 2011; Jacobs 2012), go into isolation (Mindes 1996), take medicines (Gostin 1995), etc. American courts have upheld the constitutionality of compelling people to quarantine (*Compagnie Francaise de Navigation a Vapeur v. Louisiana StateBoard of Health*, 186 US 380, Supreme Court, 1902), receive vaccination (*Jacobson v. Massachusetts*. 1905. 197 U.S. 11, (Supreme Court, 1905), and undergo civil commitment (*Kansas v. Hendricks*, 521 U.S. 346, Supreme Court, 1997).

Thus, ZU includes those parental decisions contemplated by Diekema (2004) and by Hickey and Lyckholm (2004), but extends beyond their scope. ZU includes parental actions that create a significant chance of severe tangible harm to a child, including psychological as well as physical harm (Jacobs and Arora 2018). ZU also includes parental decisions that create harms and other unreasonable burdens for individuals other than the child in question. An example not related to health is the recent spate of wealthy parents paying large bribes to secure their children's admission to prestigious universities (Henderson 2019), which disadvantaged children of less wealthy parents who are denied places.

However, government action to protect health and safety can be used as a pretext to attack disadvantaged groups. Two examples (not involving health issues) involve animal slaughter. One was enactment of laws in a Florida city that effectively barred animal sacrifice by the Santería religion without burdening anyone else; this legal regimen was overturned judicially in *Church of the Lukumi Babalu Aye, Inc. v. City of Hialeah,* 508 U.S. 520, Supreme Court, 1993. The other example involves the bans in some European nations on Muslim and Jewish ritual slaughter (Miele 2016; Siegal 2017), which kills the animal by rapidly severing its carotid arteries with a sharp blade. The laws required prior stunning in the interest of preventing animal cruelty. However, these nations permit hunting, presumably without requiring the hunters to stun their prey before they shoot.

In order to prevent such injustice in the arena of health, proposed ZU restrictions should be limited to harms that are a reasonably likely consequence of the restricted parental behavior. Furthermore, restrictions should not allow some classes of parents to subject their children to greater harm than other classes of parents do. Finally, there must be proportionality between harms and penalties, so that state practices do not cause more harm than the private behavior against which they are directed (Jacobs and Arora 2015, 2018).

Furthermore, these constraints are not specific to our characterization of substantive intervention standards. Even if one were to argue for using BIS, HP, or another intervention standard, these three constraints enhance the possibility of fairness in state treatment of minorities.

4.6 Conclusion

In this chapter, I have explained why parents should have default authority to make decisions on behalf of their children. This is not important when parental decisions are correct in the eyes of professionals and authorities. It is not controversial that the state should step in when parents' decisions threaten serious harm to their children. When this happens, states have the legitimate power to act to avert the harm, irrespective of the parents' motivations.

This leaves an area intermediate between parental good judgment and parental decisions that threaten serious harm. This has been called the Zone of Parental Discretion (ZPD). Parents may decide for their children provided their decisions fall into the ZPD. Parents may—and should—consider the non-medical interests of the child in question, as well as the interests of other members of the family, in making these decisions. At any rate, the state should not coercively reverse decisions that lie in the ZPD.

The state has at its disposal many means to influence parents that fall short of coercion. Parents may subject themselves to state influence if they make decisions that threaten important interests of their children, but not in a serious way. Minor deviations from ideal still do not merit government attention. Along with ideal behavior, they fall into a zone of acceptability. Next is a zone of state attention, in which the state can provide education and tangible support to try to improve parental judgment. Still more serious violations fall into a zone of concern, which merits non-coercive government measures, such as nudges, incentivization, and mandatory health programs with opt-out.

In judging parental actions, I am more concerned about their effect than about their motivation. My schema represents a refinement of Gillam's zone of parental discretion, titrating the intensity of state action to the concern for the effects of parental decisions and actions. More work is required to advance this project.

First, there are different viewpoints regarding the appropriate scope of state power. This will be addressed in a subsequent chapter. Second, the zones are defined operationally—by government response rather than by their intrinsic defining characteristics. This sort of conclusory definition often is the case in law. For example, a felony is a crime that can be punished by more than a year in prison, while a misdemeanor is one whose perpetrator can receive no more than a year's confinement. These definitions of misdemeanor and felony neither describe what acts fall into each category nor present a way to predict which act should be a felony and which a misdemeanor. My assignment of certain kinds of parental decisions to each zone of government action similarly was done inductively, based on what I observe to be generally considered reasonable. It would be preferable to substitute a more deductive approach, but I am not certain that this is possible because of the constraints of value pluralism.

Thus, there will be disagreement on which zone any parental decision should occupy. Koreans, Americans, and Swedes vary greatly with regard to views of corporal punishment. A light slap with the palm of the hand could be considered normal or criminal, depending on the nation in which the child is struck. Some such disagreement is cultural. Other disagreement may be based on objective environmental factors. The acceptability of corporal punishment, for example, may be related to the degree of external physical danger to children and the consequent need to physically control the child for his own safety. Some differences may be related to inertia; we tend to tolerate what we are used to. Some may relate to class bias. Professionals who consider exposure of children to tobacco smoke (smoking now is largely a working-class phenomenon) to constitute child abuse may be more tolerant of alcohol and marijuana use in youth, which are common in affluent, educated communities.

Finally, all societies have unique customs and values. Some of these include distaste for certain extrinsic practices, even if they do not threaten the nation or pose great harm to children. We have already discussed some of these, such as ritual slaughter. These cultural idiosyncrasies, which are important to most of us, may be as much of a factor in differential treatment of disfavored minorities as the 'wisdom of repugnance' that Kass (1997) proposed. It is beyond the scope of this discussion to quantify the value of national traditions. Physicians, however, should not confuse assumptions inherent in national traditions with objective evaluation of patient safety.

References

Conti, Adelaide, Emanuele Capasso, Claudia Casella, Piergiorgio Fedeli, Francesco Antonio Salzano, Fabio Policino, Lucia Terracciano, and Paola Delbon. 2018. Blood transfusion in children: The refusal of Jehovah's witness parents. *Open Medicine* 13(1). https://doi.org/10.1515/med-2018-0016; Available at https://www.degruyter.com/view/j/med.2018.13.issue-1/med-2018-0016/med-2018-0016.xml

Abramowicz, Sarah. 1999. English child custody law, 1660–1839: The origins of judicial intervention in parental custody. *Columbia Law Review* 99 (6): 1344–1392.

Andrew, Ernest, and Peter Lindsay. 2008. Are the judgments of conscience unreasonable? *Critical Review of International Social and Political Philosophy.* 11 (2): 235–254.

Annas, George J. 1994. Asking the courts to set the standard of emergency care-the case of baby K. *New England Journal of Medicine* 330 (21): 1542–1545.

Asma, Stephen T. 2013. *Against Fairness*. Chicago: University of Chicago Press.

Audi, Robert. 2011. *Democratic Authority and the Separation of Church and State*. Oxford: Oxford University Press.

Baier, Annette. 1985. *Postures of the Mind: Essays on Mind and Morals*. Minneapolis: University of Minnesota Press.

Basu, Sanjay, and Kristine Madsen. 2017. Effectiveness and equity of sugar-sweetened beverage taxation. *PLOS Medicine.* http://journals.plos.org/plosmedicine/article?id=10.1371/journal.pmed.1002327;

Beauchamp, Tom L., and James F. Childress. 2013. *Principles of Biomedical Ethics*, 7th ed. London: Oxford University Press.

Bester, Johan Christiaan. 2018. The harm principle cannot replace the best interest standard: Problems with using the harm principle for medical decision-making for children. *American Journal of Bioethics* 18 (8): 9–19.

Bross, Donald C. 1982. Medical care neglect. *Child Abuse and Neglect* 6 (4): 375–381.

Caruso Brown, Amy E., and Amy R. Slutzky. 2017. Refusal of treatment of childhood cancer: A systematic review. *Pediatrics* 140 (6): e20171951.

Buchanan, Allen E., and Dan W. Brock. 1989. *Deciding for Others: The Ethics of Surrogate Decision-Making*. Cambridge: Cambridge University Press.

Cooper, Rebecca, and Kathryn A. Koch. 1996. Neonatal and pediatric critical care: Ethical decision making. *Critical Care Clinics* 12 (1): 149–164.

Cunningham, Thomas V. 2016. A life below the threshold? Examining Conflict between ethical principles and parental values in neonatal treatment decision making. *Narrative Inquiry in Bioethics* 6 (1): 63–71.

Davis, Dena S. 2013. Ancient rites and new laws: How should we regulate religious circumcision of minors? *Journal of Medical Ethics* 39 (7): 456–458.

Dawkins, Richard. 2006. *The God Delusion*. Boston: Houghton Mifflin.

Dawson, Angus. 2011. Vaccination ethics. In *Public Health Ethics: Key Concepts and Issues in Policy and Practice*, ed. Angus Dawson, 143–153. Cambridge: Cambridge University Press.

DeMarco, Joseph P., Douglas P. Powell, and Douglas O. Stewart. 2011. Best interest of the child: Surrogate decision making and the economics of externalities. *Bioethical Inquiry* 8 (3): 289–298. https://doi.org/10.1007/s11673-011-9315-1.

Diekema, Douglas S. 2004. Parental refusals of medical treatment: The harm principle as threshold for state intervention. *Theoretical Medicine* 25 (4): 243–264.

Elwyn, Glyn, Dominick Frosh, Richard Thompson, Natalie Joseph-Williams, Amy Lloyd, Paul Kinnersley, Emma Cording, et al. 2012. Shared decision making: A model for clinical practice. *Journal of General Internal Medicine* 27 (10): 1361–1367. https://doi.org/10.1007/s11606-012-2077-6.

Epstein, Richard A. 1973. A theory of strict liability. *Journal of Legal Studies* 2 (1): 151–204.
Fineman, Martha A. 2010. The vulnerable subject and the responsive state. *Emory Law Journal* 60 (251): 1–41.
Frank, Johann Peter. 1976. *A System of Complete Medical Police: Selections*. Translated by E. Velum, edited by Erna Lesly. Baltimore: Johns Hopkins University Press.
FreeEconhelp. 2020. *Why Marginal Benefit Equals Marginal Cost in Economics ... Always!* FreeEconhelp. https://www.freeeconhelp.com/2011/10/why-marginal-benefit-equals-marginal.html
Frisch, Ragnar. 1955. From national accounts to macro-economic decision models. *IARIW Papers on Income and Wealth Series IV* (Bowes & Bowes, London), p. 2. https://www.sv.uio.no/econ/om/tall-og-fakta/nobelprisvinnere/ragnar-frisch/published-scientific-work/rf-published-scientific-works/rf1955b.pdf
Gheaus, Anca. 2018. Children's vulnerability and legitimate authority over children. *Journal of Applied Philosophy* 35 (S1): 60–75. https://doi.org/10.1111/japp.12262.
Gillam, Lynn. 2016. The zone of parental discretion: An ethical tool for dealing with disagreement between parents and doctors about medical treatment for a child. *Clinical Ethics* 11 (1): 1–8.
Goel, Sonu, Federica Angeli, Nonita Dhirar, Neetu Singla, and Dirk Ruwaard. 2018. What motivates medical students to select medical studies: A systematic literature review. *BMC Medical Education* 18: Art #16. https://doi.org/10.1186/s12909-018-1123-4
Gostin, Lawrence O. 1995. Tuberculosis and the power of the state: Toward the development of rational standards for the review of compulsory public health powers. *University of Chicago Law School Roundtable* 2 (1): 219–77. http://chicagounbound.uchicago.edu/roundtable/vol2/iss1/10
Groll, Daniel. 2014. Four models of family interests. *Pediatrics* 134 (Suppl. 2): S81–S86. https://doi.org/10.1542/peds.2014-1394C.
Hardwig, John. 1993. The problem of proxies with interests of their own: Toward a better theory of proxy decisions. *Journal of Clinical Ethics* 4 (1): 20–27.
Hazony, Yoram. 2018. *The virtues of nationalism*. New York: Basic Books.
Henderson, Cydney. 2019. *Lori Loughlin, Felicity Huffman Sued for $500 Billion (!) Over College Bribery Scandal*. USA Today. https://www.usatoday.com/story/life/people/2019/03/14/college-bribery-scandal-mom-sues-loughlin-huffman-500-b/3168445002/
Henrich, Joseph. 2016. *The Secret of Our Success*. Princeton: Princeton University Press.
Henrich, Joseph. 2020. *The WIERDest People in the World*. New York: Farrar, Giroux, Straus.
Hickey, Kenneth S., and Laurie Lyckholm. 2004. Child welfare versus parental autonomy: Medical ethics, the law, and faith-based healing. *Theoretical Medicine* 25 (4): 265–276.
Hoelscher, Deanna M., Nancy F. Butte, Sarah Barlow, Elizabeth A. Vandewater, Shreela V. Sharma, Terry Huang, Eric Finkelstein, et al. 2015. Incorporating primary and secondary prevention approaches to address childhood obesity prevention and treatment in a low-income, ethnically diverse population: Study design and demographic data from the Texas Childhood Obesity Research Demonstration (TX CORD) Study. *Childhood Obesity* 11 (1): 71–91.
Holm, Søren. 2004. The child as organ and tissue donor: Discussions in the danish council of ethics. *Cambridge Quarterly of Healthcare Ethics* 13 (2): 156–160.
Iltis, Ana S. 2010. Toward a coherent account of pediatric decision making. *Journal of Medicine and Philosophy* 35 (5): 526–552.
Jacobs, Allan J. 2012. Do belief exemptions to compulsory vaccination programs violate the fourteenth amendment? *University of Memphis Law Review* 42 (1): 73–126.
Jacobs, Allan J., and Kavita Shah Arora. 2015. Ritual male infant circumcision and human rights. *American Journal of Bioethics* 15 (2): 30–39.
Jacobs, Allan. J., and Kavita Shah Arora. 2018. When may government interfere with religious practices to protect the health and safety of children? *Ethics, Medicine, and Public Health Ethics in Medicine and Public Health* 5 (1): 86–93.
Kass, Leon. R. 1997. The Wisdom of Repugnance. *New Republic*. June 1997, 17–26.
Kerstetter, Todd. 2004. That's just the American way': The branch Davidian tragedy and western religious history. *Western Historical Quarterly* 35 (4): 453–471.

Lantos, John D. 2017. The tragic case of Charlie Gard. *JAMA Pediatrics* 171 (10): 935–936.
Leiter, Brian. 2014. *Why Tolerate Religion?* Princeton: Princeton University Press.
Lindemann, Hilde. 2014. Why families matter. *Pediatrics* 134 (2): S97–S103. https://doi.org/10.1542/peds.2014-1394E
Manchester, Colin. 1977. The origins of strict criminal liability. *Anglo-American Law Review* 6 (4): 277–83.
McDougall, Rosalind J., and Lauren Notini. 2014. Overriding parents' medical decisions for their children: A systematic review of normative literature. *Journal of Medical Ethics* 40 (7): 448–452.
Miele, Mara. 2016. Killing animals for food: How science, religion and technologies affect the public debate about religious slaughter. *Food Ethics* 1 (1): 47–60.
Mindes, Paula. 1996. Tuberculosis quarantine: A review of legal issues in Ohio and other states. *Journal of Law and Health* 10 (2): 403–428.
Henry, O. (pen name of William Sydney Porter). 1905. *The Gift of the Magi*. http://www.gutenberg.org/ebooks/7256
Post, Stephen G. 1995. Baby K: Medical futility and the free exercise of religion. *Journal of Law, Medicine, and Ethics* 23 (1): 20–26. https://doi.org/10.1111/j.1748-720x.1995.tb01326.x.
Rhodes, Rosamond, and Ian Holzman. 2004. The not unreasonable standard for assessment of surrogates and surrogate decisions. *Theoretical Medicine and Bioethics* 25 (4): 367–386.
Roache, Sarah A., and Lawrence O. Gostin. 2017. The untapped power of soda taxes: Incentivizing consumers, generating revenue, and altering corporate behavior. *International Journal of Health Policy Management* 6 (9): 489–493.
Ross, Lainie Friedman. 1998. *Children, families, and health care decision-making*. Oxford: Clarendon Press.
Rosemont, Henry, Jr. 2015. *Against individualism: A confucian rethinking of the foundations of morality, politics, family, and religion*. Lanham, Maryland: Lexington Books.
Schoeman, Ferdinand. 1985. Parental discretion and children's rights: Background and implications for medical decision-making. *Journal of Medicine and Philosophy* 10 (1): 45–61.
Semba, Richard D. 2008. Nutrition and development: A historical perspective. In *Nutrition and Health in Developing Countries*, 2nd edition, edited by Richard D. Semba & Martin W. Bloem, Totowa, New Jersey: Humana Press; Min, 1–32.
Siegal, Nina. 2107. New slaughtering rules pit Dutch religious freedom against animal rights. *New York Times* December 21, 2107. https://www.nytimes.com/2017/12/31/world/europe/netherlands-kosher-halal-animal-rights.html
Stoljar, Natalie. 2011. Informed consent and relational conceptions of autonomy. *Journal of Medicine and Philosophy* 36 (3): 375–384. https://doi.org/10.1093/jmp/jhr029.
Sullivan, Laura S., and Fay Niker. 2018. Relational autonomy, paternalism, and maternalism. *Ethical Theory and Moral Practice* 21 (3): 649–667. https://doi.org/10.1007/s10677-018-9900-z.
Thaler, Richard H., and Cass R. Sunstein. 2008. *Nudge: Improving decisions about health, wealth, and happiness*. New Haven: Yale University Press.
Tyrrell, Jessica, Samuel E. Jones, Robin Beaumont, Christina M. Astley, Rebecca Lovell, Hanieh Yaghootkar, et al. 2016. Height, body mass index, and socioeconomic status: Mendelian randomisation study in UK biobank. *BMJ* 352: I 582. https://doi.org/10.1136/bmj.i582
Walter, Jennifer K., and Lainie Friedman Ross. 2014. Relational autonomy: Moving beyond the limits of isolated individualism. *Pediatrics* 133 (Suppl. 1): S16–S23. https://doi.org/10.1542/peds.2013-3608D.
Weise, Kathryn L., Alexander L. Okun, Brian S. Carter, Cindy W. Christian, MD, and Committee on Bioethics, Section on Hospice and Palliative Medicine, Committee on Child Abuse and Neglect. 2017. Guidance on forgoing life-sustaining medical treatment. *Pediatrics* 140 (3): e20171905. https://doi.org/10.1542/peds.2017-1905
Wilkinson, Dominic. 2013. *Death or Disability? The "Carmentis Machine" and Decision-Making for Critically Ill Children*. Oxford: Oxford University Press.

Williams, Rebecca. 2012. Faith healing exception versus *Parens Patriae*: Something's Gotta give. *First Amendment Law Review* 10 (3): 692–730

Woolley, S. 2005. Children of Jehovah's witnesses and adolescent Jehovah's witnesses: What are their rights? *Archives of Diseases in Childhood* 90 (7): 715–719.

Chapter 5
What Society May Claim: Public Health

Abstract This brief chapter describes concepts that will be used as a basis to explain and justify claims by the state for itself, and for society beyond the family. Public health is a collective good that focuses on disease prevention, is consequentialist in its outlook, and frequently involves use of state power. In a liberal democracy, health must usually be defined relatively narrowly, as prevention of disease, rather than used as a broad concept to justify massive social engineering. Optimizing health is a public good and a common good; it benefits all, and requires the cooperation of all. As such, it requires a degree of societal solidarity that has been notably absent, for example, in the United States during the recent COVID-19 pandemic. Free riding must be minimized. Harm reduction as a means of mitigating harmful behavior is discussed as a public health strategy.

Actions or inactions with regard to individual children can have an impact outside the family. Similarly, legislation that affects child health also affects people besides the children and families directly involved. This chapter will describe the theoretical basis for public health as it pertains to the issues in this book.

The 2020 coronavirus pandemic highlights the power and, perhaps, the duty of governments to limit individual freedom of activity and movement in order to minimize disease and death. Some of the measures taken in democratic nations are listed in Table 5.1.Government action has limits. Nations differed in the extent to which they employed compulsory restriction to home, business closures, and use of personal electronic equipment to identify possible exposure to the virus. Other measures potentially affecting children but not related to Covid-19 include civil commitment to force people to take antimicrobial medication for diseases such as tuberculosis, vaccination as a requirement for school attendance (Arora et al. 2018), and identification and correction of lead in municipal water supply (Mantha et al. 2020). Classically, basic liberties have consisted of life, liberty and property (Edelstein 2019); or "liberty, property, security, and resistance to oppression" (National Assembly of France 1789, Art. 2). When and how can limitation of these liberties be justified to protect public health and safety?

A. J. Jacobs, *Assigning Responsibility for Children's Health When Parents and Authorities Disagree: Whose Child?*, The International Library of Bioethics 90,
https://doi.org/10.1007/978-3-030-87698-2_5

Table 5.1 Some public health measures used during the SARS-CoV-2 epidemic of 2020 and other indications

Public health restriction
Quarantine (sequestration of contacts)
Isolation (sequestration of cases)
Travel restriction
Electronic tracking
Vaccination
Mandatory vaccination (private businesses)
Mask mandates
Closure of government offices and businesses
Physical distancing

American courts term state power to legislate to protect the health and safety of its citizens *police power*. In the US police power is primarily a state, rather than federal, power (*Jacobson v. Massachusetts*. 197 U.S. Change to 11, Supreme Court, 1905). European jurisprudence invokes such power as a reason to limit otherwise guaranteed liberties (Council of Europe 1950, Art. 8–11). There is no generally accepted, comprehensive philosophical account that justifies police power (Holland 2015).

5.1 Justification for Public Health Programs

Faden et al. (2019) describe public health as (1) a collective good (2) that focuses on disease prevention, (3) is consequentialist in its outlook, and (4) frequently involves use of state power. Public health efforts begin with the goal of conferring widespread health benefits. But what is health? A holistic view is that it is the ability to achieve capacities or goals (Tengland 2016).[1] Aggressive state action based on this expansive view likely resonates less with the public than using state power to prevent or ameliorate discrete harmful conditions such as disease or environmental toxins (Verweij 2009). Capabilities theory has given rise to a number of empiric studies of health (Yeung and Breheny 2016; Bernardi 2019), leading to questions regarding how to measure capability as well as health (Karimi et al. 2016).

Though the public health perspective is consequentialist (Verweij 2009), it is difficult to balance the value of tangible benefits like disease prevention against dignitary goods such as loss of privacy inherent in such measures as widespread

[1] Tengland (2016) proposed six criteria for any definition of health. First, a definition should conform to a commonly used professional or lay understanding of what health is. Second, the definition should involve as few necessary components as possible (parsimony). Third, the definition should make it possible to measure how healthy a person or population is. Fourth, the definition should imply that practices carried out in the name of furthering health be reasonable. Fifth, the definition should be precise and coherent. Finally, the definition should enable us to address normative issues. No definitional concept of health meets all these criteria or is likely to do so in the future.

tracking of location through cell phones. How much loss of income from lockdowns is worth saving each life, or preventing each case of infection? Furthermore, no definition of health will please all. Even if health is defined narrowly as absence of disease or injury, some parental or state actions not directly related to medical treatment or to child safety may have important impact on health.

Let us consider whom police power can protect via public health measures. Hypothesize an industrial pollutant, genotox, that causes cancer. Only 2% of the population is susceptible to the carcinogenic effect, and that is because of an easily detectible genetic variation in susceptible individuals. In this case, a specific vulnerable population can be identified. Contrast this with another pollutant, idiotox, that also causes a rare form of cancer in 2% of the population. But idiotox's eventual victims cannot be identified in advance. The future idiotox victims constitute an *inchoate class* (Jacobs 2011). We know that members of this class exist. We cannot tell who they are, though, until they develop cancer. They do not know who they are. They can only be protected through measures that apply to the whole population (say, by removing idiotox from the environment). Only the government can take such measures. It is necessary to take measures that apply to the whole population since anyone may be a member of the inchoate class that will develop idiotox-related cancer (Jacobs 2011). Many risks, such as cancer from smoking or radon in residences, are risks that affect an inchoate class. Children can populate inchoate classes. During an epidemic of a communicable disease, it is not predictable who will contract a disease or who will be severely affected.

All members of the community benefit from appropriate public health measures. The state has its own interests in preventing disease. It benefits from reducing medical costs (Chang et al. 2018). A healthy population is per se beneficial to the state (Frank 1976), as it is necessary for economic productivity, internal peace, and an effective army to protect against external threat. Public health disasters can be catastrophic. The Athenian plague of 430 BCE probably set the stage for the ultimate defeat of Athens by Sparta in the Peloponnesian War (Kagan 1987). Similarly, the plague that ravaged the Byzantine Empire in 542 aborted Justinian's projects of reconquering the territories of the Western Roman Empire and reuniting the Mediterranean world (Rosen 2007).

5.2 Common and Public Goods

The consequences of public health, then, range from individual health to geopolitical repercussions. It is time to discuss some of the concepts that underly public health. Some benefits are *common goods*. These are facilities and programs that a state or community provides to directly satisfy interests that many members of the state or community possess in common (Hussain 2018). Museums and police protection are examples of common goods. *Public goods* are a subset of common goods. Dawson (2009) characterizes three properties that define public goods. First is *nonexcludability*, meaning that everyone benefits from the good. Second is *dependence on cooperation*. A large number of people must participate in some way to provide the good. Finally, there is *indivisibility*, meaning that the good cannot be broken down or apportioned among members Every member of the public enjoys every public good. Cullity (1995) adds additional criteria. *Jointness in supply* means that the good is available to all with no additional cost beyond that which made the good available to the first person to possess it. *Jointness in consumption* means that use of the good does not diminish its availability to others. *Compulsoriness* means that nobody can avoid using the good without excessive cost. The state may have more of a moral imperative to supply public goods than other kinds of common goods. This is because of the necessity for solidarity in creating public goods and maintaining them, and because of the problem of free riding.

There may be reasons for a state to decline to provide a presumptive common or public good (Arora and Jacobs 2017). First, it may not be, in fact, a good. A program of sterilization on demand, proposed as a public good, might, harm an underpopulated nation that would benefit from a pronatal policy. A second possible problem is that the priority of the good may be insufficient to warrant funding. A program to plant beautiful plants along municipal thoroughfares might have to be shelved to accommodate more urgent public needs. A third, and related hurdle is that a program may be so controversial that disruption caused by the program exceeds the program's value. Mandatory school screening for sexually transmitted infections might be too controversial to implement.

Fourth, public health programs must demonstrate continuous demonstrable benefit despite changing conditions. A nineteenth century government program to clear streets of horse manure may no longer be a public good in the twenty-first century. Fifth, a public good may cause so much harm to a few people that it seems grossly unfair to institute the program. An example found in two widely-read American works of fiction is a lottery to kill a few people for the entertainment of a large population (Jackson 1948). Sixth, the burden of a government campaign necessary to bring about a public good may be greater than the good itself. A law that imprisons double-parkers for five years would be such a measure. If this is what it takes to eliminate double-parking, it would be better to allow drivers to double-park. Seventh, a measure that is good in isolation may not be as good when many similar measures are aggregated. Childhood immunization recommendations in various Western nations include 17 diseases.[2] But recommendations for childhood vaccination against 60 communicable pathogens would be unreasonable. Eighth, the good may simply be inconsistent with the values of society. Consider a hypothetical nation in which 80% of the inhabitants adhere to a religion that believes it is mandatory to smoke. The government is likely not to support smoking cessation campaigns.

The effectiveness of possible public health measures is related to the degree of cultural tightness. Cultural tightness (Gelfand 2006) comprises the strength of social

---

[2] Diphtheria, *H. influenzae* type B, Hepatitis A, Hepatitis B, human papillomavirus, influenza, *H. mengididites* group C, measles, mumps, pertussis, pneumococcus, poliomyelitis, rotavirus, rubella, tetanus, tuberculosis (BCG), and varicella.

norms in a society and the degree to which its members are committed to enforcing them. It influences the ability of government to pursue effective policies. Tightness is said to be correlated with authoritarian government, but is useful in dealing with catastrophes such as wars and epidemics (Gelfand et al. 2011). Differential national tightness—the willingness of citizens to cooperate with preventive measures and with government enforcement of these measures—is highly correlated with incidence and death from COVID-!9 (Gelfand et al. 2021). Whether people cooperate with a public health measure is a different issue from whether people agree or disagree with the measure.

Once it is decided that a measure will effectively advance health, and that the pragmatic constraints I enumerated prove not to be a barrier, other ethical constraints remain.

5.3 Ethical Guidelines and Possible Overreach

Few believe that health benefits override all other considerations. Most agree that individual interests in privacy and liberty must constrain public health decisions. The four principles approach (Beauchamp and Childress 2013), balancing beneficence, nonmaleficence, respect for autonomy, and justice as a tool in clinical ethics, is a poor fit for ethical analysis of public health measures (Holland 2015). Other principles and guidelines must constrain exclusive reliance on health consequences in formulating public programs. Upshur (2002) proposed four such principles. First is the *harm principle*, which we have already encountered in this book. Second is the principle of *least restrictive means*. All other things (such as cost) being equal, appropriate public health goals should minimize coercion. Education and nudges are preferable to fines and imprisonment. This concept is found in the Siracusa Principles on suspension of human rights (UNESCO 1985). Third is a *compensatory* principle. When a public health measure burdens a person or group, the state should compensate the burden or injury through tangible measures or financial awards (Harris and Holm 1995). Finally, public health measures should be *transparent*, and also should seek the input of stakeholders when possible. Upshur's four principles seem to represent appropriate restraints on public health consequentialism.

Experts do not have the final say over policy in democracies. Whatever the flaws of the political leadership—and the recent coronavirus epidemic has shown the great variability in competence of democratic leaders—the people and their leadership, rather than experts, ultimately decide what to do. There are pragmatic reasons for this as well as principled reasons. These are outlined in public choice theory. Small groups with an intense interest in a single issue ('special interest groups') tend to capture administrative agencies (Mueller 1976; Larkin 2015) and legislatures (Elhauge 1991). Rule-making bodies not subject to elections, checks and balances may be more likely to succumb to inertia and undue influence than those whose decisionmakers are in the public eye and subject to challenge.

Table 5.2 The Nuffield Intervention Ladder (Nuffield Council of Bioethics 2007)

8. Eliminate choice Regulate in such a way as to entirely eliminate choice, for example by compulsory isolation of patients with infectious diseases
7. Restrict choice Regulate in such a way as to restrict the options available to people with the aim of protecting them, for example removing unhealthy ingredients from foods, or unhealthy foods from shops or restaurants
6. Guide choices through disincentives Fiscal and other disincentives can be put in place to influence people not to pursue certain activities, for example by taxes on cigarettes, or by discouraging the use of cars in inner cities through charging schemes or limitations on parking spaces
5. Guide choices through incentives Regulations can be offered that guide choices by fiscal and other incentives, for example by offering tax breaks for bicycles that are used as a means of travelling to work
4. Guide choices through changing the default policy For example, in a restaurant, instead of providing chips as a standard side dish (with healthier options available), menus could be changed to provide a healthier option as standard (with chips as an option available)
3. Enable choice Enable individuals to change their behaviours, for example by offering participation in an NHS 'stop smoking' program, building cycle lanes, or providing free fruit in schools
2. Provide information Inform and educate the public, for example as part of campaigns to educate to walk or eat five portions of fruit or vegetables each day
1. Do nothing or simply monitor the current situation

The least restrictive principle has been further characterized by the Nuffield Council of Bioethics (2007) as a ladder of increasingly intrusive interventions (Table 5.2). Dawson (2016) has criticized this schema as reducing ethical issues to the two dimensions of health and liberty. The ladder is relevant, though, to the decisions discussed in this book where the competing issues are child welfare and parental prerogatives, powers, and duties.

5.4 Solidarity

Solidarity is a term closely aligned with public health. But this word is used with various meanings, and often imprecisely. Ironically, the word originated as a Roman legal phrase conferring joint and several liability upon all debtors to a single creditor! (Roediger 2016). Hegel may have been the first to use 'solidarity' to denote social responsibility. By the end of the nineteenth century, the term was associated with socialism and trade unionism (Roediger 2016). It suggests a collective struggle against the dominant order of things. Durkheim (1893/1984), on the other hand, spoke of *organic solidarity*, the mutual dependence among people with different specialized occupational roles in a complex society. But solidarity need not be a comprehensive belief, a dominating emotion, or a powerful determinant of action. Fans at an athletic event demonstrate solidarity with regard to a 'cause' which has little consequence and which is intellectually frivolous.

'Solidarity' is no longer a Marxist concept, but its meaning is vague. It can denote a social arrangement, a cognitive state, or a justification for action. Gheaus (2017) regards solidarity as the *disposition* to cooperate with one's community to achieve what it considers fundamental to its interests (emphasis supplied). This describes a *cognitive state*. Contrast this with Prainsack and Buyx (2012, 346), who see solidarity as a *community practice* of actively assisting all members of society to try to meet egalitarian or sufficientarian goals. Finally, Roediger (2016) describes solidarity as an *alliance* among people who share a perception of oppression to fight the dominant order.

Heyd (2015) adds the additional overlay that solidarity implies loyalty towards a *subset* of humanity. We can be loyal to a community, but not to all of humanity. The group may be a state (e.g., patriotism), a class (e.g., socialism), a gender (e.g., as with feminism), etc. Heyd sees solidarity as more personal than ideological. The importance of solidarity as an influence on parental decisions will be seen in discussions of ritual genital procedures.

It would seem that successful commitment to public health requires some measure of solidarity, but not necessarily a degree of sharing that represents a commitment to egalitarianism. Solidarity stands in opposition to the next concept I will discuss—free riding.

5.5 Free Riding

A passenger boards a bus without paying fare. This passenger is, literally, a free rider. *Free riders* are people who violate rules that must be generally followed to maintain a common good. It succeeds only if practiced infrequently. Free riding is possible only if most people actually pay the cost, financial or otherwise, necessary to sustain a common or public good. The action of free riding may be one of commission or omission. People who burn leaves in their backyards or who fail to have their auto emissions checked annually (both contrary to law) are free riders. Intuitively, we do not like free riders. A common good that is subject to free riding need not be a public good.

Free riding is unfair to resource-contributing participants. Among bus riders, cooperators pay bus fare, but free riders do not. Cooperators bag their leaves and drag them to curbside; free riders burn them. Both enjoy clean air if and only if there are only a few free riders, nobody is hurt. Not all unfair advantage is free riding. Cullity (1995) proposes four criteria for free riding: (1) non-contribution to the common good; (2) benefit from the common good; (3) fairness would require contribution; and (4) general acceptance of the morality of the project or the contribution. Free riding does not require malice, or even intent. Nor do we necessarily try to suppress free riding. Consider a pension system supported by state general revenues, thus by current taxpayers. Someone who never had children is a free rider. It is currently working adults who sustain the economy and pay for current pensions. This childless pensioner never thought he or she was cheating anyone, and probably contributed to the education of other people's children while she was working.

The forms of free riding that need to be punished cannot, I think, be characterized by a moral argument. Rather, they are determined by the importance of the common good, the seriousness of the challenge to the common good, and our intuitive sense of outrage. The moral acceptability is affected by whether the free riding behavior is long-standing, whether it is sanctioned, and the motivations of the free rider. Conscientious objection to military service and unique bases for large, profitable corporations to claim tax relief are both forms of free riding authorized by law, without generating too much popular outrage. Parents that withhold vaccination from children because of its slight risks, while taking advantage of existing herd immunity provide a classic example of free riding in public health (Verweij and Dawson 2004).

5.6 Harm Reduction

One more concept that contributes to public health ethical theory, and that is germane to the book's topic, must be discussed. *Harm reduction* is substitution of a less harmful for a more harmful procedure in a public health context (Marlatt 1996). It is a controversial but effective technique in a number of circumstances. Marlatt contrasts a harm reduction model with moral and medical models. The medical and moral models seek to eliminate the harmful behavior. Harm reduction takes for granted that the harmful behavior will occur, and seeks to mitigate its adverse effects. Proponents of harm reduction strategies accept most initiatives that decrease harm, rather than tolerance of an unhealthy status quo. Harm reduction requires buy-in by those who exhibit the target behavior. Needle exchange programs for users of injected recreational drugs and programs designed to encourage moderate alcohol use among underage drinkers are examples of harm reduction efforts (Marlatt and Witkiewitz 2002).

Harm reduction strategies are consequentialist, though the virtue of compassion also has been invoked as a justification (Holland 2015). Opposition to harm reduction programs is apt to be program-specific, and can take one of several forms. First, it can be proposed that indirect costs of a program cause sufficient harm to outweigh the direct effects of a program. Often, such harms are dignitary, rather than tangible. Thus, Askew et al. (2016) claim that a vulvar nick expresses anti-female discrimination that outweighs the health advantages of avoiding infibulation. Second, it can be claimed that achieving abstinence from the harmful activity is feasible. Finally, deontic arguments against harm reduction applied to illegal activities, dispute the appropriateness of encouraging lawbreaking. Opposition to needle exchange programs for abusers of injectable drugs may take this form.

5.7 Conclusion

To address public health concerns, states may take measures that infringe on basic liberties. The harms that the measures themselves produce should be proportional to the threat. A pandemic projected to kill 1–10% of a nation's people, or major Anthropocene changes such as climate change, merit considerable acceptance of liberty infringement if that is necessary to prevent catastrophe. In such cases, everyone, including members of minority communities, must cooperate with public health measures. When considering economic burdens such as lockdowns and liberty burdens such as tracking citizens' movements using their mobile phones, states should try to minimize the burden of public health activities on the population.

Many authors addressing the state/parent conflict have focused on the triad of physician, parent, and child. Others have included the family as stakeholders. Resolution of these conflicts, though, can affect others outside this small circle. These stakeholders' interests need to be considered in shaping these decisions regarding children. Fairness requires that free rider problems be recognized, and often combatted.

Finally, many, if not most, public health solutions have harm reduction options. These should be entertained, both from the standpoint of maximizing benefit and from an outlook of willingness to cooperate with those who have different opinions.

References

Arora, Kavita Shah, Jane Morris, and Allan J. Jacobs. 2018. Refusal of vaccination: A test to balance societal and individual interests. *Journal of Clinical Ethics* 29 (3): 203–213.

Askew, Ian, Ted Chaiban, Benoit Kalasa, and Purna Sen. 2016. A repeat call for complete abandonment of FGM. *Journal of Medical Ethics* 42 (9): 619–620. https://doi.org/10.1136/medethics-2016-103553.

Beauchamp, Tom L., and James F. Childress. 2013. *Principles of Biomedical Ethics*, 7th ed. New York: Oxford University Press.

Bernardi, Andrea. 2019. Using the capability approach and organizational climate to study occupational health and safety. *Insights into Regional Development* 1 (2): 138–154.

Chang, Angela, Sue Horton, and Dean T. Jamison. 2018. Benefit-cost analysis in disease control priorities. In *Disease Control Priorities, Third Edition (DCP3): Improving Health and Reducing Poverty*, 3rd edn, vol. 9. Washington, D.C.: The World Bank.

Council of Europe. 1950. *European Convention on Human Rights*.

Cullity, Garrett. 1995. Moral free riding. *Philosophy and Public Affairs* 24 (1): 3–34.

Dawson, Angus. 2009. Herd Protection as a Public Good. In *Ethics, Protection, and Public Health*, ed. Angus Dawson and Marcel Verweij, 160–178. Oxford: Oxford University Press.

Dawson, Angus. 2016. Snakes and ladders: State interventions and the place of liberty in public health policy. *Journal of Medical Ethics* 42 (8): 510–513. https://doi.org/10.1136/medethics-2016-103797.

Durkheim, Emile. 1893. *The Division of Labour in Society*, Trans. W. D. Halls. Houndsmills: Macmillan.

Edelstein, Dan. 2019. *On the Spirit of Rights*. Chicago: University of Chicago Press.

Elhauge, Einer R. 1991. Does interest group theory justify more intrusive judicial review? *Yale Law Journal* 101 (1): 31–110.

Faden, Ruth R., Sirine Shebaya, & Andrew W, Siegel. 2019. Distinctive challenges of public health ethics. In *The Oxford Handbook of Public Health Ethics*, eds. Anna C. Mastroianni, Jeffrey P. Kahn, and Nancy E Kass, 12–20. Oxford: Oxford University Press.

Frank, Johann Peter. 1976. *A System of Complete Medical Police: Selections*. Trans. E. Velum, ed. Erna Lesly. Baltimore: Johns Hopkins University Press.

Gelfand, Michele J., Joshua Conrad Jackson, Xinyue Pan, Dana Nau, Dylan Pieper, Emmy Denison, et al. 2021. The relationship between cultural tightness–looseness and COVID-19 cases and deaths: A global analysis. *The Lancet Planetary Health* 5 (3): e135-e144. https://doi.org/10.1016/S2542-5196(20)30301-6. Available at https://www.sciencedirect.com/science/article/pii/S2542519620303016.

Gelfand, Michele, and J., Lisa. H. Nishii, & Jana L. Raver. 2006. On the nature and importance of cultural tightness-looseness. *Journal of Applied Psychology* 91 (6): 1225–1244. https://doi.org/10.1037/0021-9010.91.6.1225.

Gelfand. Michele J., Jana L. Raver, Lisa Nishii, Lisa M. Leslie, Janetta Lun, et al. 2011. Differences between tight and loose cultures: A 33-nation study. *Science* 332 (6033): 1100–1104. https://doi.org/10.1126/science.1197754.

Gheaus, Anca. 2017. Solidarity, justice, and unconditional access to health care. *Journal of Medical Ethics* 43 (3): 177–181. https://doi.org/10.1136/medethics-2016-103451.

Harris, John, and Søren. Holm. 1995. Is there a moral obligation not to infect others? *BMJ* 311 (7014): 1215–1217.

Heyd, David. 2015. Solidarity: A local, partial, and reflective emotion. *Diametros* 13 (1): 55–64. https://doi.org/10.13153/diam.43.2015.714.

Holland, Stephen. 2015. *Public Health Ethics*, 2nd ed. Cambridge, UK: Polity Press.

Hussain, Waheed. 2018. The common good. In *The Stanford Encyclopedia of Philosophy* (Spring 2018 Edition), ed. Edward N. Zalt.https://plato.stanford.edu/archives/spr2018/entries/common-good/.

Jackson, Shirley. *The Lottery*. 1948. https://sites.middlebury.edu/individualandthesociety/files/2010/09/jackson_lottery.pdf.

Jacobs, Allan J. 2011. is state power to protect health compatible with substantive due process rights? *Annals of Health Law* 20 (1): 113–149.

Jacobs, Allan J., and Kavita Shah Arora. 2017. Punishment of minor female genital ritual procedures: is the perfect the enemy of the good? *Developing World Bioethics* 17 (2): 134–140.

Kagan, Donald. 1987. *The Fall of the Athenian Empire*. Ithaca: Cornell University Press.

Karimi, Milad, John Brazier, and Hasan Basarir. 2016. The capability approach: A critical review of its application in health economics. *Value in Health* 19 (6): 795–799.

Larkin, Paul J., Jr. 2015. Public choice theory and occupational licensing. *Harvard Journal of Law and Public Policy* 39 (1): 210–331.

Mantha, Anurag, Min Tang, Kelsey J. Pieper, Jeffrey L. Parks, and Marc Edwards. 2020. Tracking reduction of water lead levels in two homes during the flint federal emergency. *Water Research* 7. https://doi.org/10.1016/j.wroa.2020.100047.

Marlatt, G. Alan. 1996. Harm reduction: Come as you are. *Addictive Behavior* 21 (6): 779–788.

Marlatt, G Alan, and Katie Witkiewitz. 2002. Harm reduction approaches to alcohol use: Health promotion, prevention, and treatment. *Addictive Behavior* 27 (6): 867–886.

Mueller, Dennis C. 1976. Public choice: A survey. *Journal of Economic Literature* 14 (2): 395–433.

National Assembly of France. 1789. *Declaration of the Rights of Man*.

Nuffield Council of Bioethics. 2007. *Public Health: Ethical Issues*. London: Nuffield Council of Bioethics.

Prainsack, Barbara, and Alena Buyx. 2012. Solidarity in contemporary bioethics—Towards a new approach. *Bioethics* 26 (7): 343–350.

Roediger, David. 2016. Making solidarity uneasy: Cautions on a keyword from black lives matter to the past. *American Quarterly* 68 (2): 223–248. https://doi.org/10.1353/aq.2016.0033.

Rosen, William. 2007. *Justinian's Flea: The First Great Plague and the End of the Roman Empire*. New York: Penguin Books.

Tengland, Per-Anders. 2016. Venkatapuram's capability theory of health: A critical discussion. *Bioethics* 30 (1): 8–18.

UNESCO. 1985. United Nations, Economic and Social Council. 1985. *Siracusa Principles on the Limitation and Derogation Provisions in the International Covenant on Civil and Political Rights*, U.N. Doc. E/CN.4/1985/4, Annex. http://hrlibrary.umn.edu/instree/siracusaprinciples.html

Upshur, Ross E.G. 2002. Principles for the justification of public health intervention. *Canadian Journal of Public Health* 93 (2): 101–103.

Verweij, Marcel. 2009. Tobacco Discouragement: A Non-Paternalistic Argument. In *Ethics, Prevention, and Public Health*, ed. Angus Dawson and Marcel Verweij, 179–197. Oxford: Oxford University Press.

Verweij, Marcel, and Angus Dawson. 2004. Collective principles for immunisation programmes. *Vaccine* 22 (23–24): 3122–3126.

Yeung, Polly, and Mary Breheny. 2016. Using the capability approach to understand the determinants of subjective well-being among community-dwelling older people in New Zealand. *Age and Ageing* 45 (2): 292–298. https://doi.org/10.1093/ageing/afw002.

Part II
The State Intervention Test (SIT) and its Theoretical Basis

Chapter 6
Political Considerations in a Liberal Pluralist State

Abstract Writers have devoted too little attention to the question of the appropriate limits of the state. There seems to be a tacit assumption that wise, well-meaning statesmen will translate philosophers' insights into good policy. I suggest that it is more likely to find that government leaders in large nations are narcissistic, power-obsessed, and corrupt. The necessity for protecting children's needs must balanced against the need to maintain the integrity of private spaces against the sorts of governments that are likely to wield authority. I propose seven principles that undergird this balance, and that will be reified in the State Intervention Test in the next chapter. These principles are *family primacy, pluralism, political realism, negotiation, limitation of government scope, diffusion of government power, and sufficientarianism.* Essentially, I seek a political process with constitutional guarantees of liberty. My vision derives from a contemporary movement in political theory known as *political realism.* Needs must ultimately be determined politically, and are reified through a political process as guarantees of minimum fulfillment of important interests. The idea that the state should provide such a floor is called sufficientarianism. The levels of sufficiency are established through a *modus vivendi.* There is no non-controversial principled justification, so I use sentiment to justify my political realist solution. First, it is based on compassion, and possibly solidarity. Second, it encompasses the notion of self-insurance; any of us may fall below a sufficient level without the state providing a floor. Finally, the existence of a social net promotes the legitimacy of societal institutions, including the state, thus promoting social harmony and order.

What are the appropriate extent and limits of state[1] action to constrain parental decision-making? Many writers on ethics tacitly assume that states should pursue any desirable objective. I disagree. I follow Robert Cover and Judith Shklar in viewing an active government as simultaneously necessary and unjust. In a pluralistic society, political, and not moral, considerations determine policy decisions. The framework

[1] A *state* is a geographically based entity with the power to enact and enforce laws and regulations. The United States, Texas, and Houston are states under this definition. A *government* is the organization (institutions and their officials) that wields state power.

A. J. Jacobs, *Assigning Responsibility for Children's Health When Parents and Authorities Disagree: Whose Child?*, The International Library of Bioethics 90,
https://doi.org/10.1007/978-3-030-87698-2_6

for decision is not provided by wise people who enjoy a consensus of trust. Rather, the basis for state action in a heterogeneous democratic society is *modus vivendi* with constitutional constraints to protect individual rights.

Much has been written about ethical aspects of parental decision-making. The competence of the state to address competing claims in this area has received far less attention. Many liberals and most progressives implicitly view the state as a *deus ex machina* that capably and wisely resolves problems that vex its citizens. If they, or people like them, were in charge, their benevolence and wisdom would lead to just and moral governance (Ypi 2020). I question states' propensity to do good things, and will call for a restrained state role in regulating family life, including decisions regarding children's health. Rather, the scope of the state vis-à-vis the family and parents should be limited to addressing gross abuses, because of the primacy of the family and the intrinsic tendency of any state to oppress.

6.1 Government as Inherently Oppressive

The tendency of governments to act unjustly has been recognized since ancient times. The Hebrew Bible attributes injustice even to the most righteous rulers. Joseph used an Egyptian famine to force most Egyptians into serfdom, displacing the population far from their original homes to consolidate their subservient status (Genesis 47:14–26). The prophet Samuel warned that kings would conscript the young men of the nation for war and the young women for his pleasure. (1 Samuel 8:14–17).

At the same time, the Hebrew Bible decries anarchy. The atrocity perpetrated by Benjaminites at Giv'a (Gibeah) during the chaotic Judges era, and the ensuing annihilation of the men of that tribe (Judges 19–20), affirmed the need for government. The Greeks also were ambivalent about strong government. Plato (1871) was enthusiastic about the power of the state to shape good citizens. He regarded reason as the appropriate source of laws. Aristotle (1995), though, appreciated the inherent problems with any form of rule, whether popular, oligarchic, or dictatorial.

Catholic social thought is suspicious but not antagonistic toward markets, envisioning government as a corrective force for upholding human dignity, advancing group solidarity, and promoting the common good (Gregg 2014). Catholic thought would limit the scope of government power to preserve the individual's freedom in service of individual flourishing. Subsidiarity, the delegation of function to the smallest feasible unit of society, is an important protection for the individual. For similar reasons, the US Constitution incorporated federalism (more or less an American term for subsidiarity) and a system of internal checks on government power of the US constitution. Cover (1986), Shklar (1989) and I are skeptical either that powerful governments will act in a benign manner, or that political leaders will generally exercise wisdom and restraint. As Cover (1986) notes, government officials lack the inhibitions and restraint usual in interpersonal interaction. Actions of executives and judges intrinsically deprive the objects of those actions of their capacity to act autonomously.

Shklar (1984), like Cover, regarded government as intrinsically dangerous and violent. Combining humanism with skepticism that rulers are motivated by reason, Shklar advocated a limited government with power divided among its officials. She regarded government coercion, even on behalf of a good end, as inherently cruel (Shklar 1989). People generally exhibit the 'ordinary vices' of cruelty, hypocrisy, snobbery, and betrayal, and this is more true of those who wield government power (Shklar, 1984). This appropriate misanthropy motivates a *liberalism of fear* (Shklar 1989). To keep cruelty in check, this liberalism of fear concentrates on limiting the power of government and of its officials through constitutional guarantees. Rational norms and tradition are insufficient to control government abuses (Shklar 1984). Although the government must be allowed to use power to protect rights (Shklar 1990), it must be prevented from violating the prerogatives and dignity of its citizens. Reduction of the potential impact of state cruelty also requires redistributing power from government to non-governmental groups (Shklar 1984), as Catholic subsidiarity also advocates. Loyalties divided between the state and groups such as religion, cultural affiliation, and the family not only are appropriate, but tend to sustain freedom. Primary social bonds, and especially the family, may take precedence over patriotism. Table 6.1 lists the heads of government and (when applicable) runners-up in the most recent elections of the 12 most populous highly-developed and very highly-developed nations. Readers can judge for themselves how likely such nations are to have leaders who are wise, competent, or trustworthy.

Leaders, including government officials, are motivated by a desire for power per se, (Caprara and Silvester 2018), affiliation (a desire for close relations with others) (Winter 2005), and achievement (or responsibility)—a desire to accomplish goals through exercise of authority. They also may be prone to personality disorders and to corruption. Positions of leadership in large, powerful organizations are attained through intense competition. Leaders in corporations (Simonet et al. 2018) and even universities (Perry and Miller 2021) often are narcissistic (Rosenthal and Pittinsky 2006). Dark Triad (Paulhus and Williams 2002)[2] characteristics seem to correlate with success in large organizations (Spurk et al. 2015). It is hard to study politicians either objectively or directly. But it seems as though government is not an exception to the rule that those with Dark traits vie for and attain leadership positions, even in liberal democracies (Lilienfeld et al. 2012). Narcissism and Machiavellianism, especially, seem to facilitate success in politics (Peterson and Palmer 2019). People with Dark Triad features are more likely to seek political careers (Blais and Pruyser 2017). We should not be surprised that people who desire power seek and attain powerful positions, or that such people frequently are not altruistic in their motivations. Even well-meaning officeholders are often concerned about keeping their positions or attaining higher office (Philp 2010). Nor should it be surprising that studies based on politicians' own responses to surveys put them in a better light (Vecchione et al. 2015) than studies based on external evaluation of their speech (Garrard et al. 2014) and on other external evaluations. David Owen (2008) described an acquired narcissistic personality disorder peculiar to leaders that he called the Hubris syndrome.

[2] The Dark Triad consists of narcissism, Machiavellianism, and psychopathy.

He and Davidson (Owen and Davidson 2009) documented its extent. Many of our leaders are people whom we would not want as our neighbors, let alone interfering in our family lives.

Corruption is another problem endemic to government officials. It is difficult to define corruption. First, governments have written laws to legalize much corrupt behavior. Second, bribery has become indirect, and hard to prove. If a president earns millions of dollars for speeches given soon after his term (Kasindorf 1990), if a president's adult child, an amateur artist, auctions his art at a high price (Samuels 2021), or if large contributions go to campaign funds and personal foundations—who, then, can definitively say that there is a *quid pro quo*? The transit of government officials into jobs with businesses (Meghani and Kuzma 2011) and NGO's (Vandenbergh et al. 2020) they have regulated, as well as into their lobbying (Blanes i Vidal et al. 2012) and law firms (Richmond 2021), is a well-known phenomenon. There is a borderline between legal corruption, as noted above, and legitimate actions to aid constituents. If a legislative leader represents a district with a large number of garden tool factories, llama ranches, LGBTQ residents, or evangelical Christians, the interests of those people will have greater representation than if a backbencher represented them in the legislature.

The notion that corruption can be defined as the subversion of public good to private interests[3] is too broad for criminal law, as is the notion that any act is corrupt in which a public official makes a decision on behalf of a surreptitious agenda (Ceva and Ferretti 2017). However, such behavior illustrates why citizens might be wary of government interference in their intimate relations. Government is powerful, and those who exercise that power are hardly wise philosopher-kings. Furthermore, those who would utilize state machinery expansively should be concerned that when their opponents come into power, they will use the power of the state to change policies. If government regulation of reproductive and sexual behavior is on the table, it can be used not only to protect women's legal rights to electively prevent or terminate pregnancies, but also to compel them either not to have children, or to carry their pregnancies to deliver live children. State interference in parental decisions regarding children's health can expand from overruling dangerous parental decisions (e.g., by members of religious groups such as the Jehovah's Witnesses not to transfuse children) to a readiness to question and punish any parental decision with which the state authority disagrees.

Indeed, governments often use their power in ways inimical to children's well-being. Some governments and groups aspiring to govern perpetrate violence against children (Chamberlain Bolaños 2014), compel them to be soldiers (Haer et al. 2020), and force separation of children from their families (Penchaszadeh 1972). This has recently occurred even in liberal democracies such as Canada (Fournier and Cray 1997) and Australia (van Krieken 1999). One must be skeptical that states will respect the interests of children and of their families, or that they will refrain from attacking

[3] Including gains for the government official, her family and friends, her reelection prospects, and those interests that are of narrow benefit to the government official's constituents but which do not promote the public good.

unpopular groups through actions against their children. Finally, some individuals that do not act for the government can function as *state agents*. These include health care workers, teachers, and certain other professionals, who are mandatory reporters of suspected child neglect, endangerment, or abuse. Such state agents can abuse their power.

6.2 State Must Have Power, Which Must Be Limited

Governments can harm children, but parents also can harm children. Classical literature abounds with bad parenting. King Agamemnon sacrificed his daughter, Iphigenia, in order that his army might sail to conquer Troy (Euripides 2013). Yiftach (Jephthah), an Israelite warlord, sacrificed his only child to thank God for a victory (Judges 11–12).

Many contemporary parents also make decisions that endanger or harm their children. This may arise out of ignorance, distraction, or beliefs that are injurious to the child. Some parents may harm or neglect their children because of the constraints of poverty or because they are overwhelmed. When possible, and parental motivation is not malicious, parents should be supported rather than punished. Removing a child from the home into a foster care situation is rarely ideal. Authorities must be careful not to regard non-conforming ideas about child-rearing as neglect or abuse. A 'free-range parent' may give her child less supervision than other parents in the community are comfortable with, such as allowing them to walk several blocks to elementary school through quiet streets (Pimentel 2016). Pimentel argues that this should be tolerated if there is no objective evidence that such a policy is likely to bring harm to the child. Other parents, though, may reject aspects of Western medical care that are necessary to save a child's life (Offit 2015). This categorically is not acceptable. In some cases, the threat may be more to the community than to the child in question, as in the parental refusal to vaccinate a child.

Parents are default decision-makers for their minor children. The primacy of the family is asserted by positive law, as well as by international declarations such as the United Nations Universal Declaration of Human Rights (1947; Art. 16 §3) and the Convention of the Rights of the Child (1990; Preamble, Art. 5, Art. 8 §1). Parental power is not absolute. All American jurisdictions have provisions for limiting parental authority or imposing criminal sanctions on parents for behavior that is damaging to children (Findlaw 2021). The criteria for sanctions usually involve abuse, abandonment, endangerment, or neglect of a child. Some statutes contain exemptions for faith healing (e.g., Indiana Code, § 35–46-1–4). If physicians seek court intervention in a dispute over parental medical decisions, they do so under the rubric of abuse or neglect.

There is no principled way to resolve many of the moral and ethical issues because of conflicting values and incommensurate metaethical approaches between families, or between families and authorities. A 'free range parent' might believe that the independence and self-reliance gained from a child's walking ten minutes to school outweighs the risk of being struck by a car; the school nurse might disagree. The two have the same values, but weigh them differently. Alternatively, a Christian Science parent might refuse to have her child vaccinated. Here, the parent and the nurse have different values, and different beliefs about the nature of health. The Ottoman *millet* system treated each cultural community as a self-governing entity, but Western democracies are not willing to withhold government protection from children whose culture decrees practices that the mainstream considers dangerous. States may intervene to protect children in danger.[4] Even scholars who would allow insular groups such as Old Amish or Chasidic Jews wide autonomy would insist that there must be reasonable opportunity for exit from the group (Galston 1996). This arguably requires that members be trained to support themselves physically and economically. Furthermore, such groups must adhere to some very basic rights. For example, such a group may not withhold life-saving medical treatment from children.

6.3 Pursuit of Justice

Justice has preoccupied liberal political thought over the last several decades. Even if justice were conceived as fairness, as Rawls advocates, fairness can be construed in multiple ways (Sen 2011). Fairness in allocating a resource can be based, for example, on most efficient use, on need, on effort required to create the resource, or on claim of existing ownership. Furthermore, there are important government considerations besides justice, such as stability, legitimacy, and effectiveness. If there were general agreement on principles there would be little controversy.

But justice is not subject to uniform definition (Kymlicka 2002). Models of distributional justice may be based on (1) *equality* of persons and equality of group recognition; (2); economic *efficiency*—usually measured as production per capita; (3), *equity* (as traditionally defined as reward based on merit); and (4) equity as defined in critical theory as equality of distribution of resources and positions among groups. Efficiency is not solely a concern of conservative scholars (Mazzucato 2018) because distribution of resources requires availability of resources. Traditional equity is the most difficult of the three principles to use, because it is hard to define merit (Walster et al. 1973). Many readers of this chapter, for example, will view the salary differential between a school teacher and a publicist for prominent actors as inequitable. This sort of visceral judgment does not provide a usable tool for comparing the value of qualitatively different skills, or outputs of goods and services. Different distributional principles apply to different goals. Organizational scholarship does not equate fairness with equal distribution, but suggests that perception of fairness can vary according to the goal of the observer (Deutsch 1975). Efficiency or equity, rather than equality or

[4] However, American jurisdictions are is not required to offer such protections (*DeShaney v. Winnebago County Dept. of Social Servs.*, 489 US 189, Supreme Court, 1989).

need, will be the dominant principle of distributive justice where economic productivity is required. Alternatively, where maintaining harmonious social relations is a common goal, equality may be the dominant objective.

If we could be certain that our normative beliefs were free of error, we could comfortably impose them on the occasional deviant who is mistaken about facts or deluded about reality. However, if there is one proposition that we can be certain of, it is that in 50 years normative views currently fashionable in the academy or in the general population will be supplanted. This likelihood does not dictate nihilism, but it should inspire humility when we consider imposing our views on others.

Finally, justice can be defined in terms of procedural fairness, rather than in terms of substantive outcome (Akbaş et al. 2019). This definition of justice requires, and may be limited to, ensuring honest, unbiased, and transparent processes.

Pursuit of justice is a valid goal of government, but this is only a prima facie principle. It is not an overriding principle. I will argue, along with a school of thinkers known as*political realists*, that stability, freedom, and governmental legitimacy are at least as important. Groups with opposing, and often incommensurate, beliefs and agendas must settle their differences through compromise. But there must be limits on political solutions. Shklar's liberalism of fear must constrain the limits of political solutions in the interests of liberty, of citizen satisfaction, and of provision of a sufficient level of capabilities to all. In the next chapter I will propose a multi-prong test to evaluate when the state should intervene against parents. The seven principles that undergird the test are *familyprimacy, pluralism, political realism, negotiation, limitation of government scope, diffusion of government power, and sufficientarianism*. I have discussed why parents are the default decision-makers for children. The primacy of the family is both a fundamental principle per se and a mechanism to limit state power through diffusion of authority. It is a rebuttable presumption that parental decisions are to be respected.

When do we allow a government to overcome this presumption of parental authority? This is a political question. The political solution must be psychologically realistic, comporting with what we know about human behavior and its malleability. The political solution must appreciate that people will differ in needs, wants, capacities and motives. Part of this variability in human motivation is that some people will be predisposed toward antisocial behavior or toward evasion of responsibility. Thus, realities of human psychology rule out utopian solutions. It belies armchair 'laws' about human psychology that run counter to empiric evidence such as Rawls' account of moral psychology (Rawls 1971). We should eschew theory in favor of realistic solutions applicable to people as they actually behave, based on the best available empiric evidence. Any political solution should promote human flourishing. Since different people have different needs, and since there is lack of unanimity regarding the definition and the requirements for flourishing, the state should exercise restraint in actively trying to shape the preferences and activities of its citizens. It should not take an expansive view of what is necessary to all people. However, the state must protect those reliant upon it against severe threats to health and safety, and must offer some protection against severe psychological damage. Finally, children must be educated to be able to be sufficiently useful to others to allow them to function in society as adults.

The state also must maintain the ability to pursue important common goods. Government must be able to protect against natural disasters and threats by humans within and outside the state. Maintenance of order and stability relies on perception by most citizens of government legitimacy (Habermas 1996). Citizens must accept that the state will sometimes infringe on their individual interests, but that it does not have unlimited authority to do so. The primarily political nature of protection of the state's citizens does not exclude a moral component. But it is easier to characterize certain circumstances as unjust than to define what is meant by just conditions (Shklar 1990). Preventable involuntary malnutrition in an affluent society, chattel slavery, and gratuitous violence are intuitively unjust. Minority or marginalized populations are likely to need state aid to ameliorate injustice. That being said, there must be proportionality in state action. The state response to injustice should not create more injustice than it eliminates (Jacobs and Arora 2017a, b).

Finally, the mechanism for resolving disputes should be as little dependent on theoretical justification as possible. Solutions that are intuitive to many, or compatible with multiple theories, are likely to be acceptable and to be generally held to be legitimate. I therefore avoid reliance on concepts such as justice or non-legal rights.

6.4 Political Realism and *Modus Vivendi*

Of the seven principles listed above for defining the scope of state action, I have yet to discuss political realism, negotiation, and sufficientarianism.

Advocates of *political realism* (using 'realism' as a term of art denoting this movement) challenge the notion that morality—and concepts of justice in particular—should prescribe political actions (Galston 2010). Realists are not monolithic, and differ regarding the role of normative values in politics (Rossi and Sleat 2014). They agree, though, that moral philosophy does not solve political problems.

Second, not all issues have an important ethical component. There may be substantial disagreements over where to place a necessary facility such as a school or a jail. Third, political philosophy is not the usual lodestone either for the populace or for government officials. Both leaders and the led may prioritize interests, loyalties, personalities, and personal benefit over abstract issues (Philp 2010). A political process is necessary to solve such problems. Realists are concerned with political processes, divorced from moral considerations.

Third, realists see political disagreement as being constant and inevitable. There is limited consensus about normative values. Some such conflicts are based on beliefs, but adversaries are not likely to change their beliefs. Also, ambitious people will use disagreement as a tool to achieve their ambitions. Other sources of conflict, such as disagreement over how to prioritize and solve concrete problems, or over competition for status, are not based on principle and cannot be resolved through ethical analysis. An example of such a conflict is where to place an unpleasant, but necessary, facility. Changing circumstances create new foci for disagreement. Even if a monolithic faction comes to power, disagreement will arise within that faction. Disagreement is a constant in political life.

Fourth, realists are interested in the resolution of conflict, rather than in exploring the features of an ideal state (Burelli 2019). They are interested in how to govern effectively. Their primary concern involves order and stability (Hall and Sleat 2017). A successful government is one that maintains order and enjoys legitimacy, which is the willingness of people to accept without coercion a political process that denies their desires. Justice is far from the only public concern besides order. Other important preoccupations of states and citizens may include liberty, prosperity, and status.

A *modus vivendi* can be *principled* or *tactical* (Cohen-Almagor 2006). Principled compromises are those that all parties consider to be a permanent resolution of differences. A tactical compromise is one which at least one of the parties intends to abandon when in a position to do so.

This leads to at least two visions. One is Carl Schmitt's vision of politics as total combat with one's enemies (Schmitt 1932). In contrast is liberal pluralism. For liberal pluralist realists, an attainable goal of politics is to achieve a *modus vivendi*—an expedient compromise of differences negotiated under the aegis of a legitimate governing body. A *modus vivendi* reflects the importance of various interests to the parties themselves, and also the relative strength of the parties. A *modus vivendi* then, is an agreement establishing a stable political framework in which parties participate for expedient reasons (Rossi 2010). A *modus vivendi* is not based on morality. Gaus (2003) regards an agreement between two (or more) entities as a *modus vivendi* when it promotes the interests and goals of both, when it gives neither everything they want, when the relative power of A and B determines how much each gains and each cedes, and when persistence of the agreement is contingent on beliefs by the parties that the agreement is worth continuing.

Consider the question of whether individuals should pay for the health consequences of their dangerous behavior—either directly or through actuarial adjustments in insurance premiums in a system such as Part B Social Security.[5] Evel may not want to subsidize Jean-Paul's smoking habit, but Jean-Paul may not want to pay for Evel's motorcycle injuries. A possible *modus vivendi* between motorcyclists and smokers might be to agree to include smoking and motorcycle riding injuries as part of covered care. An alternative *modus vivendi* may be to exclude payment for smoking-related *and* motorcycle related medical costs. If there are far more smokers than stunt motorcyclists, the *modus vivendi* might be to pay for smoking-related costs but not for motorcycle-related costs. As long as the process is achieved through a peaceful, orderly, legitimate process in which the process and the result are accepted by both sides, a *modus vivendi* exists.

Bald coercion is not *modus vivendi*. Power alone does not legitimize rules of a state, even if those under the state accept the rule as a fiat (Hall 2015). A government can rarely rely on coercion alone to enforce laws. Rather, those who are subject to

[5] This covers outpatient costs in the United States funding system for the elderly. It is funded partly by the government and partly through income-based premiums paid by recipients.

the laws must have sufficient respect for authority that they will voluntarily comply even with laws that disadvantage them (Habermas 1996). If not, the laws will be unenforceable and widely flouted. This accounts for the widespread tax evasion seen in some Southern European nations. In the United States, widespread de facto school segregation persists because of resistance to integration (National Center for Education Statistics 2020), more than 65 years after the Supreme Court declared *de jure* segregation to be unconstitutional. Appeals to moralism and philosophical conceptions of justice arguably do not win elections, form coalitions, or motivate people to obey unpopular laws. A regimen for resolving disagreements over decisions must be sufficiently acceptable to avoid widespread evasion or defiance. All this being said, there is not a sharp line between coercion and negotiating from a position of strength.

Political theorists from socialists to liberals to conservatives have embraced political realism. It is the contemporary expression of the ideas of classical theorists such as Thucydides, Hobbes, and Max Weber (Burelli 2019). To sum up, realism emphasizes.

1. Separation of politics from ethics, rejecting an ethics-first approach.
2. Focus on order as primary desideratum of politics, with legitimacy needed to achieve order.
3. A concept of psychology that holds that citizens will be motivated by their affiliations, emotions, interests and passions.
4. Deemphasis on reasoned discourse
5. Inevitability of conflict; emphasis on differences.
6. Emphasis on historicity and on needs of particular situations.
7. *Modus vivendi* as the method of resolving conflict.

6.5 Limitations on Government Action

So far, I have established several bases for scrutinizing how to approach parent/state conflicts regarding children. First is the primacy of the family. Second, state coercive power will be limited to intervening when family decisions threaten serious harm to the child. Third, political *modus vivendi* will determine state policy. I now look at the specific protections that individuals and families should have to insulate them from government overzealousness.

Without constraint, political realism is compatible with total amorality. The need for legitimacy beyond coercion, which most contemporary realists accept, rescues realism from the dog-eat-dog authoritarianism of an Antonio Gramsci or a Carl Schmitt. Even a majoritarian regime in which two wolves and a lamb get to vote on the dinner menu is inadequate to protect people and families; one does not want to be the lamb. I return, then, to Judith Shklar's demand for constitutional safeguards to protect individuals from cruelty inflicted by government and by other powerful people. I turn Rawls's concept of the original position on its head, and ask what protections against government power any of us might want, not knowing in advance our position or its political strength, before entering a negotiation to achieve a *modus vivendi*. How might we prevent a government from hurting us if we are in the minority, or prevent the strong from so hurting us if we are weak? We resort to what Shklar calls the liberalism of fear. Some of the limitations on government, though, will be structural. These include separation of powers and federalism (or its European analog, subsidiarity). Another is creation of a robust civil society to provide services as an alternative to the state doing so. It is necessary to have a constitution that guarantees the negative rights that citizens of Western democracy have come to expect. Finally, we accommodate a welfare state but limit its reach through the principle of *sufficientarianism*.

6.6 Sufficientarianism

I will characterize sufficientarianism, and then apply it to child health and safety. Sufficientarianism is a distributional arrangement that seeks to allocate *scarce resources*[6] so that everyone is allocated the quantity that society considers essential (Fourie and Rid 2017). A resource that everyone must have in sufficient amounts is called a *currency*. *Pure sufficientarianism*, as conceived by Frankfurt (1987), holds *only* that justice requires that everyone possesses the sufficient amount of any currency. If there is more than one currency, there must be sufficient distribution of each currency; currencies are not fungible. Sufficientarianism is concerned only with absolute amounts of each currency that each person holds. It is not concerned with amounts of a currency that people possess relative to one another—i.e., with equality and inequality. In pure sufficientarianism, distribution of a currency above the threshold level is morally irrelevant (Frankfurt 1987).

There are two prototypical ways to abate the need of people below the sufficiency threshold. First, one can prioritize the needs of the *worst off*, devoting relatively great resources to those in most need (Herlitz 2017). Second, policy towards those below the sufficiency level may be based on '*headcount*,' favoring minimal redistribution to many people to maximize the number of those with sufficiency. Imagine that Urinetown has $100,000 to spend on plumbing. Ten households have no indoor plumbing, while 100 have indoor plumbing, but no flush toilet. Urinetown could have a 'worst off' approach, and build indoor plumbing for the ten houses without it at a cost of $10,000 per household. Alternatively, it could use a 'headcount' approach, and upgrade houses with plumbing to install flush toilets in 100 households for $1,000 per household. If each household has four people, the 'worst off' policy will raise 40 people from a terrible situation to the sufficiency standard. The headcount strategy will raise 400 people with milder deficiencies to the sufficiency threshold, but will leave the worst-off 40 in their very bad straits.

---

[6] A scarce resource is defined as one not present in sufficient quantities to satisfy the *desire* for that resource.

Modifications have been suggested to the stark viewpoint of pure sufficientarianism. Shift sufficientarianism proposes that moral or ethical considerations still exist above the sufficiency threshold, though they are weaker above the sufficiency threshold than below. Thus, if universal sufficiency is achieved, and a surplus exists, other factors become relevant. Possible candidates include egalitarianism, economic efficiency, and laissez faire. I consider effects on economic efficiency and production as relevant as well.

A primary reason for accepting sufficientarianism is that it is practically impossible to have another model for health care distribution in a real-life system. Hypothesize a generous single-payor healthcare system in the social democratic state of Sconya. In its efforts to be egalitarian, Sconya sets a limit of $1,000,000/QALY[7] as the most it is willing to pay for treatment. A wealthy patient, Midas, wants treatment whose cost–benefit exceeds the limit for Sconyan coverage. Can Midas pay for this care out of pocket? If he can, then Sconya has a sufficientarian system, though few will fall below the limit. If Sconya is so committed to egalitarianism that it is unwilling to let Midas pay for care out of pocket, then can Midas go abroad to get his treatment? If so, Sconya's health plan arguably is still sufficientarian. Only if it forbids Midas or any other citizen to obtain any uncovered treatment anywhere can Sconya be called egalitarian. To avoid sufficientarianism in favor of egalitarianism, it is necessary to forbid all health care outside the parameters of state coverage. This might ban cosmetic procedures. It might assign doctors randomly, banning sophisticated patients (like physicians and their families) from finding the best doctors and choosing them selectively. Practically speaking, it is almost impossible to avoid some degree of sufficientarianism in a healthcare system.

6.7 Sufficientarianism Versus Equity

I will apply the concept of sufficientarian distribution of health care to state oversight of parental error. In doing so, I will contrast a sufficientarian approach with the widely accepted goal of '*health equity*.' In an articulate statement of the health equity position, Sir Michael Marmot (2007), writing on behalf of a WHO-sponsored NGO, notes that there are great disparities in health between and within nations. He asserts that inequalities in health that are avoidable, but not avoided, are inequitable and unjust. Correcting this outcome requires more than disproportionate allocation of healthcare resources for those at risk, but (according to proponents of this point of view) extensive redistribution of other resources (Braveman et al. 2018). This is

[7] A QALY, or Quality-Adjusted Life Year, is "a measure of the state of health of a person or group in which the benefits, in terms of length of life, are adjusted to reflect the quality of life. One quality-adjusted life year (QALY) is equal to 1 year of life in perfect health. QALYs are calculated by estimating the years of life remaining for a patient following a particular treatment or intervention and weighting each year with a quality-of-life score (on a 0 to 1 scale). It is often measured in terms of the person's ability to carry out the activities of daily life, and freedom from pain and mental disturbance (NICE 2001).

because disparities result from such factors as wealth and status differentials, as well as from socially-mediated circumstances such as violent or polluted environments, diet, and use of harmful substances such as tobacco and alcohol. Advocates of this position for extensive changes in education, residential arrangements, and 'health-promoting' social environments (Braveman et al. 2018) have diverted the meaning of the word 'equity' from its traditional meaning of distribution according to merit.

All other things being equal, improving the health of those who are least healthy is highly desirable. There are some concerns with use of 'health equity' as a goal. First, there seems no good reason to prioritize health to the extent that all other features of social organization (e.g., education, economic distribution, housing, etc.) are subordinate to minimizing differences in health. If the goal is a healthy mind in a healthy body, priorities have to be set. Cultural differences, personal preferences in prioritizing health, as well as differing genetic propensities to develop illness, all contribute to health disparities. Furthermore, other policy priorities, such as overall economic production and national security, must compete with redistributionist welfare goals. Resources inevitably are limited, so it is necessary to decide how much money and effort to allocate to health improvement, given competing priorities. There will always be more worthy projects than available resources, and this scarcity problem forces governments to set a de facto sufficiency level for any objective. Certainly, health equity advocates are correct in that funding of education, sanitation, and other areas of spending may be more efficient ways of improving health than investing in expensive treatment.

Second, social engineering designed to eliminate all inequality that can be eliminated is a broad use of power that is likely to seriously intrude on civil liberties. Parents might be pressured to adopt practices that the government thought maximized their children's health. This might mean, for example, mandated dietary regimens, or limiting close work (such as reading) by children to prevent myopia. In societies with high crime rates due to cultural features that encouraged violent self-help in resolving disputes, a draconian criminal justice system might be necessary to curb violence. Prohibition of alcohol or tobacco might be on the political agenda. And, when all is said and done, there will always be hierarchies, and there will always be privilege.

Third, reasonable people can disagree on health priorities. Take the simple question of playground safety. Prevention of injuries may conflict with goals of fostering fortitude and independence. What play equipment should be available? Some places have monkey bars on their playgrounds, while others have eliminated them (Jordan 2018). Policy must account for (1) health shortfalls; (2) the capacity to alleviate these through intervention (which may not always be as great as health equity activists assume it is); and (3) proportionality between the resources expended and the benefits they generate (Herlitz 2017).

Fourth, even if resources could be equalized, education, personality, status, and street smarts will produce differences in access. Suppose the child of a pediatrics professor and the child of a hospital orderly who does not speak the native language both have a serious disease that requires complex care. Even with no financial barriers, availability of efficient, cheap transportation, etc., the professor is more likely than the janitor to identify high quality care and utilize it. She has the tools to accurately judge whether care is adequate, and to take the appropriate decision as to whether to continue care from the same source. No redistributionist program can equalize education and sophistication.

Once de facto sufficiency is achieved, will affluent parents be allowed to purchase additional care for their child? Pure sufficientarianism allows this. A shift sufficientarianism that requires equality or 'health equity' above the sufficiency level may not. Health equity also has to deal with the question of medically-created enhancements, such as hormones for increased stature or orthodontia for better facial appearance, whose main function is to increase the child's current happiness and future chances for secular success. Will a health equity regime only permit those enhancements that it will pay for?

A fifth concern is that creating maximalist demands and insisting that they must be honored as a matter of right can result in politicizing patient care. Physicians taking the Oath of Maimonides[8] swear to "never see in the patient anything but a fellow creature in pain." We can, and should, work to eliminate disparities in treatment within a hospital such as those documented by Eberly et al. (2019). Doctors, however, should be uncomfortable with a program that asks them to triage care based explicitly on ethnic criteria, as Wispelwey and Morse (2021) propose.

Health and other political priorities are best addressed as individual matters in a liberal society that prioritizes individual flourishing and liberty. Heath care has improved for the most disadvantaged, and likely will continue to do so without radical restructuring of society.

6.8 Health Care Sufficientarianism and Political Reality

Although the contemporary discussion of sufficientarianism arose from philosophical literature and so treats it as a moral principle, I will treat it as a political principle—as a guideline for public policy under a system that relies on realism as its main political principle, and that depends on *modus vivendi* to settle differences. Segall's (2016) objection that sufficientarianism does not adequately rely on values then becomes irrelevant. How then, can we justify sufficientarianism in a political sense, going into a negotiation to form a modus vivendi? One argument is that we are compassionate, and want to prevent suffering if we can (Crisp 2003). A second benefit is that assuring sufficiency serves as an insurance measure for all, protecting us against consequences of future possible destitution. Crisp reads Mill as saying that our conception of justice arises out of our natural tendencies toward self-defense and toward sympathy with others. So, self-defense is the second justification for sufficientarianism, just as compassion was the first. This concept is widely called a 'safety net;' a term probably first applied to sufficientarian welfare programs by the

[8] The Oath of Maimonides was actually composed by Marcus Herz in 1783, almost 600 years after the death of Maimonides.

late American politician, Jack Kemp (Safire 1981). Finally, sufficientarianism also may benefit third parties and society as a whole. Those who know that their basic needs will be met by the government may grant that government legitimacy. They may feel connected and loyal to society, as demanded by political realism.

There are at least two problems with sufficientarianism. First, the currencies of health sufficiency may be hard to characterize. If they are known, there might be so many of them that it is impractical to use them in practical analysis. Some of these differences can be elided using management techniques such as measuring health outcome in QALY's and by applying cost–benefit analysis to health spending priorities. Second, the level of a currency required to establish sufficiency must be arbitrary, and so may be controversial. Eliminating starvation is sufficient to keep people alive, but does not require providing them with a varied diet. But an affluent nation may insist that dietary sufficiency requires a diet less monotonous and tastier than one restricted to nutraloaf (Spanos 2014) or Soylent. On the other hand, universal caviar and white truffles are beyond the level of sufficiency. Analogous problems exist in applying sufficiency doctrine to health care.

Vandamme (2017) believes that sufficientarianism can be a practical approach to justice in public policy. First, it accommodates different degrees of urgency. Second, sufficiency is more attainable in practical politics than is equality. Finally, and especially important in this context, sufficientarianism provides a way to balance goals of distributional justice against other desirable values. We can use sufficientarianism to balance children's interests against parental prerogative. Parents' prerogative ends when they do not supply a child's sufficiency currencies in adequate amounts.[9] Sufficientarianism also allows us to finesse ethical controversies over how much parents should be required to protect children. Operationally, sufficient health care either is or is not present. Parents are held responsible for this without need to invoke interests or harms. Deliberate failure to meet goals of sufficiency is neglect—a legal concept. We have thus divorced the ethical discussion from the legal discussion. This is a good thing. Alignment with putatively correct philosophical positions is not the function of the state. Rather, its job is to meet the needs and wants of the citizenry, subject to basic constraints that protect liberty and needs. The next section will discuss in the abstract how to use sufficientarianism. The next chapter will reify this as a test to be applied to specific disputes.

---

[9] If provision of sufficient quantities of any currency is impossible because there are insufficient resources (or for some other reason), there will arise a new *modus vivendi* that redefines the level of sufficiency. We cannot, for example, expect parents to provide adequate housing for their children if a hurricane has just leveled their city. Government must then define what parents must do to avoid liability for neglect.

6.9 A *Modus Vivendi* for Parents, Children, Physicians, and the State

Government interference with parental decisions as primarily a political matter. The state should seek a *modus vivendi* that respects all stakeholders. The only legitimate goal of government intervention is to attain sufficiency in a currency whose provision is under the parents' control. If parental fulfillment of a child's needs is insufficient, intervention is triggered. Such circumstances trigger a Hohfeldian state power to correct deficiencies in parental behavior. The *modus vivendi* that I propose begins with the axiom that parents are the default decision-makers. Different parents have different priorities and values, though, which inevitably affect their decisions. Furthermore, parents must balance a child's health needs against other needs of that child and against all the needs of other family members. Most parents prefer relatively relaxed government supervision. They do not want visits from the food police to make sure vegetables are on the table, or visits from the literacy police to ensure that parents read appropriate books to their children each day (Iltis 2010).

Most parents also would prefer the opportunity to teach their values to their children. They are responsible for the day-to-day shaping of the children's behavior and morality. Standards of parenting vary from place to place. For example, different nations have different norms regarding the extent to which parents must exert direct supervision over a child (Pimentel 2016). Standards also vary from parent to parent regarding the importance of education, the necessity of chores, or the desirability of participating in contact sports. State agents should seek intervention, and the government should intervene, only in situations which the consensus of responsible parents would find intolerable.

Indeterminacy is inevitable. A starting point for a useful approach is that it is easier to identify gross injustice than to characterize what is just. There should be no argument in affluent Western nations that starving children, inflicting wanton serious injuries on them, or housing them in grossly unsanitary quarters, all fall below the sufficiency level for the needs of nutrition, safety, and shelter. Legal philosophy, applied to criminal law, draws a distinction between behavior that constitutes *malum in se* (acts acknowledged to be immoral) and behavior that is *malum prohibitum* (punished because the law allows or demands it) (Maibom 2008). In a democracy, an act is *malum prohibitum* when the *modus vivendi* arising from a democratic process declares it to be so. I believe it follows from my discussion in this book to this point, that the basis for coercive restriction of parental decisions (which is quasi-criminal) should be uncontroversial *malum in se*. I propose two currencies for sufficiency in the area of parental care: *minimizing the negative consequences to children of parental actions*, and *minimizing the negative consequences to third parties of parental actions*.

Any insufficiency in either of these currencies can appropriately trigger a coercive state remedy, authorized by *modus vivendi* as constrained by constitutional limits. Limitation of parental rights and actual criminal penalties should require a more stringent conception of sufficiency than should provision of state services, non-coercive visits by health care professionals and social workers, or educational efforts. A government can appropriately overrule parental decisions if the parental decision created a substantial chance of serious compromise of a physiological function; or it the decision was likely to have another serious detrimental effect on the child's present or future welfare. Any parental decision that is likely to impede the child from ultimately functioning as a productive member of society (or at least as a productive member of an isolated subculture within a state) must be suspect. As for society, parents should not be allowed to treat their children in a way that is likely to impose an unreasonable burden on society or on individuals outside the child's family. For example, a parent who knowingly sends a child to school with a serious communicable disease, or even head lice, can legitimately be punished. Acts that violate controversial political norms, or that do not cause harm, should not result in coercive action.

Governments with too few constraints can use ostensible child welfare considerations as a pretext for attacks on minority cultures and their practices. Consequentially, the concerns of state agents must be actual, rather than hypothetical, and must be reasonably likely to occur. When harm avoidance is a justification for overruling a parental decision, the potential harm must be greater than harms typically tolerated for comparable mainstream practices. Finally, the harms to family members and the children themselves created by punishment, or of restricting or terminating parental care, should not exceed the benefits of the punitive measures (Jacobs 2013, 2015; Jacobs and Arora 2017a, b).

Having discussed the theoretical basis for the test of the appropriateness of government intervention I will now describe my test.

Table 6.1 Heads of government and electoral runners up in the 12 highly- and very highly-developed nations with the greatest population[a]

Nation	Head of government	Runner-up
China[d]	Xi Jinping	N/A
United States[c]	Joseph Biden	Donald Trump
Brazil[d]	Jair Bolsonaro	Fernando Haddad
Russia[c]	Vladimir Putin	Pavel Grudinin
Mexico[d]	A.M. Lopez Obrador	Ricardo Anaya
Japan[c]	Yoshihide Suga	Yukio Edano
Philippines[d]	Roderigo Duterte	Mar Roxas
Germany[c]	Angela Merkel	Martin Schulz
Turkey[c]	Recep Tayyip Erdogan	Muharram İnce
Iran[d]	Ebrahim Raisi	Mohsen Rezaee
United Kingdom[c]	Boris Johnson	Jeremy Corbyn
France[c]	Emmanuel Macron	Marine Le Pen

[a]Development status is based on information contained in "Human Development Report 2019—Human Development Indices and Indicators" (PDF). HDRO (Human Development Report Office) United Nations Development Programme. pp. 22–25. Available at http://hdr.undp.org/en/countries. Retrieved 23 December 2019. Population data (not supplied in table) obtained from United Nations Data. 2019. *Total Population (Both Sexes Combined)*. Available at http://data.un.org/Data.aspx?d=PopDiv&f=variableID%3a12%3btimeID%3a83%2c84%3bvarID%3a2&c=2,4,6,7&s=_crEngNameOrderBy:asc,_timeEngNameOrderBy:desc,_varEngNameOrderBy:asc&v=1

[b]Nations whose names are in **boldface** do not have popular election of the head of government. Nations *italicized* have elections that do not meet democratic standards to a great extent

[c]Very highly developed

[d]Highly developed

References

Akbaş, Merve, Dan Ariely, and Sevgi Yuksel. 2019. When is inequality fair? An experiment on the effect of procedural justice and agency. *Journal of Economic Behavior and Organization* 161 (2): 114–127. https://doi.org/10.1016/j.jebo.2019.02.014.

Aristotle. 1995. *Politics*, Trans. Ernest Barker. Oxford: Oxford University Press.

Blais, Julie, and Scott Pruysers. 2017. The power of the dark side: Personality, the dark triad, and political ambition. *Personality and Individual Differences* 113 (2): 167–172. https://doi.org/10.1016/j.paid.2017.03.029.

Blanes. 2012. Revolving door lobbyists. *American Economic Review* 102 (7): 3731–3748. https://doi.org/10.1257/aer.102.7.3731373.

Braveman, Paula, Elaine Arkin, Tracy Orleans, Dwayne Proctor, Julia Acker, and Alonzo Plough. 2018. What is health equity? *Behavioral Science and Policy* 4 (1): 1–14.

Burelli, Carlo. 2019. realistic conception of politics: Conflict, order and political realism. *Critical Review of International Social and Political Philosophy* 1–23. https://doi.org/10.1080/13698230.2019.1604045.

Caprara, Gian Vittorio, and Jo. Silvester. 2018. The personality attributes of political elites. In *The Palgrave Handbook of Political Elites*, ed. Heinrich Best and John Higley, 467–487. London: Palgrave Macmillan.

Ceva, Emanuela, and Maria Paola Ferretti. 2017. Political corruption. *Political Compass* 12 (12). https://doi.org/10.1111/phc3.12461.

Chamberlain Bolaños, Cynthia. 2014. *Children and the International Criminal Court Analysis of the Rome Statute through a Children's Rights Perspective*. Dissertation, University of Leiden. https://openaccess.leidenuniv.nl/bitstream/handle/1887/24891/MANUSCRIPT%20CHAMBERLAIN%20FINAL.pdf?sequence=3.

Cohen-Almagor, Raphael. 2006. On compromise and coercion. *Ratio Juris* 19 (4): 434–455.

Cover, Robert M. 1986. Violence and the word. *Yale Law Journal* 95 (8): 1601–1629.

Crisp, Roger. 2003. Equality, priority, and compassion. *Ethics* 113 (4): 745–763. https://doi.org/10.1086/373954.

Deutsch, Morton. 1975. Equity, equality, and need: What determines which value will be used as the basis of distributive justice? *Journal of Social Issues* 31 (3): 137–149. https://doi.org/10.1111/j.1540-4560.1975.tb01000.x.

Eberly, Lauren A., Aaron Richterman, Anne G. Beckett, Bram Wispelwey, Regan H. Marsh, Emily C. Cleveland Manchanda, Cindy Y. Chang, et al. 2019. Identification of racial inequities in access

to specialized inpatient heart failure care at an academic medical center. *Circulation: Heart Failure* 12 (11): e006214. https://doi.org/10.1161/CIRCHEARTFAILURE.119.006214.
Euripides. 2013. *Iphigenia in Aulis*, Trans. Edward Einhorn. http://www.iphigeniainaulis.com/.
Findlaw: 2021. *Child Abuse Laws by State*. https://family.findlaw.com/child-abuse/child-abuse-laws-state-by-state.html.
Fourie, Carina, and Annette Rid, eds. 2017. *What Is Enough? Sufficiency, Justice, and Health*. Oxford: Oxford University Press.
Fournier, Suzanne, and Ernie Cray. 1997. *Stolen from Our Embrace: The Abduction of First Nations Children and The Restoration of Aboriginal Communities*. Vancouver: Douglas & McIntyre Ltd.
Frankfurt, Harry. 1987. Equality as a moral ideal. *Ethics* 98 (1): 21–43. https://doi.org/10.1086/292913.
Galston, William A. 2010. Realism in political theory. *European Journal of Political Theory* 9 (4): 385–411.
Galston, William A. 1996. Value pluralism and political liberalism. *Philosophy and Public Policy Quarterly* 16 (2): 7–13. https://doi.org/10.13021/G8pppq.161996.239.
Garrard, Peter, Vassiliki Rentoumi, Christian Lambert, and David Owen. 2014. Linguistic biomarkers of hubris syndrome. *Cortex* 55 (2): 167–181.
Gaus, Gerald F. 2003. *Contemporary Theories of Liberalism*. London: Sage.
Gregg, Samuel. 2014. Catholicism and the Case for Limited Government. In *Catholic Teaching and the Market Economy*, ed. Philip Booth, 254–273. London: Institute of Human Affairs.
Habermas, Jürgen. 1996. *Between Facts and Norms: Contributions to a Discourse Theory of Law and Democracy, translated by William Rehg*. Cambridge, Massachusetts: MIT Press.
Haer, Roos, Christopher Michael Faulkner, and Beth Elise Whitaker. 2020. Rebel funding and child soldiers: Exploring the relationship between natural resources and forcible recruitment. *European Journal of International Relations* 26 (1): 236–262. https://doi.org/10.1177/1354066119850622.
Hall, Edward. 2015. Bernard Williams and the basic legitimation demand: A defence. *Political Studies* 63: 2. https://doi.org/10.1111/1467-9248.12070.
Hall, Edward, and Matt Sleat. 2017. Ethics, morality and the case for realist political theory. *Critical Review of International Social and Political Philosophy* 20 (3): 278–295. https://doi.org/10.1080/13698230.2017.1293343.
Herlitz, Anders. 2017. Indeterminacy and the principle of need. *Theoretical Medicine and Bioethics* 38 (1): 1–14. https://doi.org/10.1007/s11017-016-9393-5.
Iltis, Ana S. 2010. Toward a coherent account of pediatric decision making. *Journal of Medicine and Philosophy* 35 (5): 526–552. https://doi.org/10.1093/jmp/jhq039.
Jacobs, Allan J. 2013. The ethics of circumcision of male infants. *Israel Medical Association. Journal: IMAJ* 15 (1): 60-64.
Jacobs, Allan J., and Kavita Shah Arora. 2015. Ritual male infant circumcision and human rights. *Journal of Bioethics* 15 (2): 30-39.
Jacobs, Allan J., and Kavita Shah Arora. 2017a. Punishment of minor female genital ritual procedures: Is the perfect the enemy of the good? *Developing World Bioethics* 17 (2): 134–140. https://doi.org/10.1111/dewb.12135.
Jacobs, Allan J., and Kavita Shah Arora. 2017b. Vulvar Nick and Metzitzah B'peh: Punishment or harm reduction? In *Reproductive Ethics: New Challenges and Conversations*, ed. Lisa Campo-Engelstein and Paul Burcher, 151–70. Cham, Switzerland: Springer Nature.
Jordan, Simone Amelia. 2018. Has the world gone mad banning monkey bars? *10 Daily (Sydney, Australia)* (blog). https://10daily.com.au/news/australia/a181126bci/has-the-world-gone-mad-banning-monkey-bars-20181127.
Kasindorf, Martin. 1990. Reagan's fall from grace: The $2-Million Japan tour, Nancy's vengeful memoirs and legal battles over the Iran-Contra affair have made his retirement anything but restful. *Los Angeles Times*. https://www.latimes.com/archives/la-xpm-1990-03-04-tm-2327-story.html, Accessed 8 July 2021.
Kymlicka, Will. 2002. *Contemporary Political Philosophy: An Introduction*. Oxford: Oxford University Press.

Lilienfeld, Scott O., Irwin D. Waldman, Kristin Landfield, Ashley L. Watts, Steven Rubenzer, and Thomas R. Faschingbauer. 2012. Fearless dominance and the U.S. presidency: Implications of psychopathic personality traits for successful and unsuccessful political leadership. *Journal of Personality and Social Psychology* 103 (3): 489–505. https://doi.org/10.1037/a0029392.

Maibom, Heidi L 2008. The mad, the bad, and the psychopath. *Neuroethics* 1 (3): 167–84. https://doi.org/10.1007/s12152-008-9013-9.

Marmot, Michael. 2007. Achieving health equity: From root causes to fair outcomes. *Lancet* 370 (9593): 1153–1163. https://doi.org/10.1016/S0140-6736(07)61385-3.

Mazzucato, Mariana. 2018. *The value of everything: Making and taking in a global economy.* London: Penguin Random House.

Meghani, Zahra, and Jennifer Kuzma. 2011. The "'revolving door'" between regulatory agencies and industry: A problem that requires reconceptualizing objectivity. *Journal of Agricultural and Environmental Ethics* 24 (6): 575–599. https://doi.org/10.1007/s10806-010-9287-x.

National Center for Education Statistics. 2020. Preprimary, elementary, and secondary education—Elementary and secondary enrollment—Racial/ethnic enrollment in public schools. *The Condition of* Education. https://nces.ed.gov/programs/coe/indicator_cge.asp.

NICE. 2001. Quality-adjusted life year. Glossary. *National Institute for Health and Care Excellence (UK)*. https://www.nice.org.uk/Glossary?letter=Q#QALY. Accessed 20 June 2001.

Offit, Paul. 2015. *Bad Faith: When Religious Belief Undermines Modern Medicine*. New York: Basic Books.

Owen, David. 2008. Hubris syndrome. *Clinical Medicine (London)* 8 (4): 428–432. https://doi.org/10.7861/clinmedicine.8-4-428.

Owen, D., and J. Davidson. 2009. Hubris syndrome: An acquired personality disorder? A study of US presidents and UK prime ministers over the last 100 years. *Brain* 132 (5): 1396–1406. https://doi.org/10.1093/brain/awp008.

Paulhus, Delroy L., and Kevin M. Williams. 2002. The dark triad of personality: Narcissism, Machiavellianism, and psychopathy. *Journal of Research in Personality* 36 (6): 556–563. https://doi.org/10.1016/S0092-6566(02)00505-6.

Penchaszadeh, Victor B. 1972. Genetic identification of children of the disappeared in Argentina. *Journal of the American Medical Women's Association* 52 (1): 16–21.

Perry, Chad, and Peter Miller. 2021. Dysfunctional leadership in universities: Identifying and dealing with sociopaths. In *Management, Leadership and Marketing of Universities and Colleges of Higher Education*, Forthcoming. https://pdfs.semanticscholar.org/bfe6/bcbeef73aae62208c35e5e905c322ff58ebf.pdf.

Peterson, Rolfe Daus, and Carl L. Palmer. 2019. The dark triad and nascent political ambition. *Journal of Elections, Public Opinion and Parties*. https://doi.org/10.1080/17457289.2019.1660354.

Philp, Mark. 2010. What is to be done? Political theory and political realism. *European Journal of Political Theory* 9 (4): 466–484. https://doi.org/10.1177/1474885110374010.

Pimentel, David. 2016. Protecting the free-range kid: Recalibrating parents' rights and the best interests of the child. *Cardozo Law Review* 38 (1): 1–57.

Plato. 1871. *The Laws of Plato*, Trans. Benjamin Jowett. https://www.gutenberg.org/files/1750/1750-h/1750-h.htm#link2H_4_0004. Accessed 5 June 2021.

Plato. 1991. *The Republic of Plato*, Trans. Allan Bloom. New York: Basic Books.

Rawls, John. 1971. *A Theory of Justice*. Cambridge, Massachusetts: Belknap Press.

Richmond, Douglas R. 2021. As the revolving door turns: Government lawyers entering or returning to private practice and conflicts of interest. *St. Louis University Law Journal* 65 (2), 325–359.

Rosenthal, Seth A., and Todd L. Pittinsky. 2006. Narcissistic leadership. *Leadership Quarterly* 17 (6): 617–633. https://doi.org/10.1016/j.leaqua.2006.10.005.

Rossi, Enzo. 2010. Public reason—Modus vivendi, consensus, and (realist) liberal Legitimacy. *Public Reason* 2 (2): 21–39.

Rossi, Enzo, and Matt Sleat. 2014. Realism in normative political theory. *Philosophy Compass* 9 (10): 689–701. https://doi.org/10.1111/phc3.12148.

Safire, William. 1981. On language; safety nets. *New York Times*. https://www.nytimes.com/1981/03/29/magazine/on-language-safety-nets.html.

Samuels, Brett. 2021. Hunter Biden artwork attracts ethics scrutiny: Report. *The Hill*. https://thehill.com/homenews/administration/562021-hunter-biden-artwork-attracts-ethics-scrutiny-report.

Schmitt, Carl. 1932. *The Concept of the Political*. Chicago: University of Chicago Press.

Segall, Shlomi. 2016. What is the point of sufficiency? *Journal of Applied Philosophy* 33 (1): 36–52. https://doi.org/10.1111/japp.12062.

Sen, Amartya. 2012. *The Idea of Justice*. Cambridge, Massachusetts: Harvard University Press. https://www.hup.harvard.edu/catalog.php?isbn=9780674060470.

Shklar, Judith. 1984. *Ordinary Vices*. Cambridge, Massachusetts: Belknap Press.

Shklar, Judith. 1989. The liberalism of fear. In *Liberalism and the Moral Life*, ed. Nancy L. Rosenbaum, 21–38. Cambridge, Massachusetts: Harvard University Press.

Shklar, Judith. 1990. *The Faces of Injustice*. New Haven: Yale University Press.

Simonet, Daniel V., Robert P. Tett, Jeff Foster, Anastasia I. Angelback, and Jennifer M. Bartlett. 2018. Dark-side personality trait interactions: Amplifying negative predictions of leadership performance. *Journal of Leadership and Organizational Studies* 25 (2): 233–250. https://doi.org/10.1177/1548051817727703.

Spanos, Alexander. 2014. The eighth amendment and nutraloaf: A recipe for disaster. *Journal of Contemporary Health Law and Policy* 30 (2): 222–248.

Spurk, Daniel, Anita C. Keller, and Andreas Hirschi. 2015. Do bad guys get ahead or fall behind? Relationships of the dark triad of personality with objective and subjective career success. *Social Psychological and Personality Science* 7(2): 113–121. https://doi.org/10.1177/2F1948550615609735.

Van Krieken, Robert. 1999. The 'stolen generations' and cultural genocide: The forced removal of Australian indigenous children from their families and its implications for the sociology of childhood. *Childhood* 6 (3): 297–311. https://doi.org/10.1177/0907568299006003002.

Vandamme, Pierre-Étienne. 2017. Why not more equality? Sufficientarianism and Inequalities above the Threshold. *Law, Ethics and Philosophy* 5: 130–141. https://doi.org/10.31009/LEAP.2017.V5.11.

Vandenbergh, Michael P., Jonathan M. Gilligan, and Haley Feuerman. 2020. The new revolving door. *Case Western Reserve Law Review* 70 (4): 1121–1149.

Vecchione, Michele, Shalom Schwartz, Gian Vittorio Caprara, Harald Schoen, Jan Cieciuch, Jo. Silvester, Paul Bain, et al. 2015. Personal values and political activism: A cross-national study. *British Journal of Psychology* 106 (1): 84–106. https://doi.org/10.1111/bjop.12067.

Walster, Elaine, Ellen Berscheid, and G. William Walster. 1973. New directions in equity research. *Journal of Personality and Social Psychology* 25 (2): 151–176.

Winter, David G. 2005. Things I've learned about personality from studying political leaders at a distance. *Journal of Personality* 73 (3): 557–584. https://doi.org/10.1111/j.1467-6494.2005.00321.x.

Wispelwey, Bram, and Michelle Morse. 2021. An antiracist agenda for medicine. *Boston Record*. http://bostonreview.net/science-nature-race/bram-wispelwey-michelle-morse-antiracist-agenda-medicine.

Ypi, Lea. 2020. Democratic dictatorship: political legitimacy in Marxist perspective. *European Journal of Philosophy* 28 (2): 277–291. https://doi.org/10.1111/ejop.12500.

Chapter 7
The State Intervention Test: When to Interfere with Parental Decisions

7.1 Why the Test is Necessary

I now specify when the state may exercise power to supersede the default power of parents to make decisions on behalf of their children. I propose a two-pronged test that specifies when the state may modify, reverse, or punish parental decisions or behavior related to children's health or safety. I call this test the *State Intervention Test* (the Test). The first prong of the Test outlines the Bases for such state action. The second prong establishes Constraints limiting state action even if there is a prima facie basis for action under the first prong.

Garrett (2018) challenged those proposing ethical frameworks to evaluate parental decisions. I have accepted most of his demands. He demanded that an ethical framework apply to all aspects of decision making. I do this, and extend it to state legislation. He insisted that present and future interests be balanced. Health interests must be balanced with other interests of the child. He demanded consideration of other stakeholders' interests. Finally, Garret and I would both avoid imprecise and misleading language to the greatest extent possible. I would add an additional feature—that the evaluative framework be applicable to legal as well as ethical discourse. I have rejected Garrett's first desideratum, that analysis encompass guidance and intervention principles. Guidance principles are not relevant to state coercion of parental decisions and actions in the field of health. My overall framework elaborated in Chap. 4 relates guidance principles, intervention principles, and state action, however.

The State Intervention Test is compatible with value pluralism. It addresses the problem of illiberal cultural practices by setting a standard that is a reification of the abuse/neglect standard as applied to health and safety. Resolution of parent/state conflict must consider needs and interests of those beyond the child. This begins with the family, but extends beyond the child's immediate circle. The Test will preclude child marriage (Raj et al. 2010) and other practices that have a major secondary impact on a child's health.

A. J. Jacobs, *Assigning Responsibility for Children's Health When Parents and Authorities Disagree: Whose Child?*, The International Library of Bioethics 90,
https://doi.org/10.1007/978-3-030-87698-2_7

Now consider a vaccine for a hypothetical virus that infects all children because of its ready communicability. In 90% of children, it causes lifetime asymptomatic infection with continuous viral shedding. The other 10% of children infected with the virus develop a rapidly fatal illness. The carrier state can be prevented by a vaccine that causes serious reactions in 0.5% of those receiving it. Only potential carriers can be immunized; those susceptible to the fatal disease state cannot successfully be vaccinated. Testing can determine whether a child will develop a carrier state or a fulminant infection. This hypothetical situation demonstrates that public health considerations may require some children to be subjected to risk for the greater good of society.

The coronavirus vaccines using synthetic mRNA present a situation in which personal health and public health may be at odds. The necessity of controlling the pandemic may cause some governments to require people to receive vaccines whose long-term effects are unknown and unpredictable.[1] If the intent is to create herd immunity, the vaccine must be given to children who are at low risk of serious illness. The point is that the state is not just concerned with the welfare of the individual child when making decisions. It must consider public health and other relevant political considerations.

The Test is pragmatic; it does not require a specific philosophical approach. It reflects a commitment to pluralism, while not going to extremes of cultural relativism. It therefore tries to accommodate parental decisions and preserve familial autonomy while recognizing that some parental activities may cause so much harm as to be intolerable. In order for a test to be acceptable in an electoral democracy it must lean towards consequentialism. Voters are likely to be more swayed by the effects of a policy than by its justification. To the extent that citizens are moved by principles that do not maximize material outcomes they are likely to turn to their *leitkultur*. A *leitkultur* (literally 'leading culture,' but perhaps better translated as 'core culture') is the values, attitudes, and behavior that members of a national culture are expected to have assimilated. Thus, the *leitkultur* will influence what a society will prize, tolerate, or disfavor. All states have cultural practices and taboos that impinge on ideals of liberalism. One cannot sell dog meat for human consumption in California (*Calif. Penal Code,* §598b), but may sell it in parts of Asia (Brady 2018). An approach to parent/state conflict must be able to accommodate relatively minor deviations from ideal liberalism. Intuitively, some interventions (or refusals of intervention) seem more burdensome to children than others. Piercing the ears of an infant girl is much less harmful than is fracturing and binding her feet to keep them small. Also, some activities seem intuitively to pose more of threat to society than others. The bounds of government action must be drawn somewhere in between the trivial and the unconscionable. By using terms like 'substantial' and 'unreasonable,' the State Intervention Test allows differences in local conditions to lead to different conclusions regarding acceptability of a practice.

---

[1] Since I wrote this passage, there has been 6 months' experience with widespread vaccine administration, with safety over that time interval comparable to many other vaccines in general clinical use.

The existence of a *leitkultur* does not justify all discrimination against those with deviating attitudes and practices. I therefore demand that local practices treat harms inherent in minority practices comparably to the way they treat harms tolerated by the majority.

The State Intervention Test provides a clear framework that considers all relevant parties. The Test places greater emphasis on the interests of society than do the approaches of some who have written on the subject. This is not a criticism of previous work. Rather, it follows from my interest in non-medical cultural practices, from which the Test emerged. In contrast, the starting point for others who have worked in this area has been the medical encounter. The Test avoids the false dichotomy between parental 'ownership' versus parental duties as mere agents of the state, with no rights except for access to the resources necessary to be an effective steward on behalf of the state. The Test protects the interest of children in avoiding experiences that produce impaired of emotional or physical functioning affecting daily living. The Test therefore places the burden of justification on those who would countermand parental decisions.

The State Intervention Test is divided into two prongs. The first prong sets forth the two justifiable Bases for state-imposed limitations. The second prong imposes three Constraints upon the state that may limit state action even when application of the first prong would establish a prima facie basis for such action.

7.2 The State Intervention Test

The State Intervention Test, as formulated below, modifies previous published iterations (Jacobs 2013; Jacobs and Arora 2015; Levin et al. 2016; Arora et al. 2018; Jacobs and Arora 2018). The name 'State Intervention Test' is novel to this book; previously the test was named eponymously for the author. The test follows:

A state may limit a parental decision that jeopardizes a child's health or safety if either of the two bases in the first prong exists, but only if none of the Constraints in the second prong apply.

First prong: **Bases for limiting parental decisions**. *It is warranted for a state to overturn, a parental decision, and possibly to punish a parent for the decision, if, as a consequence of the decision, unreasonable burdens are likely to be created either for:*

1. *Children to whom the decision applies, by: creating a substantial chance of death or of major disruption of a physiological function, or creating other objectively severe harmful effects, such as malnutrition or major psychological morbidity. (In situations where both a disease and a proposed treatment carry such risk of harmful effects, intervention is permissible if parents seek care whose risk/benefit ratio greatly exceeds the risk/benefit ratio expected from the management choice proposed by health care professionals.) This Basis is called the* ***Direct Effects Basis****.*

2. *Society as a whole or members of society besides the involved child. This is called the* ***Indirect Effects Basis****.*

Second prong: Constraints on government action. *Notwithstanding the bases in the First Prong, a state* ***may not restrict****parental action if any of the following Constraints applies:*

1. The supposed harm underlying the restriction is hypothetical, rather than actual; or rare rather than likely; this is the **Likelihood of Effect Constraint**.
2. The harm that the restriction seeks to avoid is less than harms typically tolerated for comparable practices; this is the **Comparability of Effect Constraint**.
3. Harms of the restriction to all parties concerned foreseeably exceed overall benefits. This is the **Harm/Benefit Constraint**.

7.3 The Two Bases

I did not explicitly grant standing in my test to group rights, nor did I explicitly talk about authority of groups over their members. Clearly, group powers over members are deeply entrenched in the economic sphere. For example, corporations and unions have great power to create and enforce rules for the workplace. Some religious bodies exercise great control over their members' personal lives. Monistic liberal states, though, assume that states and parents engage with each other without groups such as cultural or religious bodies participating directly, unless the state stipulates otherwise. Other democracies may delegate civil authority to religious bodies (Galanter and Krishnan 2001).

7.3.1 Indirect Basis: Effect of the Practice on Society or its Members

A decision or practice can be either an affirmative act or a decision to refrain from an act. An example of an affirmative act is allowing a child to play a full-contact sport. Withholding vaccination would be an instance of refraining from an important act. The burden a decision or practice inflicts need not be directly related to health care, but may involve other safety considerations. Thus, the Canadian Supreme Court found minimal danger in a Sikh student carrying a *kirpan* (ceremonial dagger) to school, allowing the practice (Shariff 2006).

Most questionable decisions by parents do not exist in a vacuum. Rather, they are made in the context of cultural traditions, factual misunderstandings, etc. Secular states should not interpret religious and cultural norms. A recent example of a government doing precisely this is the decision of the Mumbai High Court to require a Muslim shrine to admit women, partially on the grounds that exclusion of women was not essential to Islamic faith. In the United States, government interpretation of religious norms violates the Constitution (*United States vs. Ballard*, 322 US 78, Supreme Court, 1944). Government interpretation of religious law also is forbidden by the European Court of Human Rights (ECoHR) (*Martinez vs. Spain*, European

Court of Human Rights Grand Chamber Decision, App no 6030/07, 12 June 2014).[2] States may, however, probe the sincerity of claims of conscience (*United States vs. Seeger*, 380 US 163. Supreme Court, 1965). Consider a fictional group, the Blue Jews, who claim draft exemption because they interpret Numbers 15:38[3] as requiring to wear entirely blue clothes. A state may determine whether the group actually professes this doctrine, and whether it or its members do so sincerely. It may not, however, decide whether this belief is compatible with authentic Jewish doctrine.

The Indirect Effects Basis easily solves the problem posed by the virus vaccination scenario proposed earlier in this chapter. Vaccination would be permitted or required for carriers under this Basis. That is an extreme case. I appreciate that delineating the features of an unreasonable burden creates indeterminacy. However, identical decisions may have different consequences in different circumstances, so exclusion of all indeterminacy is impossible. I believe that the Test minimizes indeterminacy of state decisions.

Limitation of a practice based on the Indirect Effects Basis is a public policy decision to be made by government, and not a bedside decision by physicians (contrary to Wispelwey and Morse 2021). A common form of ad hoc decision-making based on Indirect Effects Basis-like considerations is pediatricians' exclusion of unvaccinated children from their practices. Though popular with vaccine-accepting parents, exclusion of children from obtaining pediatric services based on vaccination status has been criticized by some scholars (Kemper and Guth 2006), and by respected professional organizations.

7.3.2 Direct Effects Basis: Effect of the Practice on Children in the Minority Group

This Basis addresses possible harms to individual children from parental decisions. These considerations impact on clinical ethics as well as on public policy.

One such dangerous practice is withholding medical care in the face of acute illness. Also, this test would cover harmful procedures done for social or economic reasons, such as the obsolete practices of binding girls' feet to keep them tiny, and the European practice of castrating boys to employ them as singers in high ranges. Forms of female genital cutting that often make intercourse painful or vaginal delivery dangerous also can be banned under this prong. The Direct Effects Basis also allows restriction if the procedure causes non-physical foreseeable and objectively severe harms. These could be, for example, major psychological morbidity, child labor and denial of education are obvious examples.

Use of the phrase 'substantial chance' introduces indeterminacy to analyses conducted under the Test. I have criticized other approaches for this indeterminacy, but total consistency of approach is impossible. Although the locomotor effects of

---

[2] But states may regulate established churches and interpret their doctrine.

[3] "[The Israelites] should make them a fringe on the skirts of their garments for their generations and place on the fringe of the skirt an indigo twist."

foot binding and the reproductive and sexual effects of child castration always occur, and always are disabling, there are some other practices whose adverse effects may vary in frequency or magnitude. When severe risks are small, they must be weighed against the likely tangible and intangible benefits. Such balancing is appropriate with cosmetic orthodontia, infant circumcision, or height enhancement using injections of human growth hormone.

7.4 The Three Constraints

The three Constraints are intended to prevent unfairness in applying the two Bases. The first two Constraints are meant to prevent the use of the State Intervention Test as a pretext to persecute minorities and dissenters. The last Constraint is intended to prevent destructive state action against parents who are causing harm that is not of great consequence.

7.4.1 The Likelihood Constraint

Not only the magnitude, but the probability of the adverse consequences of an intervention should be considered (Gillam 2016). A risk of 1 in 10,00,000 may be insubstantial regarding the possibility of a single person contracting a moderately severe illness, but is more substantial if the risk involved creating a pandemic such as the current coronavirus pandemic. The Likelihood Constraint provides that the harm must be actual, rather than hypothetical; and likely, rather than unlikely or rare.

To illustrate the Likelihood Constraint in action, consider a state that abolishes child baptism requiring brief total immersion in water. The premier fears that a vasovagal reaction to immersion may cause death. This outcome is highly improbable, though it may occasionally occur. Therefore, foreseeability and likelihood should be the benchmarks. A sensibility similar to this is at work in NRDC vs. EPA (440 F.3d 476, 483, DC Circuit Court of Appeals, 2006), which disallowed an award for possible prospective damages whose occurrence had a probability of only 1 in 4.2 billion per person per year.

7.4.2 The Comparability Constraint[4]

The Comparability Constraint mandates that, whether great or small, any harm from minority or idiosyncratic acts must be disproportionately greater than the harm from comparable acts tolerated by the *leitkultur* to warrant government interference. Suppression of minority practices that inflict no more harm than analogous widespread and legal majority practices is unjustly discriminatory. This Constraint tries to track the seminal Supreme Court ruling, *Church of the Lukumi BabaluAye,*

[4] In previous iterations of the test, I called this Constraint the Magnitude Constraint.

Inc. vs. City of Hialeah (508 US 520, 1993). Ethically, majorities should not impose restrictions on minority groups that they would not impose on ourselves. UK law permits cosmetic labial surgery for adults, but does not permit religiously-motivated labial alteration for women of any age (UK Female Genital Mutilation Act, 2003). This is inappropriate.

In discussing the importance of this Constraint, I turn to the EU Court of Justice case of *Centraal Israëlitisch Consistorie van België and Others vs. Vlaamse Regering* (2020), which does not involve health matters. This decision allowed a regional Belgian government to ban Jewish and Islamic slaughter of food animals, without first stunning the animal. Ritual slaughter kills the animals rapidly by severing the carotid arteries. The court, citing the principle of margin of appreciation (67), relegated this question to sub-EU jurisdictions. The court disingenuously distinguished relatively painless ritual slaughter from the more painful practices of hunting and sport (such as bullfighting and cockfighting). The court noted that the purpose of the Belgian law was to regulate food production, but hunting and sport are not important sources of food production. Second, the principle of proportionality, allowed governments that prohibited ritual slaughter to permit hunting and bullfighting. Third, you can't stun animals when you are hunting them, so you can't require stunning (91). The court went on to interpret Judaism and Islam. It described the (religious) purpose of ritual slaughter as (1) to kill the animal by exsanguination; and (2) to remove as much blood as possible. Stunning does not interfere with these purposes (75).

But interpretation of religious law by a secular court is impermissible in the US and in Europe (Grimm 2018). Courts may overrule religious law on the basis of secular law, but they may not set themselves up as authorities on religious law. Compounding this error, the court incorrectly stated the reasons for ritual slaughter! The religions do not justify the laws on the basis of their material effects. Rather, the basis for laws regarding slaughter is divine command, as interpreted by recognized religious authorities, as interpreted through religious hermeneutic traditions (Levin et al. 2016). Material consequences are rationalizations outside religious law.

Centraal Israëlitisch Consistorie epitomizes the sort of state that the State Intervention Test opposes.

7.4.3 The Benefit/Harm Constraint

Finally, I require a benefit/harm analysis as part of my test. Gillam (2016) emphasizes that the harms of state intervention should be considered as well as the harms of parental intervention. Such harms include disrupting relationships between parents and children, as well as the tangible harms resulting from punishing parents. These harms are no less harmful by virtue of being unintended or indirect. The principle of proportionality must apply to any restriction or punishment. The costs of punishing behavior perceived as deviant may be more harmful than allowing the behavior. That should not be permitted.

7.5 The Test in the Context of Other Approaches to State-Parent Conflict

7.5.1 General Considerations

The State Intervention Test sets a limit on parental discretion when a parental decision is likely to lead to serious effects—physical and otherwise—on children. Serious harm caused by parent fails to meet the Test's sufficientarian standard. Tighter restrictions on parents would violate bounds of family integrity that ought to be constitutionalized for the protection of liberty. Adults have a prima facie entitlement to form a family with their biological children. But parents must meet the needs of children, such as providing physical care and sufficient education to survive and thrive as adults.

Parental authority is appropriately constrained by non-governmental institutions to which parents belong, and whose norms parents accept. Such groups include community, extended family, perhaps religious and other cultural institutions. Both formal associations such as team sports and informal associations such as neighborhoods and extended families impose rules and provide moral guidance. The state, though, is the final bulwark against parental malfeasance because its government is powerful and possesses legitimacy.

Governments and parents each have an area of appropriate authority. Diekema (2004), Kopelman (1997), Ross (1998), and Iltis (2010) all note that the criterion for state intervention is not maximization of that child's welfare (as the state construes child welfare). Parents with more than one child need to balance the interests of their children. The interests of a particular child do not receive special preference because he happens to be under the active care of a doctor. Furthermore, it also is reasonable for parents to balance their own interests with those of their children. A literal application of the best interests standard leads to the *reductio ad absurdum* of granular state supervision (Iltis 2010). But there still is a zone of unacceptability from which a state may properly exclude parental behavior. Parents must provide for their children's basic needs.

There is controversy over the extent to which the state should acknowledge the importance of children's relational and spiritual interests in determining the adequacy of parental decisions. Authors such as Rawls and Audi have argued that one may use one's conceptions of the good to guide private behavior, but only public reasons, which are theoretically comprehensible and acceptable to all, are valid in public discourse. This excludes religious reasons, which are not subject to scientific or philosophical analysis. The *effects* of religious belief and practice on individual behavior and on society are comprehensible to all, and subject to scientific study. Putnam and Campbell (2010) attempt to demonstrate that these effects are, on the whole, positive. Such a demonstration is unlikely to convince political theorists who believe that religious discourse has no place in resolution of political issues or—for that matter—in bioethics (Li, 2020; Matisonn 2020). Some who wish to restrict the space for using theological motivations as a basis for decisions simply do not want religion to be present in the public sphere.

The might wielded by government seriously disadvantages religion if religion is removed as a relevant consideration in public discourse. The state can, and will, assert that public considerations trump religious practice (See, *Employment Division vs. Smith*, 494 US 872, Supreme Court, 1990). I have described the opinions Brighouse & Swift, and Dwyer, who seem to regard the family as a public institution, rather than as private space. Fineman (2019) explicitly denies that there are private areas of interpersonal relations exempt from state regulation. I have argued in earlier chapters to the contrary.

The State Intervention Test neither privileges religions nor places special burdens on religion. State action is based on the tangible situation of the child. But children are entitled to a permanent family that lives by reasonably consistent principles and values. This is endorsed by the Convention on the Rights of the Child (Preamble; Art. 2, § 2; Art. 5; Art. 8).[5] Values and standards of behavior that children assimilate as members of a family provide guidance, and perhaps default solutions, in addressing personal choices. The state seldom should interrogate parental values.

However, some parental practices and decisions are injurious to important secular interests of children. These may result in conflict between parents and state authorities regarding parental care. Areas of conflict may revolve around health and safety issues. I also emphasize the effect of parental choices on individuals outside the family, and the social context of state intervention as well as the impact on the child. Too little attention has been devoted to this topic.

State action on the basis of parental beliefs raises the specter of possible socioeconomic discrimination. Jehovah's Witnesses attract more attention for attempting to deny blood transfusions to their children than do Christian Scientists for denying children any medical care (Vaillant 2000). Unsurprisingly, Jehovah's Witnesses are disproportionately poor, non-White, and poorly educated (Pew Research Center 2016), while Christian Scientists are more prosperous and influential (Stark 1998). The Test seeks to guard against this sort of discrimination.

7.5.2 *The Harm Principle and the Test*

My test has much in common with Douglas Diekema's harm standard, described in Chap. 3. We both set a floor for parental behavior based on the likelihood of serious harm to the child. Diekema's third and sixth conditions[6] resemble the constitutional strict scrutiny test applied to government incursions on fundamental rights, requiring that a measure that limits fundamental constitutional rights "furthers a compelling interest and is narrowly tailored to achieve that interest" (*Citizens United*

[5] This citation is not intended as a normative argument, but rather to indicate that the sorts of people who draft United Nations Conventions recognize the family as a fundamental building block of society, and as entitled to protection.

[6] These conditions are (Diekema, 2004): 3. Is the intervention that has been refused necessary to prevent the serious harm? 6. Would any other option prevent serious harm to the child in a way that is less intrusive to parental autonomy and more acceptable to the parents?

vs. Federal Election Com'n, 558 US 310, 330, Supreme Court, 2010, 330). The State Intervention Test does not go this far. Its consequentialist and expedient perspective requires government restraint, but does not demand that the government choose the most narrowly tailored remedy. I believe such strict scrutiny to be impractical. The State Intervention Test, therefore, employs a standard for intervention more akin to intermediate scrutiny, which requires merely that a measure "directly advances a substantial governmental interest and is not more extensive than is necessary to serve that interest" (*Central Hudson Gas & Elec. Corp. vs. Public Serv. Com'n of NY*, 447 US 557, Supreme Court, 1980, 573). In other words, the interest needs to be substantial, but not compelling, and the state measure need not be the most narrowly tailored possible. Also, I also do not require that the harm be imminent, in contrast to Diekema.

I differ from Diekema in my emphasis on protecting society and its members. Diekema acknowledged the dual goals of protecting the vulnerable under the *parens patriae* doctrine and protecting society and its members under the police power doctrine (Diekema 2004). His emphasis, though, is on the individuals directly involved. Thus, unlike Diekema, I would require children to submit to vaccinations against serious communicable diseases even if the community enjoys herd immunity. This is because herd immunity does not prevent sporadic outbreaks, and because of my general distaste for free riding (Arora et al. 2018).

I also emphasize the context of a decision. I demand that all analogous cases be treated alike with regard to government interference, or lack of interference, with parental decisions. It is necessary to compare and contrast policies toward different procedures that somewhat resemble each other. The state should not permit those procedures that enjoy mainstream acceptance while discouraging or punishing comparably risky ones practiced by minorities.

Finally, Diekema's discussion was focused on medical decisions, while my test considers all parental decisions that may affect health and safety, such as those regarding discipline or sports participation.

In summary, my approach is not radically different from Diekema's. We both would limit restrictions based on *parens patriae* to situations in which there is a likelihood of serious harm to the child involved. There are, however, a few significant differences—my emphasis on the public's claims, and my use of an intermediate scrutiny rather than a strict scrutiny standard.

7.5.3 Family-Based Approaches and the Test

My position recognizes the child as a member of the family. I substantially agree with the approach of Lainie Friedman Ross (1998), whose position is exceptionally well developed. Ross holds that parents have responsibilities such as refraining from abuse and neglect, but these fall short of a literal best interests standard. Reasons for believing that parents should be given wide latitude have been explored in detail in Chap. 4.

Describing her stance as *constrained parental autonomy*, Ross (1998) emphasizes that different parents will prioritize goods differently, as value pluralism prevents assigning a categorical value to any good or expression of that good. Ross also stresses that parents have to balance the interests of all family members, including other children. This means that wide variation in parental decision making should be tolerated. My trigger point for state intervention is similar to that of Ross, which is that the possibility of death or serious damage be sufficiently frequent. Ross therefore does not consider the right of bodily integrity to be absolute. Ross deems it inappropriate to apply rights paradigms to the family setting except in extreme cases. In situations such as parental consent for bone marrow transplantation donation, or neonatal circumcision, parental decisions should not be overruled. My elaborations on Ross consist in my attempts to integrate ethical and legal approaches.

7.6 Potential Problems with the State Intervention Test

I identify four potential problems with the State Intervention Test. First, it is necessary to decide how to treat economic costs to society under the Indirect Effects Basis of the Test. Second, the Test does not directly address parental decisions that may limit the child's future economic potential. Third, the Test takes no account of intangible harms, such as dignitary harm and autonomy. Finally, the test does not address parental practices that are not objectively harmful but which offend the deep sensibilities of a society.

7.6.1 Economic Costs

Someone must pay for the costs of treatment. If not parents, these must be covered by others, through insurance and government benefits. Could high cost justify state reversal of parental decisions or suppression of minority practices under the Indirect Effects Basis? Consider parental demands for prolonged life support for a terminally ill child. In the United States, ethical guidance and practice standards discourage physicians from providing medically ineffective care.[7]

States might use economic metrics to limit parental choices, even when clinical futility is not an issue. They could impose a requirement on parents to accept medical decisions because of moderate economic savings. To construe all economic costs as a burden under the Indirect Effect Basis would negate the Test. On the other hand, to allow any level of cost provided parents could pay for it themselves would raise issues of equity that extend beyond the problems that the Test is intended to solve (Truog 2017). Wilkinson and Nair (2016) proposed that there be both a harm test and a cost test when parents demanded treatment contrary to medical advice.

[7] For further discussion, *see*, American Medical Association, *Code of Medical Ethics, Opinion 2.035: Futile Care*, (2015) Available at http://www.ama-assn.org/ama/pub/physician-resources/medical-ethics/code-medical-ethics/opinion2035.page?

There are at least three possible solutions to the problem of intersection of the Test with economic constraints. One is to arbitrarily exclude economic causes from harms to society that can trigger the Indirect Effects Basis. A second is to allow economic burdens to overrule parental decisions, but only if treatment is not likely to be effective. The final solution, which I endorse, is to use the Comparability Constraint to protect minorities from abuse of the Indirect Effects Basis. Sufficientarianism requires economic limits to state provision of care. These must be provided on the same basis to everyone. A government could only use economic costs as a reason for restricting minority practices if it would restrict activity by mainstream individuals and groups according to the same economic criteria in comparable situations. Health care budgeting has repercussions both for just distribution of health care resources and for other government programs, as economic resources are fungible (Truog 2017). The state should have broad authority to budget for health care. This leaves the issue of allocation of private funds for expensive or futile care, as was offered to Charley Gard (Shah et al. 2017), This is a complex topic largely beyond the scope of this discussion.

7.6.2 Decisions that Interfere with the Child's Economic Potential

Some parental decisions may interfere with the child's future economic productivity. Indeed, almost any major parental decision has ramifications for the child's income potential. Most of these decisions do not involve health and safety matters. Where the family settles, what interests they encourage, or how children are taught to dress, dine, and speak to others all have an impact.

It is a mistake to conflate income with value to society. Housework, child care, and much volunteer work contribute materially to the well-being of society. A social worker may contribute more by some lights than an intellectual property lawyer who earns 50 times her income. That being said, refusal of treatment that provides or restores functions such as sight, hearing, or speech reduces productivity. Withholding of enhancements such as growth hormones for short boys, or orthodontia and other cosmetic facial interventions, primarily affect appearance, but appearance affects economic and social prospects. Educational choices have a major impact as well. Utilizing the effects of parental decisions as a reason for government action permits the government to overrule parents virtually at will. I therefore only require that parents, insofar as possible, raise children to be productive. Operationally, this may mean that they are not likely to require permanent state support. This is a sufficientarian definition of the child's needs in this area. This, essentially, places productivity in the realm of the Indirect Effects Basis. A full description of productivity, as used in this context, has yet to be worked out.

7.6.3 Intangible Harms

The test does not support government intervention for intangible harms, primarily threats to dignity. The strong affirmations of children's autonomy expressed by some scholars do not reflect the reality of the child's dependence. Socialization of the child inevitably involves implicit or explicit indoctrination into thick values. The role of the state is not to maximize autonomy, but to further flourishing and to ensure that a child is productive. It is reasonable for the state to assure education and health care that seek to enable children, when mature, to sustain themselves materially. The Indirect Effects Basis addresses this goal.[8]

Adequate dignity is even more difficult to define than appropriate child autonomy. Dignity is not equivalent to equality, nor is either a necessary or a sufficient condition for the other. Dignity can be defined in terms of constitutional or other rights. But there are aspects of dignity related to one's humanity, one's status, one's behavior, and possibly one's capabilities. I do not know how to draw a line between legally permissible and impermissible affronts to dignity. Laws requiring confidentiality and informed consent address obvious cases. But they do not specify when a parent is affronting her child's dignity.

7.6.4 Repugnance

Leon Kass suggested, in the context of human cloning, that general repugnance to a practice indicates that the practice likely is immoral. He stated that "[r]epugnance is the emotional expression of deep wisdom, beyond reason's power to articulate it" (Kass 1998, 687). This has been called the 'yuck factor' (Fiester 2008), and may be the basis for criminalizing certain non-medical practices that cause no objective human harm, such as laws banning sale of horse meat for human consumption (*Cavel International, Inc. vs. Madigan*, 500 F3d 551, 7th Circuit Court of Appeals, 2007), blasphemy laws (*Otto-Preminger-Institut vs. Austria*, 295 Eur. Ct. H.R. (ser. A), 1994; and laws prohibiting lèse-majesté (Streckfuss 1995).

The State Intervention Test is designed for liberal political systems—that is, for societies committed to maximal opportunities for individual freedom and individual expression consistent with general order. To the extent that a state prohibits acts whose only harms consist of affronts to general beliefs or psychological comfort, that state may not be liberal. There are at least two reasons for such departure from liberalism in a liberal state. One is to combat a serious threat to the liberal democratic order; constitutional regimens that guarantee individual rights are "not a suicide pact" (*Terminiello vs. Chicago*, 337 US—Supreme Court 1949, Jackson, J (dissenting)

[8] The question of increasing power for older minors to participate in their healthcare decisions is complex, and will be addressed in later chapters.

37).[9] President Lincoln's suspension of *habeas corpus* during the American Civil War (Jackson 2004)—including the arrest and prolonged detention without trial of Maryland legislators known to support secession (Cannon 2010)—and European laws prohibiting genocide denial (Garibian 2007), may be examples of this. Such restrictions should be limited and temporary.

The more common reason for departure from liberalism is restriction in order to support features of a *leitkultur*. A state will then engage in willing departures from liberalism based on widely and strongly held attitudes. Defense of the ideal of liberalism against state legislative affirmation of thick substantive principles is beyond the scope of this discussion.

7.7 Conclusion

Parental decisions arising out of minority practices or idiosyncratic beliefs and involving the health and safety of children sometimes pose difficulty for states that desire to maximize individual liberty while ensuring child welfare. Limitation of these parental decisions should therefore be based on principles that are consistent, fair, and non-discriminatory. Policies pertaining to such limitation must acknowledge both that the interests of a child encompass considerations beyond physical health and that many majority practices also pose risks to a child. Tangible elements of a child's welfare must be balanced with a child's relational, spiritual and psychological interests, the well-being of the entire family, and the needs of society and its members. Considerations of child welfare must not be used as a pretext to attack a disfavored minority group. The State Intervention Test serves to determine when states may limit minority religious and cultural practices that involve children. The test considers the relevant interests of parent, child, and parties outside the family and related religious or cultural groups. Thus, application of this test would appropriately balance competing interests I have identified and permit the state to ensure the application of fundamental decency and justice to all children under its jurisdiction while protecting minority expression.

The remainder of the book discusses application of the State Intervention Test to specific problems pertaining to decisions regarding children's health.

References

Arora, Kavita Shah, Jane Morris, and Allan J. Jacobs. 2018. Refusal of vaccination: A test to balance societal and individual interests. *Journal of Clinical Ethics* 29(3):203–13.

Brady, Heather. 2018. Dog meat's controversial history, from the ancients to the winter Olympics. *National Geographic Online*, Feb 2018. https://news.nationalgeographic.com/2018/02/dog-meat-south-korea-olympics-explainer-spd/.

[9] This analogy to a suicide pact often is misattributed to Abraham Lincoln.

Cannon, Jessica A. 2010. *Lincoln's divided backyard: Maryland in the civil war era*. Ph.D. Dissertation, Rice University, Department of History. Available at https://scholarship.rice.edu/bitstream/handle/1911/61958/3421215.pdf?sequence=1&isAllowed=y.

Diekema, Douglas S. 2004. Parental refusals of medical treatment: The harm principle as threshold for state intervention. *Theoretical Medicine* 25 (4): 241–264.

Diekema, Douglas S. 2005. Responding to parental refusals of immunization of children. American Academy of Pediatrics, Committee on Bioethics. *Pediatrics* 115 (5): 1428–14.

Fiester, Autumn. 2008. Justifying a presumption of restraint in animal biotechnology research. *American Journal of Bioethics* 8 (6): 36–44.

Fineman, Martha Albertson. 2019. Vulnerability and social justice. *Valparaiso University Law Review* 53(2):341–69.

Galanter, Marc, Jayanth Krishnan. 2001. Personal law systems and religious conflict Gerald James Eds Religion and personal law in secular India: A call to judgment. Bloomington: University of Indiana Press Larson, pp. 270–300.

Garibian, Sevane. 2007. Taking Denial seriously: Genocide denial and freedom of speech in the French law. *Cardozo Journal of Conflict Resolution* 9(3):479–488.

Garrett, Jeremy R. 2018. Prolegomena to any future pediatric bioethics. *American Journal of Bioethics* 18 (8): 63–65.

Gillam, Lynn. 2016. The zone of parental discretion: An ethical tool for dealing with disagreement between parents and doctors about medical treatment for a child. *Clinical Ethics* 11 (1): 1–8.

Grimm, Dieter. 2018. Sovereignty and religious norms in the secular constitutional state. In *Religion, secularism, and constitutional democracy*. ed. L. Jean, 341–357. New York: Columbia University Press Cohen & Cécile Laborde.

Iltis, Ana S. 2010. Toward a coherent account of pediatric decision making. *Journal of Medicine and Philosophy* 35 (5): 526–552.

Jackson, Jeffrey D. 2004. The power to suspend habeas corpus: An answer from the arguments surrounding *Ex Parte Merryman. University of Baltimore Law Review* 34(1): 11-54.

Jacobs, Allan J. 2013. The ethics of circumcision of male infants. *Israel Medical Association. Journal: IMAJ* 15 (1): 60–64.

Jacobs, Allan J., and Kavita Shah Arora. 2015. Ritual male infant circumcision and human rights. *American Journal of Bioethics* 15(2):30–9.

Jacobs, Allan J., and Kavita Shah Arora. 2018. When may government interfere with religious practices to protect the health and safety of children? *Ethics in Medicine and Public Health* 5(1):86–93.

Kass, Leon. R. 1998. The wisdom of repugnance: Why we should ban the cloning of humans.*Valparaiso University Law Review* 32(2):679–705.

Kemper, Kathi and Caryl J. Guth. 2006. Dismissing families: A slippery slope. *Archives of Pediatric and Adolescent Medicine* 160 (4): 452–453.

Kopelman, Loretta M. 1997. The best-interests standard as threshold, ideal, and standard of reasonableness. *Journal of Medicine and Philosophy* 22 (3): 271–289.

Levin, Hillel Y, Allan J. Jacobs, and Kavita Shah Arora. 2016. To accommodate or not to accommodate: (When) Should the state regulate religion to protect the rights of children and third parties? *Washington and Lee Law Review* 73(2):915–1017.

Li, Hon Lam. 2020. Public reason as the way for dialogue. *American Journal of Bioethics* 20 (12): 29–31.

Matisonn, Heidi. 2020. Talking at cross purposes: Why we shouldn't re-establish the relationship between theological and secular bioethics. *American Journal of Bioethics* 20 (12): 45–47.

Pew Research Center. 2016. Religious landscape study: Jehovah's witnesses. http://www.pewforum.org/religious-landscape-study/religious-tradition/jehovahs-witness/. Accessed 7 Jan 2016.

Putnam, Robert D. and David F. Campbell. 2010. *Amazing grace: How religion divides and unites us*. Simon and Shuster: New York

Raj, Anita, Niranjan Saggurti, Michael Winter, Alan Labonte, Michele R Decker, Donta Balaiah, and Jay G Silverman. 2010. The effect of maternal child marriage on morbidity and mortality of children under 5 in India: cross sectional study of a nationally representative sample. *BMJ* 340:b4258.

Ross, Lainie Friedman. 1998. *Children, families, and health care decision-making*. Oxford: Clarendon Press.

Shah, Seema K., Abby R. Rosenberg, and Douglas S. Diekema. 2017. Charlie Gard and the limits of best interests. *JAMA Pediatrics* 171(10):937–938.

Shariff, Shaheen. 2006. Balancing competing rights: A stakeholder model for democratic schools. *Canadian Journal of Education/Revue Canadienne De L'éducation* 29 (2): 476–496.

Stark, Rodney. 1998. The rise and fall of Christian science. *Journal of Contemporary Religion* 13 (2): 189-214.

Streckfuss, David. 1995. Kings in the age of nations: The paradox of lèse-majesté as political crime in Thailand. *Comparative Studies in Society and History* 37 (3): 445-475.

Truog, Robert D. 2017. The United Kingdom sets limits on experimental treatments: The case of Charlie Gard. *JAMA*. 318(11):1001–1002. https://doi.org/10.1001/jama.2017.10410.

Vaillant, Daniel. 2000. Prosecution of Christian scientists: A needed protection for children or insult added to injury. *Cleveland State Law Review* 48(3):479–502.

Wilkinson, Dominic and Nair Tara. 2016. Harm isn't all you need: Parental discretion and medical decisions for a child. *Journal of Medical Ethics* 42 (2): 116–118.

Wispelwey, Bram, and Michelle Morse. 2021. An antiracist agenda for medicine. *Boston Record*, Mar 17, 2021. http://bostonreview.net/science-nature-race/bram-wispelwey-michelle-morse-antiracist-agenda-medicine

Part III
Applications of the State Intervention Test

Chapter 8
Treatment of Disease

Abstract This chapter identifies four types of situations in which parents and physicians are likely to encounter disagreement. The chapter also points toward avenues toward resolution. The first situation is one in which the parent refuses a measure proffered by a physician. The second is the circumstance in which the parent demands treatment the physician deems inappropriate. The third paradigm involves disagreement among custodial parents regarding the child. Finally, either a parent or a physician can abuse her power to undercut the appropriate authority of the other. Each of these paradigms requires different analysis, pointing to a different approach to solution. The State Intervention Test is useful in identifying the problem and pointing toward a solution. With regard to unreasonable demands for care, the traditional Roman Catholic distinction between ordinary and extraordinary care proves very useful.

8.1 Introduction

A good place to apply the State Intervention Test (the Test) is the subject of disagreement over the treatment of an illness. When a dispute between a parent and a physician over how to treat a sick child must be resolved in court, this represents a failure of shared clinical decision-making. Reasonable, well-meaning people ordinarily can accommodate each other's points of view and reach a compromise. Sometimes, though, agreement is not possible, and the dispute requires legal adjudication.

Such a dispute is argued by representatives of the parties. The child's interests are asserted by a court-appointed advocate known as a guardian *ad litem*, who, in turn, may retain legal counsel to argue the child's case in court. The parties themselves are not heard directly, save perhaps in the formal and constrained way that witnesses testify in court. The structure of court proceedings turns the child, the parent, and the medical caregivers into mutual adversaries.[1] The guardian *ad litem* theoretically speaks on behalf of the child, but likely does not have a sense of unique

[1] Article III of the US Constitution limits jurisdiction of courts to controversies between specific parties.

A. J. Jacobs, *Assigning Responsibility for Children's Health When Parents and Authorities Disagree: Whose Child?*, The International Library of Bioethics 90,
https://doi.org/10.1007/978-3-030-87698-2_8

Table 8.1 Reasons for parent refusal of treatment

Cost
Lack of parental commitment to treatment requiring parental effort
Poor quality of life for child
Suspicion of healthcare system or of physicians
Belief in non-standard treatment
Poor insight into severity of condition (denial)
Culture in which Western medicine is alternative and traditional beliefs are normative
Desire to lose child

conditions such as embeddedness in a family or community, which contributes to the child's current interests or anticipated mature desires. Furthermore, the guardian *ad litem* is not necessarily sensitive to these interests. This is especially true if the child's community is a minority group with different customs and values than the professional class from which the guardian *ad litem* is likely to be appointed. The educational and social background of a guardian *ad litem* may lead her to be more sympathetic with the opinions of health professionals than with the parents. This is especially true if the parents have limited education and means. The judicial outcome depends to a large measure on the experience and beliefs of the judge, and on the advocacy skills of the parties' lawyers (Dolgin 2019).

It generally is preferable to resolve disputes between parents and doctors through in-house ethics consultations. A sensitive, professionally independent ethics consultant oriented toward facilitation of an agreement is likely to mediate an outcome in which the parties feel that they have been heard and respected. Accommodation and reconciliation of shareholders' points of view ideally should take priority over the triumph of skillful advocacy or the imposition of the norms of the *bien pensant*.[2] Furthermore, parties are more likely to abide by a negotiated outcome than by an imposed outcome (Dolgin 2019).

Government intervention should be a last resort, and should be sought only when attempts at counseling and mediation have failed. Physicians must try to understand why parents disagree with them. Common reasons are listed in Table 8.1. Note that a parental loss in court will not necessarily ensure that a child will receive the care that physicians seek. The family may defy the court, hide, or leave the jurisdiction.

Many disputes are clouded by medical, ethical, and legal uncertainty (Dolgin 2019). Furthermore, resort to the courts may have desirable consequences. Litigation can do more than settle the dispute at hand. Judicial opinions may raise and definitively settle a frequently disputed issue with legal ramifications (Dolgin 2019). *Cruzan v. Director, Missouri Dept. of Health*, 497 U.S. 261, Supreme Court, 1990,

[2] Utilizing legal counsel in an advisory role is not incompatible with ethics consultation (Beeson et al. 2013).

for example, resolved a question regarding when a surrogate could apply to discontinue treatment of a patient. Furthermore, the state itself is a stakeholder—both on its own behalf and on behalf of its citizens. The state's only tools are legislation, administrative regulation, and judicial determination. The state can only act through these avenues. National legal systems differ regarding the appropriate balance among parent, child, and state. American law is more deferential to parental concerns than is European law. The United Kingdom's assertion of the paramountcy of children's interests (Children Act 1989, S. 108(2) may be even broader than European law, since the European Court of Human Rights (ECoHR) guarantees "the right to respect for his private and family life" (Art. 8. §1), and assigns best interests *a*, rather than *the* paramount role).

Even resort to ethics panels can be avoided by sensitive management of incipient conflict (Linney et al. 2019). Good communication among different treating physicians prevents conflicting messages being given to patients or to their parents. Designation of a lead clinician to coordinate treatment and consultation both coordinates care and prevents error. Early psychosocial support to families may avert conflict. Early conflict may be ameliorated through involving experienced senior clinicians and support staff.

Shared decision-making is the most appropriate way to avoid or resolve these conflicts (Katz et al. 2016). But not all conflicts are resolved. So, let us turn to some paradigmatic situations.

1. **Parental refusal of treatment offered by physician.** Dr. Casey and the Cleavers disagree on how often to see their child, Weaver, to monitor a stable medical condition. Casey wants to see Weaver every 3 months but the Cleavers are only willing to come every 6 months. This difference might be resolved by (1) accommodating the Cleavers; (2) Persuading the Cleavers to come more frequently; (3) the Cleavers' finding another physician who will agree to see Weaver every 6 months; or (4) ideally, discussion leading to mutual understanding. In this low-risk situation, Casey is unlikely to seek state intervention, and likely will lose if he does. But let's change the paradigm. Weaver Cleaver is diagnosed with acute lymphoblastic leukemia, which chemotherapy cures in almost 90% of children. The Cleavers decline chemotherapy in favor of vitamins and prayer. Dr. Casey now may ask a court to compel chemotherapy, and may well prevail.
2. **Parents demand treatment that physician does not consider advisable.** Eddie Haskell has brain metastases that cannot be treated effectively. Eddie has irreversible coma. His parents want their oncologist, Dr. Kildare, to keep Eddie alive as long as possible, using whatever means are necessary. Kildare estimates that Eddie can live a maximum of 2 months, and declines to order intubation. His reasons are lack of benefit to Eddie, and the moral distress experienced by the staff that has to provide physical care to the comatose child.
3. **Disagreement between parents.** Dr. Welby has told Robert and Margaret March that Meg's abscess could be treated either surgically or with percutaneous drainage. The Marches cannot agree which treatment to authorize.

4. **Parents and physicians attempt to settle disputes by disrupting the decision-making ability of the other party.** Dr. Merrin is treating Regan, who has had worsening complaints of gastrointestinal discomfort, malabsorption, and fatigue. Her mother, Chris, wishes to transfer her care to Dr. Damian across town. Merrin is the fourth physician who has treated Regan in the three years since she became ill. Mitochondrial disease (Suomalainen and Battersby 2018) and Lyme Disease have been suspected, but no definitive diagnosis has been established and no treatment has proven effective. Merrin wonders whether the symptoms are psychosomatic, and even whether Chris is poisoning Regan. He considers reporting Regan's parents to the state for suspected medical child abuse.

I will consider each of these types of disputes. I will assume for purposes of discussion that the child in question lacks sufficient capacity to be able to provide meaningful assent, or to be capable of consent.

8.2 Parents Disagree on Treatment

This problem is exemplified by the vignette involving the March family. It is the easiest of the scenarios to address, at least in principle. The identity of a child's healthcare surrogate is purely a legal matter. If parents are separated or divorced, a parent with health custody can make decisions. The standard for change of custody is whether the custodial parent is able to properly care for the child (*Marriage of Boldt*, 176 P. 3d 388, Oregon Supreme Court, 2008, 392). In the case of joint custody, an elective procedure ordinarily would not be performed unless both parents consent.

But Meg March's parents were married. They have an equal say regarding medical treatment. If they cannot agree despite mediation by the medical staff and ethics consultants, a court may have to settle the matter. A court might take into account the opinions of an expert or the mature child. The State Intervention Test would not preclude judicial intervention if the physician thought that an erroneous choice, or failure to make a choice, was likely to impose serious physiological or psychological harm.

8.3 Parents Decline Recommendations That Physicians Deem Beneficial

As noted in the vignettes involving the Cleavers, parents may not agree to treatments that their child's doctor considers beneficial, or even necessary. The parent's wishes should be overridden only if the criteria of the Direct Effects Basis are met. The parents cannot refuse a treatment that probably will save a life or prevent a major disability. If parents refuse blood transfusions for hemorrhage, appendectomy for ruptured appendix, or antibiotics for tibial osteomyelitis, then physicians should appeal to courts as a last resort, and courts ordinarily order treatment. If potential harm to the child does not rise to the level stipulated by the Direct Effects Basis, then parents should have the authority to refuse a suggested medical treatment. A situation sufficient to invoke state intervention need not be immediate or urgent. Neither dignitary concerns nor numinous issues count. A parent may not decline life-saving transfusion of their children for the sake of their salvation or for other religious benefits with no secular meaning (Beauchamp and Childress 2013; but see Redmann et al. 2018, for a minority opinion).

Scholarly literature tends to focus on legal aspects of transfusion refusal (Layon et al. 1990) rather than on ethical aspects. It prioritizes the life-saving nature of transfusion over respect for the beliefs of parents who are Jehovah's Witnesses.[3] American courts have held that "states have a compelling interest in and a solemn duty to protect the lives and health of the children within their borders" (*P.J. v. Wagner*, 603 F.3d 1182, 1189, 10th Cir., 2010). Lethality may not be necessary (*Matthews v. State,* 126 So. 2d 245, Mississippi Supreme Court, 1961); parents must obtain treatment for illnesses that endanger a child's "life or limb" (*In re Karwath,* 199 N.W.2d 147, 150, Iowa Supreme Court, 1972). In the phrase 'life or limb,' 'limb' is a metonym denoting long-term major morbidity. Threat to life or health appears to be a general standard for judicial action (*Matter of Sampson*, 29 NY 2d 900, New York Court of Appeals, 1972). All of these cases, and the State Intervention Test's Direct Effects Basis for state intervention, follow *Prince v. Massachusetts* (321 U.S. 158, 170, 1944) in assigning "psychological or physical injury" as potential reasons to limit parental actions toward their children in the face of competing rights. *Wisconsin v. Yoder* (406 U.S. 205, 230, Supreme Court, 1972) also uses "physical or mental health" as a benchmark for limiting parental action.

The Likelihood Constraint is important ethically and legally. The two component standards of this constraint are whether a harm is real or hypothetical, and, if real, whether it is relatively common or rare. 'Rarity' should be titrated to the severity of the consequences. A 0.1% chance of chicken pox may be rare, while a 0.1% chance of rabies is not. American courts ordinarily will not remove children from parental custody for hypothetical future damage (*Osier v. Osier*, 410 A. 2d 1027, Maine Supreme Judicial Court, 1980; *Matter of Cochise County Juvenile Action*, 650 P. 2d 459, Arizona Supreme Court, 1982).

[3] Jehovah' Witness doctrine at worst consigns the souls of those who do not achieve grace to postmortem obliteration rather than to damnation. The notion of incurring guilt without intent should not bother believing Christians or Jews. The Christian concept of original sin (Mann 2001) is based on guilt without intent, as are laws in the Hebrew Bible about incurring impurity (e.g., Numbers: 19). Even atheists should realize that many secular laws impose liability without culpability. Some crimes and torts do not require intent, knowledge, or recklessness (known as strict liability). I include this brief discussion because many people with whom I have discussed this issue are intuitively appalled by the notion of liability without blame, without realizing how frequently this occurs in secular contexts and mainstream religious contexts. Questions regarding Jehovah's Witnesses' decisions should be judged on their merits, and not tainted by prejudices against what many believe to be the group's *outré* ideas.

Not all disputes involve cases whose issues are as tidy as those of transfusion cases. Some tragic cases involve cancer treatment that itself is difficult to bear, and which is only sometimes successful in curing or mitigating the cancer involved. In such cases, the ethical issues are the same, but the solution may be ambiguous. Courts have resolved some such cases in favor of doctors (*Matter of Hamilton*, 657 SW 2d 425, Tennessee Court of Appeals, Eastern Section, 1983), and others in favor of parental refusal of treatment (*Newmark v. Williams*, 588 A. 2d 1108, Delaware Supreme Court, 1991). In situations where life is not at stake and the likelihood of damage is not as certain, the parent is more likely to prevail (*Matter of Martin F.*, 13 Misc. 3d 659, New York Family Court, 2006). Points of disagreement that are not monumental, such as whether to use opioids for postoperative analgesia in minors, are best solved through dialogue, and through seeking alternatives if parents strenuously object (Moreno-Galvan et al. 2020). However, if the parents' wishes to withhold pain medicine will lead to severe pain likely to create psychological problems, including habits of avoiding medical care when the child matures, then it may be warranted to seek legal intervention to allow adequate analgesia.[4] In practical terms, disagreements over outpatient care that does not involve serious diagnoses will be resolved by the parents seeking other physicians.

Unfortunately, the acceptable threshold for intervention varies across pediatric specialties. Different subspecialties currently employ different survival thresholds for requesting court intervention (Gerdes, 2019). Cardiac surgeons will accept parental refusal if the expected survival is <90%, while neonatologists use 25–50% as a survival floor. Neither the rigor of the treatment as experienced by the child nor long-term quality of life issues account for these differences. This anomaly would be alleviated by uniform application of the State Intervention Test, with greater overall consensus on the benefit/risk calculus that warrants intervention.

8.4 Parents Demand Treatment That Physicians Deem not to be Beneficial

In the Haskell paradigm, parents request treatment that the physician considers inappropriate or harmful. Recent, widely publicized, extreme examples of this involved Charlie Gard and Alfie Evans. They were both young UK children, probably without consciousness as a result of irreversible neurological conditions, and UK hospitals wished to remove life support. The UK Children's Act (1989; *subseq. amended*) establishes the "paramountcy" of the child's welfare (§1(1)). Its standard for limiting parental care is that "the child concerned is suffering, *or is likely to suffer*, significant harm" (§31(2)(a); emphasis added). Best interests always take precedence over parental judgment, and courts are highly deferential to physicians in determining

[4] This is personally meaningful. My parents did not believe local anesthesia should be used for dental work. I had multiple dental procedures as a child without analgesia, and with my mouth propped open with a clamp so the dentist could work without pausing.

best interests. In both the Gard and Evans cases there were providers outside the UK willing to accept the child for continued treatment. In both cases, UK courts (and, ultimately, the ECoHR, permitted the UK hospitals to decline transfer and to discontinue supportive care, rapidly leading to each child's death. The courts focused on the (remote) possibility of suffering and the loss of dignity of the children, which it held outweighed the value of continued life. A sceptic or cynic might say that using a vaguely defined and controversially understood characteristic like dignity as a criterion allows a court to do pretty much what it pleases.

There are multiple ethical issues in the determination of these cases (Wilkinson and Savulescu 2018), presented in Table 8.2 with some of my own additions. The

Table 8.2 Theoretical and decisional issues in parents' demand for care that physicians are unwilling to offer. Wilkinson and Savulescu (2018)

What is the right thing to do?	How should decisions be made?
Is treatment for the child at hand In the child's best interests? Likely to cause significant harm?	When should parental requests for treatment be denied?
Does the request for treatment reflect parental malfeasance?	Should parents be permitted to consent to untested or extremely uncertain experimental treatment if a child would certainly die without it?
What criteria should be used to determine whether continued life is worth living?	What constitutes "significant harm" to justify overruling parents?
Would continued life for the child at hand be worth living?	If parents are able to pay for treatment, should that change the permissibility of continuing/providing treatment?
In the best-case scenario, would the child's life be worth living?	How should decisions about allocation of resources be made for individual patients?
Should the interests of parents be taken into account?	How should divergent views about medical facts be taken into account?
Should treatment be denied on the basis of limited public healthcare resources? (When?)	Does it matter if those diverging views come from health professionals in different countries?
Are there other individual or state interests shat should be taken into account?	How should divergent views about normative issues (e.g. life worth living, parental rights) be taken into account?
	Should parents be free to take their child overseas for medical treatment unavailable in their home country?
	How should popular opinion and expertise (medical, ethical, legal, religious, etc.) be balanced in formulating policy to underlie these decisions?
	Who should make decisions? (Individuals, bodies, processes, including opportunity to appeal?)

ethical problems are both procedural and substantive.

In deciding to intervene, the state should act only when the matter is of sufficient magnitude to invoke one of the bases of the First Prong of the State Intervention Test; *de minimus non curat lex.*[5] In general, any procedure involving a matter that does not allow intervention under the State Intervention Test should be treated as a safe deposit box, requiring two keys to open. Metaphorically, the physician holds the beneficence key, while the parent holds the consent key. Both the child's surrogate and the physician must agree to act—the surrogate on the basis of the child's interests, broadly construed; and the physician on the basis of medical beneficence. Parents rarely can compel physicians to provide non-beneficial treatments. If the physician declines to provide services that she does not consider beneficial, then the parents' remedy is to try to find a physician who agrees with them.

If the decision involves an important societal interest, we turn to the Indirect Effects Basis. A possible burden to society is the cost of the treatment. The presence of moral distress and other psychological distress (Lee & Dupree 2007) among personnel engaged in long-term invasive treatment of children with dismal prognosis may also be a burden under the Indirect Effects Basis. Moral distress is an adverse psychological response to situations in which one is forced to collaborate or refrain from intervening in morally dubious enterprises. Moral distress arises when health-care professionals feel they cannot practice as they should. It is common in intensive care situations among nurses and physicians.

A third state interest is popular opinion. Charlie and Alfie touch a nerve. A non-expert might conclude that legal, and especially media, authorities, are disingenuous in attributing sensations, interests, and rights to someone with no cortical function. The medical position is particularly salient. Physicians have power over patients' lives that provokes fear of betrayal. This is a compelling theme in popular literature.[6] Nobody should be surprised that lay people are disturbed when doctors and hospitals battle to let children die against the wishes of their parents. It does not do justice to the intuitive belief that physicians ought to err on the side of preserving life to disparage lay opposition as populist (Das 2018). Gard's parents had found a physician in the US willing to take on Charlie's care at no expense to the UK; why was the hospital in which he was a patient so adamant in its refusal?

The adjudication of Gard has negative implications for parental authority and for the idea of shared decision-making between physicians and parents (Lantos 2017). Furthermore, it did not seem fair to the parents. The ECoHR opinion (*Gard* et al. *v. United Kingdom*, Application no, 39,793/17, 2017) declared without irony that Charlie Gard was "represented by an independent, professional, court appointed guardian precisely to ensure that [Charlie's] own voice can be heard" (¶ 65). Charlie Gard's guardian *ad litem* was a barrister and medical ethicist who was a leader of an organization that promoted advance directives; she was closely aligned with another organization that promoted assisted suicide (Mendick 2017). Charlie's working-class

---

[5] The law does not concern itself with insignificant matters.

[6] Depictions of physician treachery in literature can be found in Shaw, George Bernard, The Doctor's Dilemma (1906); Herbert, Frank, *Dune* (1965); and Cook, Robin, *Coma* (1977) resonate strongly.

parents reasonably surmised that the guardian may have been neither objective nor accurate in channeling Charlie's "voice." The principle that physicians should be respectful of parents and their values is key to medical trust. And such trust arguably is more important to public health than any issue pertaining to the individuals directly involved in these end-of-life situations.

Under the Test, then, there is a state interest in transferring Charlie Gard to preserve legitimacy of the government and the medical profession. The concern that prolonging Charlie's life made him suffer does not survive the Likelihood Constraint.[7]

Texas has struck a better balance among the interests of institutions, physicians, parents, and children. Texas legislation (*Texas Health and Safety Code*, Chap. 166) provides that an institutional body such as an ethics committee should evaluate the facts and issues pertinent to disagreements on maintaining life-supportive care. If the institutional body upholds the physician's position, the parents have 10 days to find an alternative institution that will accept the patient in transfer. If the parents fail to do so, then the physician's position prevails. This reasonably fair procedure still has at least two problems. First, members of the institution serving on ethics committees may sympathize with interests of the institution that employs them. Second, the Texas rule does not seem to protect against charlatans offering false hope under the cover of medical degrees and hospital certification. Texas procedures would not have prevented Charlie Gard's parents from transferring Charlie to an overseas hospital that would have treated him with expensive aromatherapy and enemas, while cleaning out his parents' assets. The Texas approach seems as fair as possible, though it should be modified to allow the state to prevent unscrupulous parties from taking advantage of desperate parents.

Let us now consider cases that are not as dramatic. Let us take as a given that physicians should not give treatment they know is futile (Wilkinson 2013). Physicians should reject parental requests—perhaps based on internet searches—for coffee enemas as primary treatment for a child's cancer. Let us also stipulate that there are certain standard treatments used frequently and effectively. These are mandatory, regardless of the wishes of the parents. Parents should not be able to compel physicians to use either unproven methods or recognized medical modalities known to be useless in the situation at hand (President's Commission 1983, 44). This has come up with regard to drugs such as ivermectin prematurely touted as effective against COVID-19. It has long been an issue with regard to Lyme disease. However, I further propose that while there is no obligation to provide such treatment if the anticipated risks and benefits are trivial, I am not certain that there is an affirmative obligation *not* to provide such treatment. The State Intervention Test is concerned with serious conditions and treatments that have possible major consequences. The Test does not address safe, inexpensive regimens or medical conditions with minor consequences. There is a 'gray zone' in between these two paradigms. Perhaps a treatment

[7] In the case of Alfie Evans, care would potentially have cost the UK a lot of money, but I arbitrarily, though tentatively, excluded such considerations from the test.

proffered by a physician is only occasionally effective. Perhaps it is experimental. Parental demands for treatment can fall into the gray zone.

Catholic ethical traditions help with the problem of this gray zone.[8] Catholic ethicists distinguished between ordinary and extraordinary treatment as early as the sixteenthcentury (González-Merado and Di Pietro 2020). Cronin (2011) defines ordinary means of preserving life as "those means commonly used in given circumstances, which this individual in his present physical, psychological, and economic condition can reasonably employ with hope of proportionate [likely][9] benefit." Ordinary treatment is ethically mandatory. Futile treatment is forbidden. Extraordinary treatment that is not futile is ethically optional. But God (or the Devil) is in the details.[10] Factors that might lead a family to reject extraordinary treatment include (modified from González-Merado and Di Pietro 2020).

1. Whether the effort in administering treatment is excessive to the family, or undergoing and bearing the effects of treatment is excessive to the patient or the family.
2. Whether physical pain or other suffering is unbearable or cannot be sufficiently relieved.
3. Whether the patient's relatives or caregivers experience a tremendous fear or a strong repugnance regarding the use of the means.
4. Whether the patient or family regards the overall risks of treatment to be disproportionate to the anticipated benefits.
5. Whether the efficacy rate for the treatment warrants its application, in the judgment of the patient or family.
6. Whether the residua, after successful treatment, are such that they prevent the patient from fulfilling the most serious and pressing duties, or maintain a satisfactory quality of life.
7. Whether the patient and family are willing to incur risks and benefits of experimental treatment,.
8. Whether the economic costs to use the treatment are overly burdensome. Depending on the organization of payment for health care, this decision is made by patients, families, insurers, or state agencies. Note that if there is a third party payor involved, both the Test's Comparability constraint and other ethical literature (Close et al. 2018) insist that there must be fair and transparent rules for denying care.

Whether a possibly efficacious treatment is extraordinary is determined partly by the patient, family, and circumstances.

---

[8] I am not a Catholic, nor do I belong to a denomination with similar beliefs or intellectual approaches.

[9] I added 'likely' before 'benefit' because no treatment is definitely beneficial, and my opinion that any term that applies more definiteness than 'likely' is incompatible with what reasonable physicians, ethicists, and families would accept.

[10] The adage, *Le bon Dieu est dans le détail* has been attributed to Gustave Flaubert (Prozesky 2013).

González-Merado and Di Pietro (2020) would have the physician decide whether a treatment is futile and impermissible. If treatment is permissible, the physician then determines whether treatment is ordinary, and therefore required. The physician's judgment, of course, is subject to error, and therefore to peer review, institutional review, and judicial or other state review. If treatment is not futile or ordinary, then it is extraordinary. In this case, the patient (or, in the case of a child, the parents as surrogates) decides whether to accept treatment, though environmental factors such as cost present constraints. If there is a contest regarding whether a proposed treatment is in the extraordinary/permissible zone, the criterion for decision will be whether the parents are making a reasonable decision, all things considered (Bester 2018).

8.5 Parents or Physicians Inappropriately Disrupt the Decision-Making Ability of the Other

Readers will recall the Regan scenario, in which a child is not improving under a physician's care, and the parent wishes to change doctors. Consider a related scenario involving Henley, a presumptively competent adult. Henley has a small malignant pancreatic tumor, and is advised to have a Whipple procedure in an attempt to cure the tumor. He wants a simple pancreatectomy, and obtains a second opinion. He is told is that he should have radiation and chemotherapy as palliative treatment. He now goes to a famous clinic in the Midwest for a third opinion to break the tie. So far he is reasonable. The Whipple operation is recommended, but Henley had hoped that the consultant would recommend a more conservative pancreatectomy. He goes to four more doctors for opinions. Getting seven opinions is *not* something a reasonable adult patient would do. Henley may be using multiple consultations to procrastinate. He may also be shopping for a doctor who will comply with his wishes, which do not conform to standard treatment options.

Henley may be the master of his fate and the captain of his soul, and he is allowed do unwise things that may cause him harm. But if he is a parent, he cannot adopt this strategy for his child. The power of the parent to seek repeated consultation is limited by what is reasonable, and can be challenged by the state. Parents should be allowed to seek opinions for their children and switch their children's care to other physicians under circumstances in which it would be reasonable for adults to do this. Multiple opinions that delay surgery, or frequent changes in caregiver before treatments have adequate opportunity to demonstrate efficacy, should prompt consideration of involving public authorities.

A difficult paradigm is the child who has chronic non-specific symptoms leading to a working diagnosis that is difficult to establish definitively, especially if psychosomatic etiology is included in the differential diagnoses. Mitochondrial disease (Parikh et al. 2017) and juvenile fibromyalgia (de Sanctis et al. 2019) are examples of such conditions. When children fail to show improvement, parents are tempted to change doctors in the hope that the next physician will find something the current doctor missed, or try a new treatment that is not part of the current doctor's armamentarium. This may involve unproven tests and remedies for uncertain diagnoses. This is common in presumptive Lyme disease (Shapiro et al. 2017).

Physicians also can abuse clinical and legal processes to constrain parents from leaving their care. Physicians consider themselves health fiduciaries of children, but have a duty to their employers and concern about their reputations. Also, physicians can make errors. Parents have a duty to their children that is broader than any fiduciary duty—consisting of primary responsibility for supervision of all aspects of a child's life. However, parents are hardly objective, and can become frustrated when their child does not improve. The standard for court interference with parental decisions is neglect or abuse in the US, and substantial harm in the UK. There is no standard limiting patients from changing their physicians. A patient, like any beneficiary of a fiduciary relationship not involving a trust, can fire her physician. Parents not infrequently change pediatricians for reasons trivial or momentous. The limitation is that they cannot endanger their child through changing physicians. Meanwhile, physicians, at least theoretically, may inappropriately characterize parental decisions as neglectful or abusive. Distinguished family law professor Maxine Eichner (2016) had a child with a rare disease that required several years and multiple consultants to diagnose. She writes (Eichner 2016) that other families with less sophistication, knowledge, and stature, have been railroaded through the threat or use of medical child abuse action into continuing care with existing providers, or even have lost custody of their children when they tried to change providers. As she describes these cases, action against the parents does not seem warranted. If we are to accept this conclusion we must depend on her objectivity.

Suspected parental injury to children to obtain medical attention, sometimes called Munchausen's syndrome by proxy, or caregiver-fabricated illness (Flaherty et al. 2013/2018), is a form of medical child abuse. Professional guidelines are vague in setting standards for diagnosing medical child abuse (Stirling 2007), in contrast to their recommendations to vigorously attempt to remove children from offending parents. The hallmark of medical child abuse is that the parent instigates unnecessary medical care (Roesler and Jenny 2008), regardless of the magnitude of the effect or of any actual underlying illness. This standard is breathtakingly overbroad. It could find a parent guilty of medical child abuse if she asks a pediatrician for antibiotics to treat a cold, or for an x-ray when a child has a minor injury. However, this standard gives doctors a legal basis with which to combat parents who reject treatment suggestions, or who seek second opinions (Eichner 2016). If disagreement with a physician can be criminalized, then the parent is effectively shut out of the decision process. Courts may be prone to give more credibility to hospital experts than to parental experts, (Howe 2017). If it is the physician who demands treatment and the parent who demurs, the parent can be accused of medical child neglect, with the same potential consequences as with medical child abuse. Either way, parents are likely to be persuaded to accede to medical recommendations if a possible alternative is imprisonment or removal of the child from the family. Jenny and Metz (2020, 50) assign diagnostic criteria that would implicate many parents.

These include anticipated harm without treatment, the existence of a beneficial treatment, and a determination that reasonable parents would accept the treatment. Their approach does not consider choice among alternate treatments. Furthermore, it is not clear whether Jenny and Matz would allow parents to obtain additional pediatric consultations. Indeed, some medical neglect cases have been filed when parents sought second opinions from respectable physicians. The criteria proposed by Jenny and Matz also make no allowance for possible missed diagnoses, erroneous diagnoses, or poor treatment decisions by physicians. It is impossible to eliminate all diagnostic error. Determining the etiology of vague, chronic, serious conditions may be difficult. Certainly, parental harm to the child is part of the differential diagnosis in some of these cases. It can be tragic, though, when parental action is falsely blamed for a child's illness.

The medical literature contains case reports of parents losing custody because of a disagreement with doctors. One mother was convicted of murder after physicians failed to diagnose a rare genetic disorder in which a child accumulated a substance (methylmalonic acid) that a forensic laboratory mistakenly identified as ethylene glycol (Hoffman 1991). Another child's parents lost custody because a physician misread a weight chart and reported the parent to civil authorities for underfeeding the child (van Gemert et al. 2018).

When it is difficult to determine whether a disease is present, establishment of responsibility is difficult. Furthermore, statements of fact in judicial opinions (and in press reports) often omit details that are relevant to assessing whether parties acted appropriately. The standard should be whether parents' seeking different medical care would be reasonable if an adult were making a similar decision for herself. Otherwise, prosecution of parents for changing physicians constitutes abuse of the legal system. In difficult cases in which the diagnosis is unclear, courts ideally should seek independent expert evaluation rather than relying on expert testimony provided by the adversaries. This may not be possible within the constraints of specific jurisdictional rules that govern introduction of evidence. It appears that litigation in this area has effectively reversed the burden of proof from the physician to the parent.

This should be corrected. Standards for demonstrating medical child abuse and neglect should be more objective, and the process for resolving disputes should not be stacked in favor of physicians.

8.6 Conclusion

This chapter, like the rest of the book, is not about how parents should best care for their children; it is about when states should restrict parents who provide grossly inadequate care. The State Intervention Test standard is not parental perfection. Rather, there are strict limits to permissibility of state action, since there are possible harms from state intrusion.

The State Intervention Test allows us to decide when we ought to interfere with parental refusal of treatment for their children. When considering parental demands for continued treatment, we ask two questions. First, can the treatment bring about the desired physiologic effect. If the treatment is not futile to all intents and purposes, we look at the odds of therapeutic effectiveness. We then use some ethical intuitions half a millennium old and determine whether the proffered treatment is ordinary or extraordinary in the context of the index patient's situation.

Disagreement between parents is primarily a legal matter. Finally, when parents seek additional professional opinions, they may be performing a parent's due diligence or they may be procrastinating or using the time spent getting consultations as a passive-aggressive way to refuse treatment. The benchmark for intervention in parental medical treatment decisions should be whether such consultation patterns would be reasonable for an adult patient to obtain.

References

Beauchamp, Tom L., and James F. Childress. 2013. *Principles of Biomedical Ethics*, 7th ed. Oxford: Oxford University Press.

Beeson, Tishra, Brittany Dawn McAllister, and Marsha Regenstein. 2013. *Making the Case for Medical-Legal Partnerships: A Review of the Evidence.* George Washington University, National Center for Medical-Legal Partnership. https://medical-legalpartnership.org/wp-content/uploads/2014/03/Medical-Legal-Partnership-Literature-Review-February-2013.pdf.

Bester, Johan Christiaan. 2018. The Harm Principle Cannot Replace the Best Interest Standard: Problems with Using the Harm Principle for Medical Decision-Making for Children. *American Journal of Bioethics* 18 (8): 9–19.

Close, Eliana, Lindy Willmott, and Ben White. 2018. Charlie Gard. In Defence of the Law. *Journal of Medical Ethics* 44 (7): 476–480. https://doi.org/10.1136/medethics-2017-104721.

Cook, Robin. 1977. *Coma.* New York: Signet.

Cronin, Daniel A. 2011. *Ordinary and Extraordinary Means of Conserving Life.* Philadelphia: The National Catholic Bioethics Center.

Das, Ranjana. 2018. Populist Discourse on a British Social Media Patient-Support Community: The Case of the Charlie Gard Support Campaign on Facebook. *Discourse, Context & Media* 24 (1): 76–84. https://doi.org/10.1016/j.dcm.2017.11.005.

de Sanctis, Vincenzo, Vincenzo Abbasciano, Ashraf T Soliman, Nada Soliman, Salvatore Di Maio, Bernadette Fiscina, and Christos Kattamis. 2019. The Juvenile Fibromyalgia Syndrome (JFMS): A Poorly Defined Disorder. *Acta Biomedica* 90(1): 134–148. https://doi.org/10.23750/abm.v90i1.8141.

Dolgin, Janet L. 2019. Resolving Health Care Conflicts: A Comparative Study of Judicial and Hospital Responses. *Wake Forest Journal of Law and Policy* 9 (3): 495–580.

Eichner, Maxine. 2016. Bad Medicine: Parents, the State, and the Charge of Medical Child Abuse. *University of California Davis Law Review* 50 (1): 205–320.

Flaherty, Emalee G., Harriet L. MacMillan, and American Academy of Pediatrics Committee on Child Abuse and Neglect. 2013, reaffirmed 2018. Caregiver-Fabricated Illness in a Child: A Manifestation of Child Maltreatment. *Pediatrics* 132 (3): 590–597. https://doi.org/10.1542/peds.2013-2045.

González-Merado, Fermín Jesús, and Di Pietro, María. 2020. The Therapeutic Proportionality Standard: A New Content for the Best Interests Standard. *Cuadernos de Bioética* 31 (101): 19-42. https://doi.org/10.30444/CB.50.

Herbert, Frank. 1965. *Dune.* New York: Penguin.

Hoffman, Michelle. 1991. Scientific Sleuths Solve a Murder Mystery. *Science* 254 (5034): 931. https://doi.org/10.1126/science.1948075.

Howe, Janet. 2017. De-Junking MSBP Adjudication. *Arizona Law Review* 59 (2): 201–234.

Jenny, Carole, and James B. Metz. 2020. Medical Child Abuse and Medical Neglect. *Pediatrics in Review* 41 (2): 49–60. https://doi.org/10.1542/pir.2017-0302.

Katz, Aviva L., Sally A. Webb, and The Committee on Bioethics, American Academy of Pediatrics. 2016. Informed Consent in Decision-Making in Pediatric Practice. *Pediatrics*. 138(2): e20161485.

Lantos, John D. 2017. The Tragic Case of Charlie Gard. *JAMA Pediatrics* 171 (1): 935–936.

Layon, A. Joseph, Arthur D'Amico, Donald Caton, and Chris J. Mollet. 1990. And the Patient Chose: Medical Ethics and the Case of the Jehovah's Witness. *Anesthesiology* 73(6): 1258–1262.

Linney, Mike, Richard D W. Hain, Dominic Wilkinson Peter-Marc. Fortune, Sarah Barclay, Vic Larcher, Jacqueline Fitzgerald, and Emily Arkell. 2019. Achieving Consensus Advice for Paediatricians and Other Health Professionals: On Prevention, Recognition and Management of Conflict in Paediatric Practice. *Archives of Disease in Childhood* 104 (5): 413–416. https://doi.org/10.1136/archdischild-2018-316485.

Mann, William E. 2001. Augustine on Evil and Original Sin. In *The Cambridge Companion to Augustine*, edited by Eleonore Stump & Norman Kretzmann. Cambridge, UK: Cambridge University Press, 40–48.

Mendick, Robert. 2017. Charlie Gard's Parents Angry That Baby's Lawyer Is Head of Charity That Backs Assisted Dying. *The Telegraph* July 18, 2017. https://www.telegraph.co.uk/news/2017/07/16/charlie-gards-parents-angry-babys-lawyeris-head-charity-backs/#:~:text=Victoria%20Butler%2DCole%2C%20who%20speaks,called%20the%20Voluntary%20Euthanasia%20Society.

Moreno-Galvan, Anna, Jonathan Michael Marron, and Angela Maree Marsiglia. 2020. How Should We Approach Parental Refusals of Opioids on Behalf of Children in The Perioperative Setting? A Practical Approach Based on Ethical Theory. *Pediatric Anesthesia* 30 (8): 852–858. https://doi.org/10.1111/pan.13941.

Parikh, Sumit, Amy Goldstein, Amel Karaa, Mary Kay Koenig, Irina Anselm, Catherine Brunel-Guitton, John Christodoulou, et al. 2017. Patient Care Standards for Primary Mitochondrial Disease: A Consensus Statement from the Mitochondrial Medicine Society. *Genetics in Medicine* 19 (12): 1380–1397. https://doi.org/10.1038/gim.2017.107.

President's Commission. 1983. President's Commission for the Study of Ethical Problems in Medicine and Biomedical and Behavioral Research. *Deciding to Forego Life-Sustaining Treatment: Ethical, Medical, and Legal Issues in Treatment Decisions.*

Prozesky, Detlef. 2013. *Le bon Dieu est dans le detail*—Reflections on Being a Beaver. *African Journal of Health Professions Education* 5 (2): 50–55.

Redmann, Andrew J., Melissa Schopper, Judith Ragsdale, Michael J. Rutter, Catherine K. Hart, and Charles M. Myer. 2018. Posttonsillectomy Hemorrhage in a Pediatric Jehovah's Witness and the Decision to Transfuse. *Otolaryngology–Head and Neck Surgery* 159(2): 238–41.

Roesler, Thomas A. and Carole Jenny. 2008. *Medical Child Abuse: Beyond Munchausen Syndrome by Proxy*. New Hyde Park, New York: American Academy of Pediatrics.

Shapiro, Eugene D., Phillip J. Baker, and Gary P. Wormser. 2017. False and Misleading Information About Lyme Disease. *American Journal of Medicine* 139 (7): 771–772. https://doi.org/10.1016/j.amjmed.2017.01.030.

Shaw, George Bernard. 1906. *The Doctor's Dilemma*. http://www.online-literature.com/george_bernard_shaw/doctors-dilemma/

Stirling, John, and The Committee on Child Abuse and Neglect. 2007. Beyond Munchausen Syndrome by Proxy: Identification and Treatment of Child Abuse in a Medical Setting. *Pediatrics* 119(5): 1026–30.S. https://doi.org/10.1542/peds.2007-0563.

Suomalainen, Anu, and Brendan J. Battersby. 2018. Mitochondrial Diseases: The Contribution of Organelle Stress Responses to Pathology. *Nature Reviews: Molecular Cell Biology* 19 (1): 77–92.

van Gemert, Martin J.C., Marianne Vlaming, Eric Osinga, Cornelis M.A. Bruijninckx, H.A. Martino Neumann, and Pieter J.J. Sauer. 2018. Pediatric Condition Falsification Misdiagnosed by Misjudged Weight Growth from the Curve of Measured Weights. *American Journal of Case Reports* 19: 752–756. https://doi.org/10.12659/AJCR.908770.

Wilkinson, Dominic. 2013. *Death or Disability? The "Carmentis Machine" and Decision-Making for Critically Ill Children*. Oxford: Oxford University Press.

Wilkinson, Dominic, and Julian Savulescu. 2018. Hard Lessons: Learning from The Charlie Gard Case. *Journal of Medical Ethics* 44 (7): 438–442. https://doi.org/10.1136/medethics-2017-104492.

Chapter 9
Prevention and Screening

Abstract The question of prevention and screening differs from treatment of disease in its greater impact on society. Prevention and early detection of serious illness has major human and financial implications. Motivated in part by observation of widespread lack of social concern during the recent COVID-19 pandemic, I argue that states have broad power to compel screening and preventive measures. Using vaccination as an example, I describe four paradigmatic cases. In one case, the disease (tetanus) is grave, but not communicable or common. In the second (common cold), it is common and communicable but not serious. The third type of disease (polio) is grave and highly communicable. In the fourth case, the state seeks to vaccinate people not at high risk of serious illness to prevent serious disease in another subpopulation. I maintain that the third and fourth sorts of cases warrant compulsory vaccination of children over parents' wishes. I also argue that compulsory screening is acceptable if the screening procedure itself does not violate the Direct Effects Basis—i.e., is unlikely to cause serious harm. Finally, I explore, without definitive conclusions, the question of children living in environments in which they are taught unhealthy practices.

Prevention and screening present ethical problems different from those that occur in treatment of disease. To treat a child to cure or ameliorate disease is paternalistic. But fathers (and mothers) are supposed to be paternalistic (they are parents, after all!). They are responsible for protecting their children from harm. Prevention and screening measures may be directed toward other ends. Kraaijveld (2020) described four types of screening and prevention based on who authorizes the test and who receives the test (Table 9.1). Children most commonly are objects of paternalistic measures, as when a parent has a child vaccinated or tested. Unlike treatment, prevention and screening often follow a government mandate that applicable to a class of people. When the child is ill, it is the parent that initiates a request for care, but much prevention and screening is either mandated or conducted by the state. Another difference is that treatment of disease is focused on an obvious problem. With prevention and screening, though, there are a vast number of potential targets, so decisions must

A. J. Jacobs, *Assigning Responsibility for Children's Health When Parents and Authorities Disagree: Whose Child?*, The International Library of Bioethics 90,
https://doi.org/10.1007/978-3-030-87698-2_9

Table 9.1 Four types of preventive or screening measures (after Kraaijeveld 2020)

		Beneficiary	
		Object of test	Someone else
Decider	Object of test	Ordering a test for oneself Woman opts to get mammogram	Altruistic Pregnant woman receives pertussis vaccine to protect newborn baby
	Someone else	Paternalistic Primary school provides visual and auditory screening for students	Indirect Hospital mandates tuberculosis screening of health care workers to protect patients and staff

be made as to which diseases to screen for, and which to target with prevention campaigns.

9.1 Screening for Childhood Illness

Some interventions aimed at early detection of disease have much the same ethical profile as disease treatment. Consider, for example, neonatal pulse oximetry screening for critical congenital heart defects (CCHD). This consists of briefly placing a pulse oximeter on the infant's foot without breaking the skin. If blood oxygen saturation is low, more specific and invasive tests are recommended to diagnose or exclude CCHD. Pulse oximetry is painless, risk-free, and inexpensive. If diagnosed and treated promptly, the 0.2% of children born with CCHD promptly can be treated surgically with good results. However, delayed diagnosis results in greatly increased morbidity, and mortality doubles (Eckersley et al. 2016) Pulse oximetry is a sensitive, specific, and cost-effective screening test for CCHD (Thangaratinam et al. 2012). It is part of the United States Department of Health and Human Services Recommended Uniform Screening Panel for newborns (DHHS 2018).

The reason for most parental refusal of pulse oximetry is general objection to medical care (Jacobs and Arora 2018). The relevant Hohfeldian ethical relationship is that newborns have a claim on their parents and the state for protection of health. Parents have a corresponding obligation to meet the claim is not absolute, but have the power to make decisions on behalf of their children. They must take both medical and non-medical considerations into account and can make decisions that they believe best resolve conflicting needs and interests of the stakeholders. Physicians have an obligation to safeguard children's health, and an obligation to children under their care, to parents, and to the state to exercise this power according to professional rules and standards. The state has the power to further the health and safety of its citizens. The state also has the power to protect vulnerable persons such as children against any serious threats. States may have an ethically justified power to compel their citizens to engage in practices that protect their health (Frank 1976). Each of these Hohfeldian relationships pulls in a different direction. The State Intervention Test can help resolve these conflicts and propose when government may intervene in parental refusal of pulse oximetry.

There are empiric issues involved in deciding when to screen. Wilson and Jungner (CDC 2011) proposed ten criteria that justify screening for early detection of disease as a public health measure:

(1) The condition sought should be an important health problem.
(2) There should be an accepted treatment for patients with recognized disease.
(3) Facilities for diagnosis and treatment should be available.
(4) There should be a recognizable latent or early symptomatic stage.
(5) There should be a suitable test or examination.
(6) The test should be acceptable to the population.
(7) The natural history of the condition, including development from latent to declared disease, should be adequately understood.
(8) There should be an agreed policy on whom to treat as patients.
(9) The cost of case-finding (including diagnosis and treatment of patients diagnosed) should be economically balanced in relation to possible expenditure on medical care as a whole.
(10) Case-finding should be a continuing process and not a "once and for all" project.

Dobrow et al. (2018) recently refined and expanded these criteria, which are paraphrased in Table 9.2).

Most states mandate screening for most or all of the conditions in the Recommended Uniform Screening Panel, usually allowing parental opt-out. This, as we shall see, contrasts with state rules concerning vaccination.

Pulse oximetry meets standard screening criteria. Other such measures include universal school testing of vision and hearing. However, despite ample evidence of effectiveness of screening for amblyopia, parents frequently fail to take advantage of ophthalmologic correction, even when it is free (Solebo et al. 2015). There is comparable lack of compliance with follow-up recommendations after auditory screening. These conditions, if not treated, may limit the educational accomplishment and general social adaptability of affected children. When severe, they arguably constitute serious physiological deficits, and invoke the Direct Effects provision of the State Intervention Test.

9.2 Vaccination

Failure to vaccinate against communicable disease has broad social and ethical impact. Failure to prevent communicable diseases can have an impact on unvaccinated children, on their families, and on strangers. It also can result in large economic costs to society. Polio vaccination saved the US economy $180 billion in direct treatment costs between 1955 (when the first polio vaccine was introduced) and 2005

Table 9.2 Final refined set of consolidated screening principles. Modified from Dobrow et al. (2018)

Domain	Consolidated screening principles (after systematic review and modified Delphi consensus process)
Disease/condition principles	1. Epidemiology: The epidemiology of the disease or condition should be adequately understood. The disease or condition should be an important health problem 2. Natural history: The Juengner disease or condition is well-defined, its course should be understood, and there should be a detectable preclinical phase 3. Target population: The target population for screening should be clearly defined
Test/intervention principles	4. Screening test performance characteristics: Screening test performance should have adequate specificity, sensitivity, and positive predictive value) It should be acceptable to the target population and it should be possible to perform or administer it safely, affordably and efficiently 5. Interpretation: Screening test results should be clearly interpretable, with agreed cut-off points, to identify those who should (and should not) be offered diagnostic testing 6. Post-screening test options: There should be an agreed-on course of action for screening participants with positive screening test results that involves diagnostic testing, treatment or intervention, and follow-up care. This should improve outcome. The effect of false-positive and false-negative tests should be minimal

*Components of a screening program include recruitment, testing, information access, diagnosis, referral, treatment, follow-up, patient education and support, staff training and program management and evaluation

(Thompson and Duintjer Tebbens 2006). This figure does not include lost economic productivity due to polio infection. Mass vaccination saves billions of dollars even in less serious diseases such as measles and mumps. Mass vaccination also reduces non-economic costs such as fear, disease symptoms, residual disability, and mourning. The current novel coronavirus pandemic illustrates the tremendous social, economic, and political costs of epidemics of serious diseases. Measures such as isolation, quarantine, and tracking are not specific to children, so I shall focus on vaccination, and on routine vaccination rather than vaccination for epidemic control.

Resistance to vaccination requirements arose as soon as the first such requirement—for smallpox vaccination—was introduced at the end of the eighteenth century. In the past 35 years, an anti-vaccine movement has proliferated as many new vaccines emerged and were mandated for school attendance (Conis 2015). Parental refusal to allow vaccination of their children (henceforth, 'vaccine refusal')[1] may have secular or religious motivation. Much secular vaccine refusal originated from second wave feminism (Navin 2013), which inspired reaction against perceived

[1] I prefer the term 'vaccine refusal' to the euphemism, 'vaccine hesitancy.' 'Hesitancy' does not describe the phenomenon of a child not receiving a vaccine against a serious illness.

authoritarian and disrespectful attitudes of physicians. Vaccine resistance may be rationalized as part of a desire to avoid technological medicine. It may be based on exaggerated concerns regarding vaccine risk (Pierek 2017), fueled in part by publicity given to rare vaccine complications. Concerns regarding encephalitis following pertussis vaccination are obsolete, as whole cell vaccines have been replaced with an acellular vaccine. The manufacturing problems that resulted in cases of polio following vaccination have been corrected. A discredited report that associated measles-mumps-rubella (MMR) vaccination with autism and inflammatory bowel disease still influences vaccine-refusing parents.

Perceived disingenuousness on the part of the medical establishment has weakened trust in vaccination. After introduction of each vaccine against a common childhood disease, medical communication to the public through mass media suddenly emphasized danger from that disease (Conis). Measles, which was previously considered a bothersome childhood rite of passage, now was a major threat. Perhaps this was just change in emphasis. Reassurance is more appropriate when active alternatives do not exist, but a different emphasis is appropriate when active measures are feasible. However, the perceived revision of the medical party line regarding measles affected the credibility of the profession, especially for those already inclined to doubt medical authority.

Another group of parents appreciates that vaccines have minimal risk, but understands that those who are not vaccinated never experience vaccine complications. By not vaccinating their children, these parents are free riders, relying on other children's vaccination to protect their children from infection. This offers good protection most of the time (Navin 2013). This strategy of free riding, aside from being unappealing, does not always work. First, if enough people pursue this strategy, herd immunity is lost. Second, it does not protect children against contracting a disease in a sporadic, self-limiting outbreak resulting from introduction of the disease from outside the geographic confines of the community with herd immunity. Herd immunity does not imply that nobody in a community will acquire disease, despite the rhetorical analogy to individual immunity. Rather, it means that if the disease is introduced into a community, any outbreaks will be self-limited (see below).

Religious objections also have been an important source of vaccine refusal (Offit 2015). Religious refusers often belong to the Christian Science church or to various small evangelical denominations.

9.3 Risks and Benefits of Vaccination

Severe vaccine complications are unusual (Institute of Medicine 1994). The trend to acellular vaccines, and to those produced through recombinant DNA technology, has made vaccines safer. There is no scientific support for the notion that vaccines overwhelm the infant immune system. Most additives in vaccines are safe except for rare allergic reactions. Mercury-containing preservatives no longer are used. No reputable study has suggested a link between autism and any vaccine.

The protective effects of vaccinations apply to the entire community. This is because of phenomena of herd immunity and (absent herd immunity) relative herd protection (Fine et al. 2011). The mean number of people to whom a person with a communicable disease transmits her infection is expressed as R. R varies according to the communicability of the infectious agent, the number of people who are already immune, precautions against transmission, etc. If $R > 1$, the disease will persist in the population. If $R < 1$, the infectious agent will disappear from the population. *Herd immunity* is defined as a situation in which $R < 1$, leading to inability of the infectious agent to establish itself permanently. Even without herd immunity, if many are vaccinated or have antibodies through infection, R will be less than if the entire population were susceptible (*herd protection*). The percentage of immunized individuals required to attain herd immunity is different for each disease and is positively associated with R. One is the ease with which the disease is transmitted (Fine et al. 2011). Measles requires a vaccination rate >95% to attain herd immunity. Herd immunity from diphtheria requires an 80% vaccination rate. Another factor in herd immunity is vaccine efficacy. Measles vaccination protects 99% of those receiving the vaccine, compared with rates $\leq$ 50% for influenza vaccines.

Even with herd immunity, introduction of the pathogen from outside the community will infect susceptible exposed individuals. The outbreak may be self-limiting, but some people will become ill. Outbreaks will affect children whose parents would like to vaccinate them but who cannot receive, or will not benefit, from vaccine. These children may be those who are too young to be vaccinated, who do not develop immunity after receiving a vaccine, or who cannot be vaccinated for medical reasons (Galazka et al. 1984), During outbreaks children of vaccine refusers will transmit the disease to them. A 2015 California outbreak of measles ended because of herd immunity, but not before 113 cases were reported (CDC 2015).

Vaccine refusal not only exposes children to vaccine-preventable infection, but increases the severity of these infections. Herd protection effect raises the average age of those who contract the disease in question. Many diseases such as measles are more severe in adolescents and adults than in young children. In the pre-vaccination era, the average age of a patient with measles was just under five years old. However, modeling suggests that if vaccination coverage were 20% below the threshold for herd immunity, the average age of a case of measles would be 19.1 years. This would increase the risk of serious complications by a factor of 4.5 (Fefferman and Naumova 2015).

In most states, vaccine refusal enjoys legal protection. All but five states[2] allow religious exemptions to laws requiring vaccination for attending school or group childcare (NVIA 2020).

[2] California, Maine, Mississippi, New York, and West Virginia. In addition, Washington has no personal exemption for mandatory measles/mumps/rubella vaccination.

9.4 Ethical Issues in Vaccination

There are more relevant Hohfeldian relationships pertinent to vaccination programs than to newborn screening. Parties affected both by vaccination programs and by screening programs, include the index child, parents, and the state, through its economic interests. Medical personnel may have some interest because of moral distress in caring for children with preventable serious disease. In addition, all children susceptible to infection are interested parties, as are their families. They have a claim on other parents in the community to vaccinate their children, and a prima facie claim on the government to ensure that this is done (Jacobs 2012). The state has the power to enforce vaccination of all children in whom this is not medically contraindicated.

The effectiveness of widely used vaccines and the very favorable benefit/risk calculus require that the state mandate childhood vaccination for many serious diseases.[3] But the availability of a vaccine does not automatically imply a requirement to vaccinate. Health always must be balanced against other considerations. The risk of serious injury from football is probably greater than the risk of major consequences from varicella. Nonetheless, for a variety of reasons schools often mandate varicella vaccination while encouraging contact sports.

Davies and Savulescu (2019) argue that in a state that provides universal health care as a solidaristic policy, individuals have a responsibility to care for their own health. Otherwise, they willingly sap state resources through their need for more health care than people who lead a healthy life style. Perhaps they should be penalized, and even denied medical care. Whether we accept this or not, we cannot penalize children for their parents' mistakes. We can, however, override parental decisions inimical to children's health.

9.5 General Ethical Issues in Prevention Programs

The index child may be the only person whose health is jeopardized by neonatal screening. However, when a parent refuses to vaccinate her child against a communicable disease, both the index child and others are endangered by this decision. The range of people who are harmed is key to whether the measure is required, rather than the severity of failure to comply. Thus, even though there is likely greater public health benefit of some screening (e.g., screening for vision, hearing, or autism) than of immunization against varicella, visual screening is not mandatory while vaccination is.

How can one formulate a broad, consistent, fair, and widely acceptable state policy regarding public health measures to prevent or ameliorate childhood illnesses?

---

[3] A mandatory requirement requires vaccination as a condition for obtaining some sort of benefit, such as school attendance or boarding an airplane. Compulsory vaccination requirements, on the other hand, are categorical.

We must begin with several established legal and ethical principles. State power to compel screening or vaccination is based on the *parens patriae* doctrine, state police power, and the interest of the state in a healthy population. These are in tension with individual and group assertion of liberty, expressed in Hohfeldian terms as immunities against application of the state power to compel vaccination. *Individual* liberty—the prerogative to pursue one's own visions and acting upon one's own beliefs—includes rearing children in accordance with one's beliefs and values. The *centrality offamily* and the default power of parents to make decisions for children are established in US constitutional law and in ethical literature (Iltis 2010). Finally, there are cultural claims, expressed as *multiculturalism*. This concept grants individuals the prerogative of associating together as minority communities, in which they can realize values and practice customs that deviate from national *leitkultur*. Five conflicting prima facie principles—*majoritarianism*, *protection of the vulnerable*, *protection of the community*, *liberalism*, the *value of the family*, and *multiculturalism*—are impossible to reconcile and difficult to balance. Prevention and screening programs have a more communitarian focus than does clinical ethics. However, a program that is inconsistent in balancing minority values against considerations related to health and safety of children is likely to discriminate against the marginal and the unpopular (Levin et al. 2016).

Legally, police power grants American states the authority to "protect the lives, health… comfort and general welfare of the people" (*Manigault v. Springs*, 199 U.S. 473, Supreme Court, 1905, 480). Governments have asserted this power for at least 4500 years (Hammurabi 2250 B.C.E.). Governments have at least six tools at their disposal when exercising police power: *educationand persuasion*, *provision of services*, *nudging*, *incentivization*, *disincentivization*, and *compulsion* (Arora et al. 2018). Compulsion should be a last resort. The State Intervention Test deals only with this extreme measure. I consider, therefore, under what circumstances government may mandate or compel vaccination.

Marcel Verweij (2009) identifies the harm principle and the consequentialist viewpoint as foundational ethical principles in public health. Flanigan (2014) uses the harm principle to assert that policies requiring vaccination are appropriate provided that the illness is communicable, vaccination is effective at reducing transmission, and people are not given a vaccine if there are sound medical reasons not to. However, driving with minimal ethanol levels meets Flanagan's criteria, but would rarely create harm. Flanigan accepts that there is a threshold of risk, but does not analyze what constitutes an undue risk. The Likelihood Constraint of the Test does some of this work, but leaves some room for indeterminacy.

Verweij (2009) relies on consequentialism in suggesting that benefits to a community or to society as a whole can be greater than the sum of individual benefits. Vaccination is a public good when it achieves herd protection or herd immunity. This benefits vaccinated and unvaccinated people alike. Herd immunity benefits all, regardless of individual contribution or any person's desire to enjoy its benefits. Herd immunity thus meets the criteria of a public good (Dawson 2009). However, some public goods are more valuable than others. A water purification system is more important than a sculpture in front of a public building, though each is a public good. I suggest that vaccination programs meet the eight conditions I proposed in Chap. 5 for adopting a program that creates a public good.[4] This has been a problem in COVID-19 vaccination in the US, where voluntary compliance is low, but mandates are politically impossible. Mistrust of government has already caused loss of legitimacy on both the Left and the Right. The recent use of lockdowns to arrest the spread of COVID-19 and the resulting economic dislocation made the government more unpopular. Instituting anti-COVID-19 measures readily accepted in other democracies have been political non-starters in the liberty-conscious US. Such measures include guarded quarantine and isolation facilities (Fu and Lee 2020), closing national borders (Mallapaty 2021), or mandating physical tracking through mobile phones (Park et al. 2020). Vaccine refusal by Americans seems to be due to concerns regarding government motives and competence, fatalism, and fears about vaccine safety (Chou and Budenz 2020).

To summarize: protection of most individuals and provision of herd immunity is possible through comprehensive vaccination. It is generally accepted that sovereign states have some power to restrict freedom in order to improve the health and safety of their citizens. The interests of various parties must be balanced in formulating vaccine policy. These include the index child, those close to that child, other children, society, and the state.

9.6 Applying the State Intervention Test to Screening

I now apply the State Intervention Test to preventive measures, bearing in mind that the State Intervention Test only applies to coercive state actions. The Direct Effect Basis addresses the effect on parties that are the subject of the intervention. It allows government interference with parental decisions only when there is a threat or actuality of serious harm. The Indirect Effects Basis addresses public health and other matters related to the polity.

Let us begin with screening that only has health implications for the index child. We start with Direct Effects, and ask whether parental refusals of tests such as pulse oximetry, or screening for visual and hearing deficiencies can create severe consequences for the child. Indeed, they can. Failure to promptly diagnose CCHD can lead to death or permanent disability. Failure to diagnose hearing and visual deficits may have less dire outcomes, but still can severely disadvantage a child educationally, socially, and, ultimately, economically. Major visual or hearing impairments may

---

[4] These are (1) that the result actually be a good; (2) that the good must have high enough priority to deserve state resources; (3) the negatives inherent in controversy and disruption caused by the program should not exceed the program's positive value; (4) the public must actually benefit; (5) the program must not unduly burden a minority; (6) the program must not cause undue secondary harm, such as a vaccination program causing people to leave the healthcare system entirely; (7) aggregated goods may, taken collectively result in harm; a childhood program of 15 vaccinations is reasonable, but 150 vaccinations would be unreasonable; and (8) the program must be consistent with the basic values (*leitkultur)* of society.

even constitute health damage sufficient to trigger the Direct Effects Basis. Looking at the Indirect Effects Basis, these sensory deficits would constitute sufficient damage to society's interests if they resulted in the individual being dependent on the state for care. Amblyopia or myopia sufficient to affect reading acquisition, but not so severe as to impair ability to carry out normal life functions such as finding one's way from place to place, is a borderline case. There are deaf people who decline to correct their children's deafness because they consider themselves and their children to be members of a 'Deaf culture' (Tucker 1998). Accepting the legitimacy of this position for argument's sake, refusal of treatment still would not apply to a deaf child of parents who consider deafness to be a negative feature, but who do not want their child to receive medical intervention. Nor would it apply to a deaf child of parents with good hearing, as they are not part of Deaf culture. Multiculturism does not require that the state permit recruitment of outsiders into a culture, and a deaf child outside the culture should not have to wait until adulthood to decide if he wants to be deaf or not. Furthermore, deafness as a cultural manifestation may be unacceptable under the Indirect Effects Basis if that culture is dependent on state largesse for physical sustenance (Tucker 1998).

I now consider the State Intervention Test's three Constraints. The Likelihood Constraint precludes states from interfering with a procedure because of hypothetical or rare considerations. It is, among other things, a limit on the precautionary principle, which requires that advocates of applying technology, and especially new technology, demonstrate the safety of the technology Resnik (2004). This Constraint assigns to the state the burden to prove that the practice is dangerous, rather than requiring the parent to prove that it is safe.

The Benefit/Harm Constraint would titrate the magnitude of the public good against the human and material cost of overcoming resistance. Perhaps vaccine refusers in a community are few in number, do not feel strongly, or their concerns can be assuaged by education. In this circumstance, it might be reasonable to have vaccination mandates for a relatively benign disease such as varicella. However, it would not be ethical to pursue criminal penalties for refusers if the overall harm to refusers and their children from putting the parents in prison exceeded the overall harm caused by not vaccinating the children. Furthermore, if a large minority of the population would defy forced vaccination of their children against a disease that rarely causes death or major disability, such enforcement would be inappropriate ethically and prudentially. Under these circumstances the government would be imprudent to try to enforce vaccination against all but lethal diseases capable of pandemic outbreaks. Finally, the Comparability of Effect Constraint asks whether minority parents or those with idiosyncratic views are being treated differently than mainstream parents.

Hom et al. (2016) argued, based on the harm principle, that parents should be allowed to decline neonatal pulse oximetry because harms entailed by alienating the parents outweigh the benefits of pulse oximetry. This point of view was opposed by Shelton and White (2016), writing from a consequentialist perspective. They state that the benefit/burden calculus favors mandatory testing. Shelton and White conclude that, since there is no rational secular reason for granting exemptions, religious exemptions should not be granted. Using a slightly different version of what I now call the State Intervention Test, Arora and Jacobs (2018) agreed that testing should be compulsory. We concluded that neither the Likelihood nor the Comparability Constraints applied to pulse oximetry screening. The Harm/Benefit Constraint is more complex, as those being coerced to obtain screening might avoid prenatal care and medical involvement delivery. This is unlikely to happen on a large enough scale to invoke this Constraint against compulsory pulse oximetry.[5]

9.7 Applying the State Intervention Test to Vaccination

The case for vaccination requirements is even stronger than for screening. The Direct Effects Basis justifies mandatory vaccination of children against relatively common diseases that pose a substantial chance of death or of major disruption of a physiological function. The Indirect Effects Basis provides justification for required vaccination against less severe diseases that still can present an unreasonable burden on children other than index children. Infectious mononucleosis (for which there is no vaccine) and hepatitis A cause prolonged school absence with rare serious sequelae, and are examples of such diseases. The financial burden on society of epidemics of serious childhood diseases also provides a justification for vaccination requirements.

Vaccination differs from screening in several respects. First, vaccination carries more risks. Second, vaccination, unlike screening, is a definitive approach to the relevant health problem. Third, vaccination benefits individuals other than the index child. Even live virus vaccines rarely cause illness in contacts of children vaccinated with these vaccines (Kamboj and Sepkowitz 2007). However, vaccination has beneficial effects on others, through herd immunity and herd protection. Herd protection is sufficient reason to require vaccination against serious illness under the Indirect Effects prong.[6] The vast economic benefit to society of preventing serious illnesses also may justify government intervention under the Indirect Effects Prong.

The benefits to children under the Direct Effects Basis are disease-dependent. Consider four archetypical diseases. Tetanus immunization is required for school attendance in most American states even though tetanus is not communicable. Though tetanus is a devastating disease, it is rare in developed nations, with an incidence under 1 per 1,000,000 (Wilson and Jungner 1968). Tetanus is rare even in unvaccinated children (CDC 2011). This low incidence, combined with other options to prevent tetanus in children at risk from puncture wounds, suggests that tetanus does not overcome the Likelihood Constraint, as applied to the Direct Effects Basis. Thus, state tolerance of conscientious exemptions for tetanus vaccination is reasonable. In practice, however, the tetanus vaccine is combined with those for diphtheria and

---

[5] Furthermore, the State Intervention Test would allow the state to prevail over the parents in demanding that corrective surgery be performed for CCHD diagnosed through a process initiated by a finding of an abnormal pulse oximetry result.

[6] Screening for asymptomatic carriers of communicable diseases such as tuberculosis has effects, albeit indirect, that benefit people other than the index child.

pertussis, which are serious. Mandates for diphtheria and pertussis vaccination are clearly permissible under the State Intervention Test. Thus, this issue is effectively moot.

Coryza—the common cold—is the opposite of tetanus in relevant respects. Assume, counterfactually, that an effective vaccine against coryza is available. Coryza is highly communicable. However, coryza's effects are mild. It consists of a few days of discomfort, and possibly of absence from school or work. Coryza is common, so that, unlike tetanus, it passes the Likelihood prong. However, increasing the chances of one's child catching cold does not subject the child to unreasonable risk under the Direct Effects Basis. The societal impact of coryza is not substantial enough to require vaccination under the Indirect Effects Basis. As with tetanus, but for a different reason, parents should not be compelled to vaccinate their children against coryza.

Polio is readily communicable and carries high mortality. It often results in severe, permanent neuromuscular deficits, both immediate and delayed. Polio is readily communicable in children (Fine and Carneiro 1999). The Direct Effects Basis permits compulsory immunization. Factors that might lead to outbreaks, such as vaccination refusal, affect society and its members, and permit compulsory immunization under the Indirect Effects Basis. Some children whose parents are not vaccine refusers can acquire polio because they are too young to be vaccinated, cannot be vaccinated for medical reasons, or fail to acquire immunity through vaccination. Vaccination refusal creates an unreasonable risk to children of non-refusers as well as to children of refusers. Polio was common prior to availability of vaccination, so the Likelihood Constraint does not apply. The magnitude of the harm caused by failure to vaccinate is greater than the magnitude of the harm caused by any permissible practice in society, so the Comparability Constraint does not apply. The external costs incurred in enforcing compliance are unlikely to be worse than the effects of foregoing herd protection. Governments may, therefore, ethically require vaccination for polio over all non-medical objections.

Finally, there is the example of Covid-19. This appears to be mild in children, but serious in adults.[7] With the caveat that childhood Covid-19 may be more serious than generally believed, I will assume that Covid is genrally mild in children. We then have a fourth paradigm. Here, we are considering mandating pediatric immunization primarily for the public health benefit of preventing a severe illness in adults who live in the community. Kraaijeveld called a situation in which S tests C to benefit third party T 'altruistic' testing, appreciating that this does not reflect the common use of 'altruistic.' Verweij and Dawson (2020) apply the same term to Covid vaccination of children. We are vaccinating children primarily to protect adults (who get more seriously ill from Covid) through herd immunity or herd protection. When a disease is mild in children but severe in adults, is it ethical to immunize children to protect the

---

[7] In a large literature review of children diagnosed with Covid-19, only 3% of 1124 cases were severe or critical (de Souza et al. 2020). However, 36% were diagnosed with pneumonia. It is possible that these studies overestimated the severity of disease, as children requiring hospitalization are more likely to have serious complications than those treated as outpatients, and there are many asymptomatic cases that are only diagnosed by aggressive testing.

adults in the community? The answer to this question is governed by the Direct Effects Basis, as controlled by the Likelihood Constraint. If the vaccine is likely to produce severe complications in children, it should not be given to them. Adults should be encouraged to receive it, especially in an epidemic. If the vaccine is demonstrated to be safe, it can be required in children, based on the ethical analysis conducted in this chapter. If the vaccine is new, and especially if (as in several coronavirus vaccines) it uses a novel technology such as injection of mRNA that codes for spike protein, the precautionary principle argues against its use in children until safety has been demonstrated in adults. The criteria for allowing use in children are beyond the scope of this discussion.

These four paradigms allow similar analyses of any proposed vaccination program.. Importantly, the terms ‘rare’ and ‘substantial’ used in the Test are intentionally left without absolute numerical qualifiers. A democratic, liberal society, society (through elected representatives, administrative agencies, and the judiciary) should set the threshold values for determining when to require vaccination.

Roland Pierek (2020), a European legal scholar, uses an approach somewhat similar to mine, though with slightly different conclusions. He contrasts what he terms parental and state fiduciary relationships. He says these are based, respectively, on what is best for the child, and on the child’s basic interests. Basic interests are determined by the public. The government, acting on behalf of the public, is constrained by a harm principle. The legal principle of proportionality determines whether the state or the parent prevails. Pierek concludes that it is appropriate to allow free riding if the prevalence of free riding will not endanger herd immunity. My own intuition is that behavioral memes such as free riding can spread, so non-medical exceptions to mandatory vaccination should not be permitted. Giubilini et al. (2018), also offer several persuasive ethical reasons why people should be compelled to vaccinate themselves and their children against severe communicable diseases. Like these authors, I am prepared to prevent parents from refusing vaccination for such diseases, except when the vaccine is dangerous to the proposed recipient. Even the most sincere and committed religious objectors and vaccinophobes should be compelled to accept vaccination if necessary to protect children under the terms of the State Intervention Test. This would be especially true to prevent or to break an epidemic.

9.8 Life-Style Interventions

So far, I have discussed medical interventions. Now I turn to life style interventions, beginning with a prototypical but (fortunately) hypothetical group of refugees from an ancient nation, who have become a significant minority in Spokane, Salzburg, and Salamanca.

> The Ehrniks have an honor code with elaborate, non-intuitive rules. Violations of honor among Ehrniks must be settled by dueling. When Ehrniks consider themselves dishonored, the dispute is brought before an Ehrnik duelmaster. Based on the severity of the alleged

> offense and the relative fighting strengths of the duelers, the duelmaster dictates a mode of combat that creates a relatively equal chance for victory between the combatants. The chance of death in the duel is proportionate to the seriousness of the alleged offense. The mode of combat may range from arm wrestling to combat with battle axes. The duelmaster's adjudication and the ensuing duel have religious overtones. Most offenses only affect honor if inflicted by cult members. If an outsider eats food from an Ehrnik's plate, however, an Ehrnik must respond with physical retaliation. This rarely involves more than a fistfight. Exogamy, though, calls for murder of both parties to the marriage by the Ehrnik party's parents. The Ehrnik age of responsibility is 12. Because of the complexity and importance of the honor code, though, education in rules of honor begins at age 5.

This example was framed to illustrate several problems. First, outsiders may be subject to harm for certain violations they do not recognize as blameworthy. Second, the Ehrniks teach their children to engage in physical retaliation from a young age. Third, adolescents within the group engage voluntarily in battles that may maim or kill them. Fourth, all of this is sanctioned by a well-established religio-cultural entity. Finally, Ehrnik customs are highly unappealing to their neighbors.

Should the state deter parents from teaching their young children the Ehrnik honor code, which mandates activities prohibited by both Bases of the Test? On the one hand, most agree that parents have wide latitude in teaching their values. On the other hand, education and other interaction that physically endangers children may amount to abuse. In the real world, actual families are not constrained by the state for teaching their children to bully, to fight back when bullied, to aspire to be soldiers, prison guards, firefighters, etc. We regard some of these activities as more praiseworthy than others, but there is probably widespread disagreement on where parents should draw the line.

The Ehrnik practice of training children in their code of honor and dueling is likely to result in many serious injuries to minors. But his may be true in families given to feeding children extremely unhealthy diets. This includes both diets that result in malnutrition and to diets that allow children to become extremely obese. Varness et al. (2009) describe two cases of very ill children with a BMI > 50 kg/m^2 and propose that children should be removed from the home if it is likely that serious harm is imminent, that it is likely that the state can provide an environment in which the child is treated effectively, and if all reasonable attempts have been made to solve the problem without disrupting the family. This three-pronged test corresponds with the prevailing American legal standard for removing children from their home (Weaver 2011). Garrahan and Eichner (2012) suggest that the standard of an unreasonable risk of harm be substituted for the imminent danger standard. 'Unreasonable risk of harm' as a standard is compatible with the standards of the Test. In the Ehrnik scenario, the risk to the safety of others would allow government to forbid Ehrnik physical retaliation against outsiders for slights recognized only by the Ehrnik honor code. In the actual world, the Indirect Effects prong would allow the state to work with parents to the point of coercion to prevent even internal physical retaliation of a degree that inflicts unacceptable physical or psychological damage. The same would be true of other antisocial behavior that is likely to make school environments unsafe or otherwise pose danger to children's health. Appropriateness of state interference with indoctrination of children into the Ehrnik social code is not as clear. The actual outcome of a government attempt to ban parents from teaching Ehrnik norms would vary from nation to nation.

The Test extends to public health measures. Excise taxes on sugary drinks, which contribute to childhood obesity and its health consequences, have been instituted widely (Muth et al. 2019). There have been proposals that states restrict marketing of foods whose caloric load is disproportionate to their overall nutritional value. This seems permissible if achieved by political *modus vivendi* rather than by administrative fiat. Indeed, analogous government action is so common as to be barely noticeable. With or without parental permission, and regardless of parental encouragement, minors may not drive, purchase tobacco products, or consume alcoholic beverages. The caveat in the dietary realm is that it is easy to selectively target cultural eating practices.

9.9 Conclusion

Conflicts between parents and states regarding a child's health can include disagreements regarding prevention and screening. I have reviewed the ethical basis for such programs. I conclude that it is are permissible under the State Intervention Test tor states to mandate extensive health screening measures, as well as preventive measures, at the individual and public health level.

References

Arora, Kavita Shah, Jane Morris, and Allan J. Jacobs. 2018. Refusal of Vaccination: A Test to Balance Societal and Individual Interests. *Journal of Clinical Ethics* 29 (3): 203–213.

CDC. 2011. Centers for Disease Control and Prevention. Tetanus Surveillance—United States, 2001–2008. *MMWR Morbidity and Mortality Weekly Report*, vol. 60, no. 12, pp. 365–369. https://www.cdc.gov/mmwr/preview/mmwrhtml/mm6012a2.htm [pii].

CDC. (2015). Centers for Disease Control. *Measles Cases and Outbreaks*. http://www.cdc.gov/measles/cases-outbreaks.html.

Chou, Wen-Ying Sylvia., and Alexandra Budenz. 2020. Considering Emotion in COVID-19 Vaccine Communication: Addressing Vaccine Hesitancy and Fostering Vaccine Confidence. *Health Communication* 35 (14): 1718–1722. https://doi.org/10.1080/10410236.2020.1838096.

Conis, Elena. 2015. *Vaccine Nation*. Chicago: University of Chicago Press.

Davies, Ben, and Julian Savulescu. 2019. Solidarity and Responsibility in Health Care. *Public Health Ethics* 12 (2): 133–144. https://doi.org/10.1093/phe/phz008.

Dawson, Angus. 2009. Herd Protection as a Public Good: Vaccination and Our Obligations to Others. In *Ethics, Prevention, and Public Health*, ed. Angus Dawson and Marcel Verweij, 160–178. Oxford: Oxford University Press.

de Souza, Tiago H., José A. Nadal, Roberto J. N. Nogueira, Ricardo M. Pereira, and Marcelo B. Brandão. 2020. Clinical Manifestations of Children with COVID-19: A Systematic Review. *Pediatric Pulmonology* 55(8): 1892–1899. https://doi.org/10.1002/ppul.24885.

DHHS. 2018 United States Department of Health and Human Services. Recommended Uniform Screening Panel. https://www.hrsa.gov/advisory-committees/heritable-disorders/rusp/index.html.

Dobrow, Mark J., Victoria Hagens, Roger Chafe, Terrence Sullivan, and Linda Rabeneck. 2018. Consolidated Principles for Screening Based on a Systematic Review and Consensus Process. *CMAJ: Canadian Medical Association Journal* 190(14): E422–E429. https://doi.org/10.1503/cmaj.171154.

Eckersley, Luke, Lynn Sadler, Emma Parry, Kirsten Finucane, and Thomas L. Gentles. 2016. Timing of Diagnosis Affects Mortality in Critical Congenital Heart Disease. *Archives of Disease in Childhood* 101 (6): 516–520. https://doi.org/10.1136/archdischild-2014-307691.

Fefferman, Nina H., and Elena N. Naumova. 2015. Dangers of Vaccine Refusal near the Herd Immunity Threshold: A Modelling Study. *Lancet Infectious Diseases* 15 (8): 922–926.

Fine, Paul, and Ilona A. M. Carneiro. 1999. "Transmissibility and Persistence of Oral Polio Vaccine Viruses: Implications for the Global Poliomyelitis Eradication Initiative. *American Journal of Epidemiology* 150 (10): 1001–1021. https://doi.org/10.1093/aje/kwi188.

Fine, Paul, Ken Eames, and David L. Heymann. 2011. Herd Immunity: A Rough Guide. *Clinical Infectious Diseases* 52 (7): 911–916. https://doi.org/10.1093/cid/cir007.

Flanigan, Jessica. 2014. A Defense of Compulsory Vaccination. *HEC Forum* 26 (1): 5–25.

Frank, Johann Peter. 1976. *A System of Complete Medical Police: Selections*, Translated by E. Velum, edited by Erna Lesly. Baltimore: Johns Hopkins University Press.

Fu, Yang-chih, and Hsuan-Wei. Lee. 2020. Daily Contacts Under Quarantine amid Limited Spread of COVID-19 in Taiwan. *International Journal of Sociology* 50 (5): 434–444. https://doi.org/10.1080/00207659.2020.1786636.

Galazka, A.M., B.A. Lauer, R.H. Henderson, and J. Keja. 1984. Indications and Contraindications for Vaccines Used in the Expanded Programme on Immunization. *Bulletin of the World Health Organization* 62 (3): 357–366.

Garrahan, Shauneen M., and Andrew W. Eichner. 2012. Tipping the Scale: A Place for Childhood Obesity in the Evolving Legal Framework of Child Abuse and Neglect. *Yale Journal of Health Policy, Law, and Ethics* 12 (2): 336–370.

Giubilini, Alberto, Thomas Douglas, and Julian Savulescu. 2018. The Moral Obligation to Be Vaccinated: Utilitarianism, Contractualism, and Collective Easy Rescue. *Medicine, Health Care and Philosophy* 21 (4): 547–560. https://doi.org/10.1007/s11019-018-9829-y.

Hammurabi. 2250 B.C.E. *Code of Hammurabi*. http://www.constitution.org/ime/hammurabi.pdf.

Hom, Lisa A., Tomas J. Silber, Kathleen Ennis-Durstine, Mary Anne Hilliard, and Gerard R. Martin. 2016. Legal and Ethical Considerations in Allowing Parental Exemptions from Newborn Critical Congenital Heart Disease (CCHD) Screening. *American Journal of Bioethics* 16 (1): 11–17.

Iltis, Ana S. 2010. Toward a Coherent Account of Pediatric Decision Making. *Journal of Medicine and Philosophy* 35 (5): 526–552.

Institute of Medicine (US). 1994. Vaccine Safety Committee. Adverse Events Associated with Childhood Vaccines: Evidence Bearing on Causality. http://www.ncbi.nlm.nih.gov/pubmed/25144097.

Jacobs, Allan J. 2012. Do Belief Exemptions to Compulsory Vaccination Programs Violate the Fourteenth Amendment? *University of Memphis Law Review* 42 (1): 73–110.

Jacobs, Allan J., and Kavita Shah Arora. 2018. Use of a Balanced Test to Resolve Competing Best Interest and Liberty Claims When Parents Refuse Consent for Neonatal Pulse Oximetry. *American Journal of Bioethics* 16 (1): 28–29.

Kamboj, Mini, and Kent A. Sepkowitz. 2007. Risk of Transmission Associated with Live Attenuated Vaccines Given to Healthy Persons Caring for or Residing with An Immunocompromised Patient. *Infection Control and Hospital Epidemiology* 28 (6): 702–707. https://doi.org/10.1086/517952.

Kraaijeveld, Steven R. 2020. Vaccinating for Whom? Distinguishing between Self-Protective, Paternalistic, Altruistic and Indirect Vaccination. *Public Health Ethics* 13 (2): 190–200. https://doi.org/10.1093/phe/phaa005.

Levin, Hillel Y., Allan J. Jacobs, and Kavita Shah Arora. 2016. To Accommodate or Not to Accommodate: (When) Should the State Regulate Religion to Protect the Rights of Children and Third Parties? *Washington and Lee Law Review* 73 (2): 915–1017.

Mallapaty, Smriti. 2021. What the Data Say About Border Closures and COVID Spread. *Nature* 589 (7841): 185. https://doi.org/10.1038/d41586-020-03605-6.

Muth, Natalie D., William H. Dietz Sheela N. Magge, and Rachel K. Johnson, The American Academy of Pediatrics, Section on Obesity, Committee on Nutrition, and The American Heart Association. 2019. Public Policies to Reduce Sugary Drink Consumption in Children and Adolescents. *Pediatrics* 143(4): e20190282. https://doi.org/10.1542/peds.2019-0282.

Navin, Mark. 2013. Competing Epistemic Spaces: How Social Epistemology Helps Explain and Evaluate Vaccine Denialism. *Social Theory and Practice* 39 (2): 241–264.

NVIA. 2020. National Vaccine Information Center. *State Law & Vaccine Requirements*. 2020. http://www.nvic.org/vaccine-laws/state-vaccine-requirements.aspx.

Offit, Paul. 2015. *Bad Faith: When Religious Belief Undermines Modern Medicine*. New York: Basic Books.

Park, Sangchul, Gina Jeehyun Choi, and Haksoo Ko. 2020. Information Technology-Based Tracing Strategy in Response to COVID-19 in South Korea—Privacy Controversies. *JAMA* 23 (21): 2129–2130. https://doi.org/10.1001/jama.2020.6602.

Pierik, Roland. 2017. Mandatory Vaccination: An Unqualified Defense. *Journal of Applied Philosophy* 35 (2): 381–398. https://doi.org/10.1111/japp.12215.

Pierik, Roland. 2020. Vaccination Policies: Between Best and Basic Interests of the Child, between Precaution and Proportionality. *Public Health Ethics* phaa008. https://doi.org/10.1093/phe/phaa008.

Resnik, David B. 2004. The Precautionary Principle and Medical Decision Making. *Journal of Medicine and Philosophy* 29 (3): 281–299. https://doi.org/10.1080/03605310490500509.

Solebo, Ameenat Lola, Phillippa M. Cumberland, and Jugnoo S. Rahi. 2015. Whole-Population Vision Screening in Children Aged 4–5 Years to Detect Amblyopia. *Lancet* 385 (9984): 2308–2319.

Shelton, Wayne N., and Bruce D. White. 2016. Putting Children at Risk in the Name of Religion. *American Journal of Bioethics* 16 (1): 32–33.

Thangaratinam, Shakila, Kiritrea Brown, Javier Zamora, Khalid S. Khan, and Andrew K. Ewer. 2012. Pulse Oximetry Screening for Critical Congenital Heart Defects in Asymptomatic Newborn Babies: A Systematic Review and Meta-Analysis. *Lancet* 379 (9835): 2459–2464. https://doi.org/10.1016/S0140-6736(12)60107-X.

Thompson, Kimberly M. and Radboud J. Duintjer Tebbens. 2006. Retrospective Cost-Effectiveness Analyses for Polio Vaccination in the United States. *Risk Analysis* 26(6): 1423-1440.

Tucker, Bonnie Poitras. 1998. Deaf Culture, Cochlear Implants, and Elective Disability. *Hastings Center Reports* 28 (4): 6–14.

Varness, Todd, David B. Allen, Aaron L. Carrel, and Norman Fost. 2009. Childhood Obesity and Medical Neglect. *Pediatrics* 123 (1): 399–406.

Verweij, Marcel. 2009. Tobacco Discouragement: A Non-Paternalistic Argument. In *Ethics, Prevention, and Public Health*, ed. Angus Dawson and Marcel Verweij, 179–197. Oxford: Oxford University Press.

Verweij, Marcel, and Angus Dawson. 2020. Public Health Ethics in a Pandemic. *Public Health Ethics* 13 (2): 125–126.

Weaver, Jessica Dixon. 2011. The Principle of Subsidiarity Applied: Reforming the Legal Framework to Capture the Psychological Abuse of Children. *Virginia Journal of Social Policy and the Law* 18 (2): 247–318.

Wilson, James Maxwell Glover and Gunnar Jungner. 1968. Principles and Practice of Screening for Disease. Public Health Papers 34. Geneva: World Health Organization.

Chapter 10
Enhancement of Function

Abstract There is good evidence that height is socially and economically beneficial to males. Consider two parents with otherwise healthy sons. One wants to obtain medical treatment to change her son's ultimate projected height from 150 (4′11′) to 160 cm (5′3″). The other would give similar medication to increase her son's projected final height from 190 (6′3′) to 200 cm (6′7″). This chapter explores some of the theoretical and practical considerations in (1) using biomedical technology to change a characteristic of a child from socially disfavored to typical; or (2) to change a characteristic from excellent to outstanding (in terms of societal norms). Prospects are poor for changing norms themselves with regard to important features of interpersonal competition such as mating desirability or markers of social dominance. It is necessary to directly confront the question of when (if ever) it should be permissible to change the child's body, or even the child's genotype, to allow him to better succeed within his culture. This leads to interesting ways to frame problems that do not necessary lend themselves to definitive recommendations.

10.1 Introduction

Medicine does not only treat and prevent disease. It seeks, in many cases, to improve lives in ways that do not cure or prevent disease. This has been called enhancement of function. This may mean bringing people who in some way are below average, closer to the mean. Or, it may mean improving attributes which already are normal. There is no bright line between these two goals. Applying the State Intervention Test (the Test) to elective biomedical interventions, I ask to what extent parents may use medical tools to change their children's life prospects.

Height differences are partially due to genetic propensities (Judge and Cable 2004), but also are related to health and other environmental influences (Schultz 2002). The United States has a presidential election every 4 years. Table 10.1 shows that since the beginning of the twentieth century, the taller candidate has won nine of 10 elections in which an incumbent was not running. The consistency with which

A. J. Jacobs, *Assigning Responsibility for Children's Health When Parents and Authorities Disagree: Whose Child?*, The International Library of Bioethics 90, https://doi.org/10.1007/978-3-030-87698-2_10

Table 10.1 Height of winning and losing presidential candidates since 1900, with no incumbent running

Open election (no incumbent running)				
Year	Victorious candidate	Height (cm)	Losing candidate	Height (cm)
1908	Taft	182	Bryan	180
1920	Harding	183	Cox	168
1928	Hoover	182	Smith	180
1952	Eisenhower	179	Stevenson	178
1960	Kennedy	185	Nixon	182
1968	Nixon	182	Humphrey	180
1988	GHW Bush	188	Dukakis	173
2000	GW Bush	182	Gore	185
2008	Obama	185	McCain	175
2016	Trump	191	H Clinton	165

American voters select the taller candidate is striking. Height correlates with occupational success in many other areas, both in men and women, even correcting for socioeconomic factors (Judge and Cable 2004). Height is correlated with income (Schultz 2002), power, and status (Schubert 2020). Hierarchical relationships are present in all societies (Fiske 1992). Along with other correlates of physical strength, including facial appearance and expressions (Lukaszewski et al. 2016), height is a factor that contributes to high status (Schubert 2020). *But short stature is not a disease.*

Height also aids males in that fierce and unending struggle—mating competition (Sugiyama 2016).[1] Across many cultures, there is a strong tendency for men to prefer shorter women and for women to prefer taller men (Buss andSchmitt 2019). This height preference appears to be innate (Sugiyama 2016). Mating preference based on physical attributes is not necessarily conscious. Ovulation may change mate-seeking behavior both of women themselves and of men with whom they are in contact (see, for example, Haselton et al. 2007; Miller et al. 2007).[2,3]

If tallness furthers male mating and occupational success,[4] a parent wishing to maximize her son's options for success may want to maximize his height. May adults ethically put their finger on the scale here by having doctors alter the height of healthy children? Is the etiology of shortness relevant? Does it matter whether a

[1] The effect of height on non-cis-heterosexual attraction has not been well-studied.

[2] Mating success does not necessarily translate into greater reproduction, due to conscious desires to limit childbearing both by men and by women.

[3] For purposes of disclosure, I am a man whose height is 178 cm.

[4] In females, there may a trade-off between occupational and social success, at least at taller height ranges. For girls, there is the dilemma that adult height may have opposite effects on occupational and mating success.

boy's shortness is due to a growth hormone deficiency or to short parents? Regardless, *short stature is not a disease.*

I turn now to a personal anecdote. When I was 8 years old, I fractured a front tooth in a fight, losing half the visible tooth. I resisted my parents' entreaties to have it repaired because of my fear of dentists. When I was 17 years old and a university student, an eccentric uncle tricked me into visiting a dental office. He correctly insisted that the tooth would be a major liability in any professional or business career. He persuaded me (well, he was paying most of my college tuition) to have a crown placed on my fractured tooth. I had been satisfied with my appearance, and hated the procedure, but I had no strong feelings about having the crown, once it was completed. Because of the stress on this incisor (a 'biting tooth') the crown had to be replaced several times over the years. After further complications, including an abscess, the tooth had to be extracted. On the positive side, there is little question that a broken tooth in front of my mouth would indeed have been a social and professional liability.

My uncle's conduct may have been problematic; he undoubtedly committed some crime by taking me for dental work without my parents' knowledge or consent. But I use this story as paradigmatic of medical enhancement for esthetic reasons. Does the nature or extent of the deviation from typical—or ideal—morphology matter? Orofacial problems, including dental abnormalities, can be caused by genetic factors, by teratogens and infections in utero, and postnatal conditions such as injury (like my fractured tooth) or disease. Is the etiology relevant to correction? What is the role of the minor's own wishes? And, can the decision of an affected juvenile ever be free of undue influence? Paradoxically, I suspect that many people would intuitively say that my parents could have authorized my procedure over my objection when I was 8, but that my assent (or consent) should have been necessary at age 17. That probably would the case in the UK, where the age of competency to make medical decisions is 16, and mature minors under 16 may consent to procedures, but may not refuse them over parental consent.

I will suggest a parental role based on my previous arguments in this volume. First, the primary goal of medical care is the child's flourishing. Second, flourishing requires life in a community; the child's community may adhere to practices or beliefs that may not be aligned with the national *leitkultur*. Third, the child's parents are the default decision-makers. Finally, the state's role is to avoid gross departure from the child's interests, rather than to maximize the child's interests as the state sees them.

10.2 The Disability Rights Perspective

Two publications (Parens 2006; Ouellette 2010) present arguments in favor of limiting parents' power to authorize surgery that is not directed toward important physiologic ends.[5] The Parens volume is primarily written by ethicists, clinicians, and activists. The Ouellette paper is written from a legal perspective. Strikingly, both Ouellette and Parens contributors describe such surgery as 'shaping.' This metaphor is used to imply that the children involved are being treated as less than persons. 'Shaping' brings to mind the unprocessed material to be used in a sculpture, as opposed to 'treating' a human with a problem. The myth of Pygmalion carving a statue, which a god turned into his wife Galatea, personifies this outlook. Parens's contributors focus on cleft lip without physiological consequences; achondroplasia (dwarfism); and surgery for intersex conditions. Ouellette provides four examples of 'shaping': eyelid surgery to Westernize the eyes of an adopted Asian child; administration of human growth hormone (hGH) to increase boys' height, liposuction for an obese 12-year-old girl; and removal of the ovaries and uterus in a girl with a severe cognitive disability.

Use of some of these treatment options as paradigms stacks the deck against medical intervention. First, it is rhetorically effective to describe a shocking or ineffective example, and to generalize from that case. Second, most of the conditions discussed are unusual or rare, making measurement of therapeutic efficacy difficult. There are insufficient numbers to permit clinical trials. Surgery must be partially individualized, so progress occurs through creative innovation rather than through systematic clinical research. Furthermore, it is obvious that some of these interventions will not confer benefit. Few people would regard characteristic East Asian eyelids in a young girl as a problem needing resolution. The principles of beneficence and nonmaleficence requires that anticipated benefits of an intervention warrant its risks, discomforts, and intrinsic harms. Removal of a hypertrophic clitoris in a child with otherwise normal female genitalia is likely to diminish sexual sensation without obvious therapeutic advantage. However, this may not be the final approach to surgical correction. Creation of typical female anatomy may eventually be possible without degrading sexual or reproductive function.

On the other hand, surgery for cleft lip and palate as currently practiced usually corrects the anomaly, with few complications and a high rate of parental satisfaction. Children themselves appear to be satisfied as well. In this condition, early correction will be safest, most effective, and causes least disruption of the child's life. Growing up with a relatively normal appearance reduces the social disadvantages that derive from facial deformities. This procedure is more akin to my front tooth repair than to clitoral removal.

Surgical limb-lengthening for achondroplasia presents an intermediate case. Limb-lengthening surgery requires multiple painful operations over several years, with uninterrupted intensive, painful rehabilitation between operations (Sanford 2006). The treatment program adds almost a foot to the height of these children, but they remain short of stature and display atypical bodies and facies. Not all of the problems caused by achondroplasia are related to height. Many have reduced

[5] The multiauthor Parens volume presents diverse points of view, most of which are skeptical towards parental authority in this area, and some of which would reject treatment of children who cannot consent.

lifespan, and most experience pain as adults (Fredwall et al. 2020). Pain may be lower in adults who have been surgically treated. The rarity of the condition and variations in treatment preclude the large studies that would be definitive. Achondroplasia treatment is not enhancement, but treatment of a condition that causes pain and medical complications besides short limbs. Treatment of talipes equinovarus (clubfoot) (van Praag et al. 2018), rather than limb lengthening, might be a better model for those who may want to consider deontic objections to enhancement for skeletal conditions causing physical disability.

Even when a procedure unquestionably improves physiological function and quality of life of children with reasonable safety and without excessive discomfort, some still raise deontic objections. Such objections are based on the child's putative rights to autonomy (Hodges et al. 2002), protection of bodily integrity, protection of an open future (Ouellette 2010), and preserving the authenticity of the child's personality (Parens 2015). I find these arguments unconvincing for reasons explained earlier in this book. Some authors go further, and view disabled persons as a vulnerable minority whose diminution of function should be accepted and accommodated, rather than reversed (Fine and Asch 1988). The course of action that follows from such objections is to defer until legal maturity any medical actions that are not directed against immediate, severe threats to health. This would seem to delegitimize such interventions as cleft lip repair, clubfoot correction, or even ear piercing and my dental crown. I have argued that the goal of medicine is to promote flourishing, that flourishing is determined empirically, that autonomy and maximization of choice do not seem to enjoy high priority with most people. Interests should be determined empirically. The most reliable way to determine what will lead to a child's flourishing is to obtain informed consent from parents.

Another misconception in the literature is what Tooby and Cosmides (2005) call the "standard social science model." This model suggests that human neural pathways have little intrinsic programming adapted to specific situations, except for perception. Adaptive behavior is learned only through external sources—experience, education, etc. Social or cultural behavior is not connected to intrinsic evolved psychological mechanisms. Evolutionary psychologists maintain, to the contrary, that there are specific evolved pathways adapted in the past to cope with different kinds of situations, such as threats, coalition-building, care of the young, or mate selection. An example of such neural adaptation is the apparent innate fear of snakes in many mammalian species (Bjorklund and Ellis 2014). These neural mechanisms may no longer be adaptive. Furthermore, their functioning is largely below the conscious level.[6] The standard social science model regards attitudes and behavior as more

[6] How is it possible to explain preservation of genes that seem maladaptive, such as genes that determine Tay-Sachs disease, or that enhance the odds for schizophrenia? Evolution results in group, or kin, adaptation, and not individual adaptation (Del Giudice and Ellis 2016). Keller and Miller propose three reasons for persistence of deleterious genes. First, a changed environment may remove the adaptiveness of the allele. Second, the heterozygous state may have survival advantage, though the homozygous state is deleterious. Third, the characteristic or disease in question may be polygenetic. Some allelic combinations of relevant genes may be beneficial, and others deleterious.

malleable than is actually the case. This can lead to wishful thinking regarding society and people with disabilities.

The standard social science error occurs repeatedly throughout the Parens (2006) volume (Parens 2006) Contributors such as Aspinall, Sanford, Asch, and Dreger deplore societal values or personal choices that disfavor people for differences in appearance. They consider it preferable that society change its attitudes than that individuals change their bodies. However, it is unlikely that people will alter responses to the physical cues involved in mate selection such as tall stature, or physical factors, interpreted consciously as attractiveness,[7] that predispose to choosing a mate. Wholesale change in response to appearance as a cue in interpersonal interaction is unrealistic. Nor is it clear that people should be judged only by their characters, as Dreger (2006) would have it. In choosing friends, let alone mates, most of us are influenced by interests, cultural similarities, intelligence, and physical condition. Character is not enough. A musician may prefer friends who also make music, and a mountaineer may want a spouse who also climbs mountains. It is reasonable for parents to have their children's bodies altered in a way that does not violate the Direct Effects Basis of the State Intervention Test, in order to enhance their social (in the broadest sense) prospects.

10.3 Enhancement for Excellence

I have so far discussed amelioration of conditions perceived as worse than typical. Some parents want to make their children better than typical. Is there an ethical difference between adding 4 inches to the height of a boy whose height is second percentile in order to improve his social acceptability and self-image, and adding 4 inches to the height of a boy whose height is 98th percentile so he will be an outstanding tennis or basketball player rather than merely excellent?

Parents should prepare children for a productive adulthood. This entails, among other things, preparing them to successfully cope with a world characterized by competition for respect, material goods and mates. Success in some or all of these competitions enhances flourishing, other things being equal. Imparting the overt and tacit skills that lead to academic and social success is not a display of parental 'ownership.' Neither is it usually parental self-dealing based on parents' deriving prestige in the community or vicarious pride or respect through their children's public success. Knowing the advantage that height confers on boys, parents might decide whether to give them weekly injections for a few years to add 5–10 cm to their height, at a cost of about $8,000/cm. Should the child participate in the decision? A prepubescent child may not have good sense of the consequences of short stature, at a time when mating and other adult competition is not in the forefront of his

In addition, epigenetic factors may determine whether a genetic allele is beneficial or harmful (Del Giudice and Ellis 2016).

[7] Some features of attractiveness are cultural, while others are innate.

consciousness. Short boys are more prone to being bullied (Sommer et al. 2017), and this problem is ameliorated by growth-enhancing hormone treatment (González Briceño et al. 2019).

Not all interventions with health consequences are instituted by doctors. Parents might, for example, incorporate large amounts of animal protein into the child's diet to promote growth. Social interventions may also have overall impact on the child's life greater than a physical intervention. Is it ethical to send children to a tennis-oriented boarding school in which a child practices tennis several hours a day, also studying and living exclusively with other children that have a serious interest in tennis? Or does this introduce skewed values, and unduly limit the sorts of acquaintances the child will meet? A desire to maximize the secular success of one's child is not equivalent to undue influence, nor does it necessarily reflect undue possessiveness. And a desire that one's children remain attached to their culture and close to their family is not tantamount to oppression. We do not want to see our adult children hungry, lonely, or vulnerable to the unjust power of others. We also want them to flourish in their relationships and remain close to us and their other close relatives. However, forcing them to devote themselves to narrow interests may detract from flourishing as well.

But is it moral for parents to feel personal pride in their children's accomplishments? An extreme example is the 'stage parent' whose ego is deeply invested in the accomplishments of her child. Parents may want their children to exceed their own accomplishments or, alternatively, to mirror them. This may be unrealistic, or harmful to the child. Children may be unable to achieve their parents' wishes for secular success, or may not be interested in doing this. At the other extreme, parents might feel no pride whatsoever in a child's accomplishments. But if parents should not live vicariously through their children, they still should provide them with the tools to develop their capabilities. Unfortunately, absent intervention, children may come to see their disabilities as part of their identity (Miller 2006). They may even regard their specific disability (Tucker 1998), or disability in general (Brown 2002) as a culture. Are these mature, autonomous, uncoerced judgments? Or are they psychological adaptations to a disadvantageous situation to which parents have consigned them by declining intervention? Is it acceptance of necessary limitations, or is it 'false consciousness' (Jost and Banaji 1994)? We all have limitations in capability. We may react to our limitations by embracing them, resenting them, combating them, or adopting some other intermediate responses. We all know people without major disability who define themselves by what they cannot do. Children growing up with a disability can be quite resilient. They may assign themselves a higher quality of life than their physicians perceive they have (Barata et al. 2017), though not all do. Individuals with obvious bodily atypicality may perceive the difference more positively than do observers, including physicians (Dey et al. 2017). Interestingly, if this condition (e.g., a colostomy) is reversed, the patient's utility rating of the condition may fall dramatically (Smith et al. 2006). Parental attitudes toward their children, the instability of a child's judgment, and the maturity of the child's judgment imagining themselves later in life, all make it difficult to assess motives and needs. On the one hand, delay to allow greater maturity may result in learned acceptance of the status quo, foreclosing options that would have led to greater flourishing. On the other hand, the child who brings reduced or average capacities to the table may adopt a self-image of inferiority or averageness. That child may learn submissiveness.

In this complicated moral environment, it is parents who are best equipped to make decisions on behalf of younger children, constrained by the limitations imposed by the State Intervention Test. Parents should make these decisions based on the child's own flourishing, the needs of all family members, and the material and non-material resources of the family. When medical decisions are involved, parents should have the benefit of expert counseling. It is useful to obtain advice from people who have seen similar children, and who have no personal or ideological investment in a decision. This is especially true when parents have to decide on a treatment plan in which the benefit/harm calculus is not clear.

Parens relies heavily on the idea of authenticity, which he takes to mean that we have an obligation to ourselves to be true to ourselves (Parens 2015). He would permit interventions that fall under the umbrella of this ideal, calling them true enhancement. He would deny interventions that separate us from our true selves. He hopes, I think, that this distinction will clarify difficult decisions regarding enhancement. Miller (2006), for example, states that his identity is connected to his achondroplasia, and is not interested in growing taller. In general, though, I do not believe that authenticity is a very helpful concept. Authenticity is malleable. Someone born without legs might regard their absence as being part of her identity. But a professional athlete who loses her legs in an accident might feel otherwise. That said, if she lives for an additional 30 years she might then come to identify with her legless state. Even so, we would not confidently predict that this individual would reject an opportunity to receive bionic legs even after decades without legs. I do not understand what authenticity means in the context of identification with one's anatomy. To use a more trivial example, if my fractured tooth had been part of a face that I felt attached to at age 12, does that mean my parents should not have compelled me to repair it against my will? Another problem is that one might not have a clear sense of what is truest to oneself. I might not appreciate until after I saw the effects of repair, that my visibly fractured tooth had frustrated other capabilities and goals closer to the essence of my authentic self. Furthermore, our 'true self' is unstable. My grandfather fought in the army of a Central Powers nation in World War I, but later became a devoted American citizen. Did his true self change, or is nationality not part of the 'true self,' no matter how strongly one feels about it at the time? The direction of causality between atypicality and 'authenticity' may not be obvious. The arrow of causation between authenticity and physical state may point in either direction, or even may be bidirectional.

Finally, being true to oneself might not be a good thing. Jeffrey Dahmer' career of serial killing, necrophilia, and cannibalism was associated with obsessions that had begun by adolescence (Davis 1991). If Dahmer's antisocial proclivities could have been detected when he was 12 years old and changed through biomedical intervention, should this have been permissible without his consent?[8] Or would that have violated his authenticity?

I conclude, then, that authenticity is not a reliable guide to permissible enhancement. Clearly, however, there are putative enhancements that seem to be beyond the pale. We have seen that major injustice is easier to define than justice. An example is surgical lobotomy, whose devastating effects on cognition, affect and experience of emotions would preclude its use even if it were effective in treating psychosis—which it is not (Gostin 1980). But extreme examples frequently do not apply to less clear-cut cases.

Enhancement comes in many forms. Some is physical and some pharmacologic. Some uses prostheses, such as eyeglasses. Some involves environmental manipulation, such as immersion from early childhood in a world devoted to an activity such as tennis. Psychotherapy is an enhancing intervention. So is health education. We should not confuse the modality with the magnitude of the intervention. Surgery can mean either simple removal of a sixth finger or extensive spinal surgery for scoliosis. Removal of an extra digit is less drastic than many forms of social intervention.

There are two other aspects of enhancement of minors that I want to address before discussing the needs of society. First, acceptability of enhancement for aesthetic and athletic reasons is somewhat arbitrary. Some societies readily accept certain aesthetic interventions. Children have their ears pierced, wear contact lenses so they don't have to wear eyeglasses, and undergo cosmetic orthodontia. As early as 20 years ago, 4.5 million Americans had braces—mostly children between 6 and 18. The primary reason for orthodontic care is aesthetic. We would not allow parents to have their children's teeth filed to a point, however, even if their subculture regarded this as beautiful. Attention deficit hyperactivity disorder (ADHD) has been diagnosed in about 8% of American children.[9] Almost 2/3 of these children receive medication, usually amphetamine/dextroamphetamine (Adderall®) or methylphenidate (Ritalin®)—both Schedule II stimulants with abuse potential. Although these drugs are given to millions of children to enhance academic performance, it is criminal to use them to enhance athletic performance. We accept enhancement modalities in some situations that are not permitted in other situations wo comparable importance.

Aesthetic procedures may signify social class or ethnic hierarchy of acceptability. Orthodontic treatment is expensive, with limited availability to children from poor households. So, having straight, evenly aligned teeth is a marker of social class in the United States (Paiva 2015). Rhinoplasty involving reduction in the size of the nose, and straightening the nasal contour used to be common. A 'Jewish nose,' characterized by prominence and convexity, was described in some twentieth century

[8] Macdonald's (1963) triad of enuresis, animal cruelty and fire-setting in children as a predictor of violent crime (Hellman and Blackman 2006) is widely accepted, but the importance of the presence of all elements of the triad is controversial. It is not far-fetched to speculate that highly predictive future discovery of childhood behavioral markers (or even biological markers) highly sensitive for subsequent serial violent behavior could transpire, and invite intervention.

[9] The prevalence of ADHD is somewhat lower in Europe (2–7%), perhaps because of underdiagnosis (Sayal et al. 2018). Unlike in North America, medicine is used as second-line treatment, after behavioral therapy, but the use of stimulants is increasing.

medical texts as a 'deformity' (Preminger 2001). Rhinoplasty was common among well-to-do Jewish adolescent girls for about two decades after World War II (Schrank 2007). The popularity of cosmetic rhinoplasty has declined as social acceptance of Jews has increased.

10.4 The State and Parental Desire for Medical Enhancement of Children

There are at least four state interests under the State Intervention Test that apply to enhancement. First, the state has an interest in preventing an unreasonable risk of major physical or psychological hardship, consistent with the Direct Effects prong of the Test. Second, the state has an interest in providing its citizens with the tools to allow them to be productive. Third, the state has a duty to regulate novel modalities. Widespread introduction of novel technology can reduce or alter the genetic composition of the population in a way that can be positive or negative, and can include unanticipated effects. Fourth, enhancement might have social consequences that the state considers to be poor social policy. These state interests, through the Test's indirect Effects Basis, can limit parental choices that are appropriate under the Direct Effects Basis.

10.4.1 Avoiding Harm to Children Other Than the Index Child

The state has an interest in protecting both the index child and uninvolved parties against indirect harm. How a minor's enhancement can hurt another minor is provided by the following example. High school students compete for places on varsity athletic teams, and for starting positions. Achilles wants to start on his high school's football team. If 15-years-old Achilles takes anabolic androgenic steroids (AAS) (Pope et al. 2014) he will have greater strength and speed than otherwise. 'Juicing up' with an AAS may even make it possible for Achilles to pursue a lucrative career as a professional athlete. Achilles and his parents understand the adverse health consequences of using AAS, which include mood disorders, aggression, atherosclerosis, cardiomyopathy, and addiction to other drugs as a result of injuries caused by overtraining. Everyone in this family values a short, heroic life over a long, uneventful life. The problem of interest to the state is that other boys have to compete with Achilles for athletic success. So Hector, who does not wish to use AAS, is under pressure to do so to make the team, become a starter, etc., if Achilles does so. He is forced to either use AAS like Achilles or to risk losing out to Achilles in athletic competition. The parental choice to provide Achilles with AAS unreasonably harms Hector, and the state may reasonably use criminal penalties to attempt to prevent this sort of pharmacologic arms race.

10.4.2 Fostering a Productive Population

The state has an interest in providing its citizens with the tools to allow them to be productive, rather than economically dependent on charity or the state itself (*Wisconsin v. Yoder*, 406 U.S. 205, Supreme Court 1972, 224–225). The state has no further interest in the child's career. The *Yoder* Court rejected Justice Douglas's dissenting position that the state might legitimately employ compulsory education to augment the attractiveness of the outside world to Amish youth to encourage them to succeed in the secular world (*Yoder*, 244–245). The Test goes no further than the *Yoder* majority. The majority suggested, at least in *dicta* that the government could interfere with parents whose concept of education would result in an avoidable dependency on welfare or charity. By analogy, the state is justified in intervening when parents' refusal to address an atypical condition would have a good chance of rendering the child economically dependent for life, but where intervention would likely allow the child to function productively. The State Intervention Test Indirect Effects Basis adopts this point of view.

10.4.3 Safety of Population and Environment

Adopted efficiently and on a large scale, any forms of genetic selection can reduce genetic variability, rendering the entire population vulnerable to altered environmental conditions. This has been a major problem in agriculture, as has happened with banana cultivation. One, cultivar predominates and is falling victim to a fatal *Fusarium* pandemic, endangering this crop worldwide. A permissive version of the precautionary principle states that "[W]here there are threats of serious or irreversible damage, lack of scientific certainty shall not be used as a reason for postponing cost-effective measures to prevent environmental degradation [or threats to public health]" (Rio Declaration 1992). In other words, agencies should be conservative in introducing new technology but should be proactive in using technology to confront major threats. The precautionary principle cannot stipulate how to weigh risk against benefit (Fischer and Ghelardi 2016) because one of the concerns that underlies the precautionary principle is that risks of novel technologies are indeterminate. Koplin et al. (2020) propose a new sufficientarian version of the precautionary principle. If adopting a technology will bring people to the level of sufficiency in a given currency, a less stringent form of the precautionary principle will apply than for a technology that will improve the lot of those who are already sufficient. This is compatible with the Indirect Effects Basis in the State Intervention Test, and I would apply it to potentially dangerous interventions. For example, mandatory widespread vaccination of the entire population using innovative mRNA technology to achieve herd immunity might be appropriate for the novel coronavirus that causes COVID-19 but should not be introduced to prevent toe fungus infection.

10.4.4 Socially Unacceptable Outcomes

Society may disapprove of some potential enhancements. An example of this might be prenatal selection for genetic traits. Consider the possibility that a woman may induce maturation of multiple ova and creating embryos from each of them through in vitro fertilization. Genetic testing already allows screening for sex and for some genetic disease. Suppose such testing also allows prospective parents to select the embryo with the most traits that are likely to confer high status (Jacobs 2000).[10] Allowing selection of those embryos for pregnancy may harden class divisions and reduce social mobility in at least two ways. First, such manipulation will be available only to the affluent. Second, some people's genomes may have a larger collection of alleles encoding for traits (such as height or cognitive ability) that contribute to secular success. This is not to suggest crude genetic determinism, but only to imply that genetic variations contribute to variation in socially desirable traits. The ability to exploit advantages inherent in one's genome to increase one's offspring's chances of success seems disruptive to the ideals of a democratic society in which social mobility is an important value.

The permissibility of using prenatal diagnosis to diagnose and abort fetuses with genetic diseases already leads to social coercion to use this technology. People in certain circles are criticized by their peers for bringing into the world a child with Down's syndrome (Davis 2010). It is not the obligation of the state, though, to shield people from all social pressure. In adopting this position, I accept the distinction between disease and enhancement, though I am not sure of how to draw this distinction. More work needs to be done in this area.

10.5 Conclusion

The State Intervention Test is applicable not only to treatment of disease, but also to elective enhancement. There should be a rebuttable resumption in favor of parental decisional and moral authority. As long as parental decisions do not seriously jeopardize the child or harm society, decisions regarding their use in young children should be left to parents, and to parents with the assent of older children. Other things being equal, a procedure that will be performed at some point is best performed when it will contribute most to the child's flourishing. There are two corollaries of this maxim. First, the procedure should be done in childhood if the benefits can only be realized

[10] The possibility of genetic surgery makes this hypothetical even more powerful.

in childhood. Second, all other things being equal, the procedure should be done in childhood if it is safer in childhood than in adulthood.

Important state considerations may constrain parental decisions. These include the future productivity of the child, the safety of other members of society, possible adverse environmental impact, and the possibility of creating social outcomes that will be detrimental to society or incompatible with its values.

References

Barata, Anna, Rodrigo Martino, Ignasi Gich, Irene García-Cadenas, Eugenia Abella, Pere Barba, Javier Briones, et al. 2017. Do Patients and Physicians Agree When They Assess Quality of Life? *Biology of Blood and Marrow Transplantation* 23 (6): 1005–1010. https://doi.org/10.1016/j.bbmt.2017.03.015.

Bjorklund, David F., and Bruce J. Ellis. 2014. Children, Childhood, and Development in Evolutionary Perspective. *Developmental Review* 34 (3): 225–264. https://doi.org/10.1016/j.dr.2014.05.005.

Brown, Steven E. 2002. What Is Disability Culture? *Disability Studies Quarterly* 22 (2): 34–50.

Buss, David W., and David P. Schmitt. 2019. Mate Preferences and Their Behavioral Manifestations. *Annual Review of Psychology* 70: 77–110. https://doi.org/10.1146/annurev-psych-010418-103408.

Davis, Dena S. 2010. *Genetic Dilemmas: Reproductive Technology, Parental Choices, and Children's Futures*, 2nd ed. New York: Oxford University Press.

Davis, Donald. 1991. *The Jeffrey Dahmer Story: An American Nightmare*. New York: Hellman, Macmillan.

Del Giudice, M., and B. Ellis. 2016. Evolutionary Foundations of Developmental Psychopathology. In *Developmental Psychopathology, vol. 1: Theory and Method*, 3rd ed., ed. Dante Cicchetti, 1–58. New York: Wiley.

Dey, Jacob K., Lisa E. Ishii, Jason C. Nellis, Kofi D. O. Boahene, Patrick J. Byrne, and Masar Ishii. 2017. Comparing Patient, Casual Observer, and Expert Perception of Permanent Unilateral Facial Paralysis. *JAMA Facial and Plastic Surgery* 19 (6): 476–483. https://doi.org/10.1001/jamafacial.2016.1630.

Dreger, Alice. 2006. What to Expect When You Have the Child You Weren't Expecting. In *Surgically Shaping Children: Technology, Ethics, and the Pursuit of Normality*, ed. Erik Parens, 253–266. Baltimore: Johns Hopkins University Press.

Fine, Michelle, and Adrienne Asch. 1988. Disability Beyond Stigma: Social Interaction, Discrimination, and Activism. *Journal of Social Issues* 44 (1): 3–21.

Fischer, Alastair J., and Gemma Ghelard. 2016. The Precautionary Principle, Evidence-Based Medicine, and Decision Theory in Public Health Evaluation. *Frontiers in Public Health* 4: 107. https://doi.org/10.3389/fpubh.2016.00107.

Fiske, Alan Page. 1992. The Four Elementary Forms of Sociality: Framework for a Unified Theory of Social Relations. *Psychological Review* 99 (4): 689–723.

Fredwall, Svein, Grethe Maanum, Heidi Johansen, Hildegun Snekkevik, Ravi Savarirayan, and B. Ingeborg. Lidal. 2020. Current Knowledge of Medical Complications in Adults with Achondroplasia: A Scoping Review. *Clinical Genetics* 97 (1): 179–197.

Briceño, González, G. Laura, Magali Viaud, Jacques Beltrand, Isabelle Flechtner, Yamina Dassa, Dinane Samara-Boustani, Caroline Thalassinos, Christian Pauwels, Kanetee Busiah, Graziella Pinto, et al. 2019. Improved General and Height-Specific Quality of Life in Children with Short Stature after 1 Year on Growth Hormone. *Journal of Clinical Endocrinology and Metabolism* 104 (6): 2103–2111. https://doi.org/10.1210/jc.2018-02523.

Gostin, Larry O. 1980. Ethical Considerations of Psychosurgery: The Unhappy Legacy of the Pre-frontal Lobotomy. *Journal of Medical Ethics*. 6 (3): 149–154.

Haselton, Martie G., Mina Mortezaie, Elizabeth G. Pillsworth, April Bleske-Rechek, and David A. Frederick. 2007. Ovulatory Shifts in Human Female Ornamentation: Near Ovulation, Women Dress to Impress. *Hormones and Behavior* 51 (1): 40–45. https://doi.org/10.1016/j.yhbeh.2006.07.007.

Hellman, Daniel, and Nathan Blackman. 2006. Enuresis, Firesetting and Cruelty to Animals: A Triad Predictive of Adult Crime. *American Journal of Psychiatry* 122 (12): 1431–1435. https://doi.org/10.1176/ajp.122.12.1431.

Hodges, Frederick M., J. Steven Svoboda, and Robert S. van Howe. 2002. Prophylactic Interventions on Children: Balancing Human Rights with Public Health. *Journal of Medical Ethics* 28 (1): 10–16.

Jacobs, Allan J. 2000. Liberty, Equality and Genetic Selection. *Pharos* 64 (1): 15–20.

Jost, John T., and Mahzarin Banaji. 1994. The Role of Stereotyping in System-Justification and the Production of False Consciousness. *British Journal of Social Psychology* 33 (1): 1–27.

Judge, Timothy A., and Daniel M. Cable. 2004. The Effect of Physical Height on Workplace Success and Income: Preliminary Test of a Theoretical Model. *Journal of Applied Psychology* 89 (3): 428–441. https://doi.org/10.1037/0021-9010.89.3.428.

Koplin, Julian J., Christopher Gyngell, and Julian Savulescu. 2020. Germline Gene Editing and the Precautionary Principle. *Bioethics* 34 (1): 49–59. https://doi.org/10.1111/bioe.12609.Fko.

Lukaszewski, Aaron W., Zachary L. Simmons, Cameron Anderson, and James R. Roney. 2016. The Role of Physical Formidability in Human Social Status Allocation. *Journal of Personality and Social Psychology* 110 (3): 385–406. https://doi.org/10.1037/pspi0000042.

Macdonald, John M. 1963. The Threat to Kill. *American Journal of Psychiatry* 120 (2): 125–130. https://doi.org/10.1176/ajp.120.2.125.

Miller, Geoffrey, Joshua M. Tybur, and Brent D. Jordan. 2007. Ovulatory cycle effects on tip earnings by lap dancers: Economic evidence for human estrus?. *Evolution and Human Behavior* 28 (6): 375–381. https://doi.org/10.1016/j.evolhumbehav.2007.06.002.

Miller, Paul Steven. 2006. Toward Truly Informed Decisions about Appearance-Normalizing Surgery. In *Surgically Shaping Children: Technology, Ethics, and the Pursuit of Normality*, ed. Erik Parens, 211–226. Baltimore: Johns Hopkins University Press.

Ouellette, Alicia. 2010. Shaping Parental Authority Over Children's Bodies. *Indiana Law Journal* 85 (3): 955–1002.

Paiva, Marianne. 2015. What Your Teeth Tell Me About Your Social Class. *Ethnography.com*. http://www.ethnography.com/2015/09/what-your-teeth-tell-me-about-your-social-class/. Accessed 30 Sep 2015.

Parens, Erik, ed. 2006. *Surgically Shaping Children: Technology, Ethics, and the Pursuit of Normality*. Baltimore: Johns Hopkins University Press.

Parens, Erik. 2015. *Shaping Ourselves: On Technology, Flourishing, and a Habit of Thinking*. Oxford: Oxford University Press.

Pope, Harrison G., Jr., Ruth I. Wood, Alan Rogol, Fred Nyberg, Larry Bowers, and Shalender Bhasin. 2014. Adverse Health Consequences of Performance-Enhancing Drugs: An Endocrine Society Scientific Statement. *Endocrine Review* 35 (3): 341–375. https://doi.org/10.1210/er.2013-1058.

Preminger, Beth. 2001. The 'Jewish nose' and Plastic Surgery: Origins and Implications. *JAMA* 286 (17): 2181.

Rio Declaration. 1992. *Rio Declaration on Environment and Development*. http://www.unep.org/Documents.Multilingual/Default.asp?documentid=78&articleid=1163.

Sanford, Emily Sullivan. 2006. My Shoe Size Stayed the Same. In *Surgically Shaping Children: Technology, Ethics, and the Pursuit of Normality*, ed. Erik Parens, 29–42. Baltimore: Johns Hopkins University Press.

Sayal, Kapil, Vibhore Prasad, David Daley, Tamsin Ford, and David Coghill. 2018. ADHD in Children and Young People: Prevalence, Care Pathways and. Service Provision. *Lancet Psychiatry* 5 (2): 175–186.

Schrank, Bernice. 2007. 'Cutting Off Your Nose to Spite Your Race': Jewish Stereotypes, Media Images, Cultural Hybridity. *Shofar* 25 (4): 18–42.

Schubert, Thomas W. 2020. Grounding of Rank: Embodiment, Space, and Magnitude. *Current Opinion in Psychology* 33: 222–226.

Schultz, T. Paul. 2002. Wage Gains Associated with Height as a Form of Health Human Capital. *American Economic Review* 92 (2): 349.

Smith, Dylan M., Ryan L. Sherriff, Laura Damschroder, George Loewenstein, and Peter A. Ubel. 2006. Misremembering Colostomies? Former Patients Give Lower Utility Ratings Than Do Current Patients. *Health Psychology* 25 (6): 688–695. https://doi.org/10.1037/0278-6133.25.6.688.

Sommer, Rachel, Monika Bullinger, John Chaplin, Juky Do, Mick Power, Andreas Pleil, and Julia Quitmann. 2017. Experiencing Health-Related Quality of Life in Paediatric Short Stature—A Cross-Cultural Analysis of Statements from Patients and Parents. *Clinical Psychology and Psychotherapy* 24 (6): 1370–1376. https://doi.org/10.1002/cpp.2105.

Sugiyama, Lawrence S. 2016. Physical Attractiveness: An Adaptationist Perspective. In *The Handbook of Evolutionary Psychology: Foundations*, 317–384, ed. David M. Buss. New York: Wiley.

Tooby, John, and Leda Cosmides. 2005. Conceptual Foundations of Evolutionary Psychology. In *Handbook of Evolutionary Psychology*, ed. David M. Buss, 1–67. New York: Wiley.

Tucker, Bonnie Poitras. 1998. Deaf Culture, Cochlear Implants, and Elective Disability. *Hastings Center Report* 28 (4): 6–14.

van Praag, Veroniek M., Magdalena Lysenko, Barbara Harvey, Rosanna Yankanah, and James G. Wright. 2018. Casting Is Effective for Recurrence Following Ponseti Treatment of Clubfoot. *Journal of Bone and Joint Surgery* 100 (12): 1001–1008. https://doi.org/10.2106/JBJS.17.01049.

Chapter 11
The Maturing Minor

Abstract Rational cognitive capacity is mostly completely acquired by the mid-teens. However, the auto-regulatory mental processes necessary to convert rational understanding to wise decisions—known as executive function—mature 10 years later. Legal capacity tends to be linked to ability to comprehend a problem rationally. In the US, the age of medical decisional competence is usually 18, though not in areas that have been carved out for public health reasons. In the UK it is 16, but earlier if rational understanding is demonstrable. Certainly, the question of deferring legal competence until the age of emotional maturity is a political non-starter in all developed nations, regardless of the emotional maturity of the older adolescent or the young adult. This chapter discusses important facets of decision-making under these conditions. This includes the role of parents.

11.1 Introduction

Aristotle wrote:

> …while young men become geometricians and mathematicians and wise in matters like these, it is thought that a young man of practical wisdom cannot be found. The cause is that such wisdom is concerned not only with universals but with particulars, which become familiar from experience, but a young man has no experience, for it is length of time that gives experience. (Nichomachean Ethics, Book VI, Chap. 8)

Many disputes and ethical quandaries arise with respect to adolescent patients. These individuals may be articulate and may evince understanding of the issues regarding medical treatment. They may not see eye to eye with parents regarding medical care involving lifestyle decisions such as sexuality. And they may make irrational decisions regarding their serious illness. This chapter considers why adolescents and young adults are inclined to make rash decisions with potentially high rewards. It will proceed to ethical and legal approaches to adolescent medical decision-making. This chapter is vital background for the chapters on sexuality, gender, and reproduction.

A. J. Jacobs, *Assigning Responsibility for Children's Health When Parents and Authorities Disagree: Whose Child?*, The International Library of Bioethics 90,
https://doi.org/10.1007/978-3-030-87698-2_11

11.2 Scientific Considerations

A person's intrinsic capacities place constraints on his or her moral responsibilities. One cannot be held morally responsible for things that one cannot control, including neuropsychological immaturity. Development of executive function lags behind maturation of intellectual comprehension alone. This has implications for adolescent decision-making.

Executive functions are a family of mental processes needed concentrate, to solve problems, to plan, to prioritize, and to reflect on facts and one's immediate desires (Diamond 2013). They are essential for success in group efforts, whether school, work, or life, Basic executive functions are based on inhibitory control such as self-control over behavior and attention; and cognitive flexibility (Lehto et al. 2010). These form the basis of more complex executive skills such as planning and problem solving (Diamond 2013). Well-developed executive functions are important for success in sports, academics, and music. Executive functions do not inhibit creativity. They make realization of creative goals possible. They are associated with the frontal lobe, though this is an oversimplification (Alvarez and Emory 2006).

Making decisions regarding one's medical care requires informed consent. The three elements of informed consent relate, respectively, to the consenter, the subject of consent, and the environment (Coughlan 2018). The consenter must have *capacity* to render consent. Capacity is the ability to understand and to reasonably assess the material factors that pertain to the clinical decision. Capacity classically has four requirements: the ability to choose; understanding of the facts relevant to the choices; an appreciation of the decision and the consequences of each choice, and the ability to assess information rationally (Diekema 2020). Almost everyone has some ability to choose. Conveying material information so that consent is *informed* is the responsibility of the physician who proffers a test or treatment. It is the third and fourth criteria that may be problematic with adolescents and, even more, with younger children. Appreciation of consequences implies not only intellectual *understanding*, but the ability to react in an appropriate manner to the information. This requires adequate executive function. Finally, consent must be *voluntary and free of coercion*. We all are exposed to external influence, and most of us welcome some of it. But what influence is appropriate, and at what point does influence become excessive? An uncoerced act does not require a Dr. Stockmann, who said, "the strongest man in the world is he who stands most alone" (Ibsen 1882). At the other extreme, is a severe threat such as a parent threatening to throw a teen out of the house.

Most people can rationally understand material facts by age 14. Most teens can understand the nature of their disease, the risks, the benefits and the alternatives to proposed treatment as well as can adults (Alderson 2017), People of this age can express choices and weigh options (Grootens-Wiegers et al. 2017). The capacity to apply these skills to one's personal situation usually matures later, though. The midbrain centers that seek reward and peer approval mature before the centers in the prefrontal cortex responsible for executive function and suppressing emotional reactions. These higher neural systems that are active in self-regulation do not fully mature until the mid-20's. In other words, adolescents mature intellectually before they mature emotionally and socially (Steinberg 2013). Maturation as a social being is complex and subtle, and understandably takes longer than maturation in perception of non-relational situations. But this differential maturation results in adolescents' greater risk-taking and susceptibility to peer pressure. Risk-taking and strong peer relations are developmentally natural (McCarthy 2018) and important (Diekema 2020) as children distance themselves from their parents. One can speculate that group survival is enhanced when young people show valor in combat and in hunting large animals, while older leaders show wisdom in managing battles and the hunt.

Rational analysis is impaired in a highly charged situations (Diekema 2020). This manifests in immature executive functions, leading to insufficient decisional capacity. Furthermore, when decisions are markedly altered by peer pressure, their voluntariness is in question. The recent fad of eating detergent capsules (McCarthy 2018) is a case in point.

The second question is when a child is being coerced. This is inevitable in a complex society. Minors are dependent on parents for physical and emotional support, which may be inherently coercive.

In short, adolescents are more susceptible to peer influence, less future-oriented, more impulsive, more likely to overestimate rewards and underestimate risks, as compared to adults. This has implications for the way we should regard adolescent decisional capacity. Furthermore, adolescents also are vulnerable to the wishes of adults with power over them, such as parents, teachers, and coaches.

11.3 Legal Constraints

Physicians who wish to keep their medical licenses must conform to legal rules. These rules differ in the US and the UK.

The bases for English and Welsh law is the well-known Gillick case ([1986] AC. 112). Young adults already could consent to medical procedures beginning at age 16. *Gillick* extended the prerogative of consent to younger minors who displayed sufficient intelligence and understanding of the procedure in question. These minors could consent to care, but they could not refuse care if their parents consented (*Re R* (*A Minor*) (*Wardship: Consent to Treatment*) [1992] Fam 11). Thus, either the rational minor or the parent can activate a doctor's medical decision. If both child and parent refuse, the physician still may seek legal redress.

The US legal system cannot adopt the British approach. First, American law is more deferential to parental rights. Second, American parents, unlike British parents, usually are responsible for some fraction of the child's medical costs.

The American starting point is that parents are health surrogates for their children until majority—18 years of age in almost all states. There are four exceptions to the exclusive parental power of consent. First is the *emancipated minor*—a chronological minor who does not live with his or her parents and is financially independent of them (Lane and Kohlenberg 2012). Another straightforward carve-out is *emergency care*, which does not require parental consent. Emergency care is supported by the common law doctrine of *implied consent* (Lee et al. 2018), and is required by the Emergency Medical Treatment and Active Labor Act (Katz et al. 2016).

The *mature minor* doctrine allows a minor (who is dependent on his parents) to make a decision because someone authorized by law—often a physician (Silber 2011)—has decided the minor is mature enough to do so. In 2015, only 17 of 50 states had adopted the mature minor doctrine (Coleman and Rosoff 2015). A decision that a child has capacity is based on clinical judgment, and not on formal neuropsychological evaluation. The mature minor doctrine is usually invoked when the minor is close in age to maturity; and the risks of the procedure are not extreme (Benston 2016). The mature minor doctrine creates, where it is in effect, a legal regimen for minors similar to *Gillick*-based UK system. As in England, courts are more likely to allow consent to medical proposals than to refuse them (Dickens and Cook 2015). Indeed, most state courts have declined to side with adolescents who refuse blood transfusions, e.g., *In re J.J.*, 582 N.E.2d 1138, (Ohio Court of Appeals 1990). Cherry (2013) argues that mature reasoning ability in the absence of mature executive functions does not confer capacity. This argues against the mature minor doctrine. Indeed, the Supreme Court has ascribed diminished responsibility for criminal acts to adolescent immaturity (Cherry 2013).

Italy takes a position between those of the US and UK. It grants children the right to be heard, and to have their views considered (Binato 2019). This means in practice that Italian law gives parents presumptive authority to make decisions on behalf of their children. However, children have some right to express their own view of their interests to rebut parental decisions.

The final exception to parental power of decision is that there are *specific legal set-asides* allowing minors to solicit, consent to, or refuse treatment. These include issues of sexuality, reproduction, psychiatric therapy, and treatment for drug dependency. Such legislation has been justified on the basis of the possibility of parental action that is contrary to the child's interest (Weithorn 2020). Also, parental consent is said to interfere with an adolescent's entitlement to confidentiality. There also is empirically justified concern that a parental notification or consent can deter adolescents from seeking sensitive services (Reddy et al. 2002). This has public health as well as individual implications. Indeed, Diekema (2020) believes that public health considerations motivate these condition-specific cutouts, and that concerns about individual minors is pretextual. With the exception of abortion (which is controversial in the US), there is broad consensus that society and minors themselves both benefit from minors' having access to these services (Weithorn 2020).

I now turn to general issues of decision-making for adolescents.

11.4 Making Decisions for Adolescent Patients

Especially with older children, shared decision-making is an increasingly accepted model in pediatrics in the US (Katz et al. 2016; Kon and Morrison 2018), Canada (Coughlan 2018), and Europe (Badarau et al. 2017). The goal is to do what the patient would want if she had the physician's knowledge.

The parent is the surrogate for minors without legal competence to consent. As we have seen, adolescents have rational capacities approximating those of adults, but lag in acquiring the executive function and perspectives to apply their understanding to the situation at hand. The "*rule of sevens*," ascribing no competence under 7 years, a rebuttable presumption of incompetence between 7 and 14; and a rebuttable presumption of competence between 14 and 21; was elaborated for purposes of criminal liability in *The Queen v. Smith*, 1 Cox CC 260 (1845). This rule later was extended to medical decisional competence in some jurisdictions (*Cardwell v. Bechtol*, 724 SW 2d 739, Tennessee Supreme Court 1987, 745). This rule acknowledges the differential development of capacity, albeit in a rigid way that should make thoughtful clinicians uncomfortable.

If most adolescents have good understanding and some ability to rationally apply this understanding to their healthcare decision, then shared decision making will involve the older minor as well as the physician and the parents (Alderson 2017). In any case, the decision process should point toward what the patient and family would do if they had the doctor's knowledge and experience. Shared decision-making is more complicated when the decision involves a child without decisional capacity. Those who believe that parents should wield decisional power (e.g., Diekema 2020), are impressed by data suggesting that immature emotional capacities trump mature capacities for rational understanding. Others, such as Alderson (2017) rely primarily on the cognitive capacity of minors of any age as the hallmark for legal decisional competence. Article 12, Sect. 1 of the CRC reads:

> (1) States Parties shall assure to the child who is capable of forming his or her own views the right to *express those views freely* in all matters affecting the child, the *views of the child being given due weight in accordance with the age and maturity of the child*. (Emphasis supplied)

Those nations that use CRC and related documents as precedent allow children the authority to accede to medical treatments that they cognitively understand. This is something close to the *Gillick* doctrine. It does not extend, however, to refusal of treatment that physicians deem important. Here, the best interest standard prevails over decisional prerogatives of minors, except for the cut-outs described above. Western professional organizations universally hold that adolescents should be consulted and taken seriously, and that, at a minimum, their desires should be accommodated when feasible.

Salter (2017) raises a provocative and convincing point that bypasses the capacity argument. She argues that the authority parents have over children derives from parental responsibility, rather than from lack of decisional ability by the minor. If a minor is physically, financially, and emotionally dependent on adults, then the adults are responsible for protecting that minor. Consider this analogy (which I, not Salter, have framed): Orville, a qualified pilot, is a passenger on a commercial flight flown by Wilbur. Orville cannot supersede Wilbur's judgment as to how to fly the plane, no matter how capable a pilot he is, or how inexperienced Wilbur is. Flying the airplane is Wilbur's responsibility, morally and legally. Of course, parental status is not arbitrary or accidental. Parents are likely to be more experienced at making judgments than their adolescent children. They are more likely to have mature executive functioning. On the other hand, while Orville and Wilbur have the same interest in arriving safely, an adolescent and her parents may have different views of the adolescent's own interest. Furthermore, the parent will not directly experience the effects of a bad decision, but the child will. On the other hand, a reader who has been a parent, spent many hours awake with a distressed child, changed many diapers, and who has helped the child navigate the physical and emotional trials of childhood, will appreciate the anguish most parents experience when they see even adult children making self-destructive choices.

Another facet of parental responsibility, according to Salter, is that parents are in the best position to consider the effects on the entire family of a medical decision for one child. Even if the state covers health care costs, there are parental expenditures of time and emotions that follow from significant medical decisions. A medical decision involving one member of the family—even an adult—can have a powerful impact on other family members. The Direct Effects Basis provides a floor that constrains parents' decisions; a parent cannot allow one child to die or become severely disabled merely to allow another child to maximize his talents.

One last general consideration is that the British system allowing either a *Gillick*—capable child or a parent to consent to a procedure may grant too much power to the physician. First, a physician's views of children's reasonableness may be based on whether the children take her advice. In fact, there may be cases in which there are reasonable differences in judgment. Indeed, physicians themselves can err. Adolescents' sensitivity to pressure may make them easily susceptible to undue influence, even from a physician. There is an opportunity for self-dealing when physicians who treat a minor also determine whether that minor has decisional capacity. In the event of disagreement, it's 'heads I win, tails you lose' for aggressive physicians. If the minor agrees with the physician and the parent does not, the minor has Gillick capacity and the parent is overruled. If it is the parent who agrees with the doctor rather than the minor, the minor may be deemed to lack *Gillick* capacity.[1]

11.5 Privacy and Confidentiality

Adolescents may avoid seeking medical care out of fear that their parents will find out. Though not ideal, this situation is not rare. When the state considers bypass of

[1] If neither the minor or his parents agree with the physician, the physician has the option of litigation.

parental consent to be good public policy, it must shield the parents from knowledge of the treatment, and from the costs of treatment. If parents are billed for the treatment, they thereby become aware of it.

The principles of privacy and confidentiality are closely related.[2] They are keystones of law and ethics. Privacy—the right to be let alone (Warren and Brandeis 1890)—is the basis for American constitutional entitlement to extensive sexual and reproductive liberties (*Griswold v. Connecticut*, 381 U.S. 479, Supreme Court, 1965). Medical information is the patient's private property, protected by unconsented release (Department of Health and Human Services 2020). Similar legal rights to medical privacy exists in most Western nations. This right to privacy is enjoyed by patients, but not by those treating them. Patients generally are free to disclose information or to subject facts about them to scrutiny.

Confidentiality is the obligation of the recipient of information not to disclose it to a third party. It is, more or less, the professional duty that arises from the patient right of privacy. It dates back at least 2,500 years, to the time of Hippocrates. The British Medical Association defines confidentiality as "keeping secure and secret from others, information given by or about an individual in the course of a professional relationship" (Marsh and Reynard 2009, 164). It is undergirded by at least three ethical bases. First is consequentialist; patients are more likely to divulge embarrassing information important for their care if they know it will be kept confidential. Second is fidelity and virtue; secrecy is part of a physician's professional obligation and skill. Finally, confidentiality is said to be part of individuals' autonomy.[3]

State legislation may give parents access to information about adolescents that adolescents might prefer to keep confidential. Many states allow breaches of minors' medical privacy by parents in various circumstances (Pathak and Chou 2019). When a minor is covered under a parent's insurance policy, the parent policyholder will be notified of all claims and payments, including care of the minor.

The upshot is that physicians have to answer both to ethical duties and to laws governing their practice. Furthermore, physicians do not have total control over their records if they work for institutions. It might be ethically and legally advisable for

[2] Privilege is a third related concept, tangential to this discussion. Privilege is the legal right of a patient to keep information obtained by professionals or their agents out of legal proceedings. American Federal rules of procedure do not provide for physician privilege at all, except for psychotherapists. Most states, though recognize a fairly weak medical privilege.

[3] The confidentiality of medical records is not as strong as is generally supposed. Medical privilege can be breached in many legal actions, both civil and criminal, and including malpractice suits or a billing dispute that reaches litigation. Indeed, in a product liability dispute that reached the US Supreme Court over a technical issue regarding pretrial summary judgment (*Celotex Corp. v. Catrett*, 477 US 317, Supreme Court 1986), Louis Catrett's name and alleged medical condition have come to the attention of at least hundreds of thousands of people, as the Court's opinion has been cited over 184,000 times! Medical information can even be disclosed in lawsuits in which the patient is not involved (*Orthopedic Associates v. HIG*, 124 P. 3d 930, Hawaii Supreme Court, 2005). Legal breaches of confidentiality may involve information regarding minors, though the name of the minor may be shielded, as by using initials. One such case, *Parham v. JR*, 442 US 584—Supreme Court, 1979, has been cited in over 5,000 sources, and is cited in this book.

physicians to inform a minor in advance about the extent and limits of medical confidentiality and privacy. If court action can be anticipated, the limits of privilege should be discussed. Unless a physician is certain of her obligations, she should consider ethical and legal consultation if there is a significant possibility that someone will request that confidentiality be breached. Medical records should contain information necessary for continuity of care for the patient by any other physician, but should not contain extraneous information that could injure the patient if unsealed.

11.6 Specific Medical Decisions

I now turn to a brief discussion of several representative decisional situations.

11.6.1 Serious Illness

In the case of an immediately threat to life or limb, a physician may treat a minor without parental consent (NDAA 2013). The legal and ethical basis for this is the doctrine of *implied consent*—that a reasonable patient or parent would consent to the treatment (*Stafford v. Louisiana StateUniversity*, 448 So. 2d 852, Louisiana Court of Appeals, 1984). Otherwise, shared decision-making among patient, parent, and physician is most satisfactory. In the event of disagreement, some variant of the *Gillick* doctrine may apply in many jurisdictions. In the US, a pediatrician's priority should be beneficence rather than autonomy—to seek the best outcome rather than to allow even an older adolescent without legal decisional competence to make decisions (Diekema 2020). Regardless of legal necessity, it is best to obtain buy-in from the minor patient if possible. Furthermore, it usually is possible to grant some power to older minors in choosing options compatible with appropriate treatment. For example, patients could decide which arm to use for venipuncture, or what time of day to take a medication (Ungaru 2011). This is good medicine, if nothing else. As the next section shows, parental buy-in is vital to successful treatment of an ongoing problem.

11.6.2 Compelled Treatment

Cases such as *in re Cassandra C.* (112 A.3d 158, Connecticut Supreme Court 2015) are exciting to lawyers and ethicists, thought fortunately are rare. Cassandra, age 17, had Hodgkin's disease which initially could probably have been cured using chemotherapy. Cassandra's diagnosis, evaluation, and treatment were delayed at length because of resistance by Cassandra and her mother. Cassandra ultimately accepted home chemotherapy, but changed her mind when this entailed insertion of a long-term venous catheter. The state Supreme Court ordered the catheter placed, but Cassandra received no further treatment. The disease recurred, likely because of initial delays and interruptions in treatment, all with the encouragement of Cassandra's mother. Cassandra died at age 22. *Cassandra C.* illustrates that parents as well as physicians can exert deleterious coercive influence, and that even a 17-year-old may be too dependent on a parent to be capable of independent judgment. Court-fashioned remedies take time, and, in any event, parents frequently do not comply with court ordered treatment (Caruso Brown and Slutzky 2017). Litigation is a clumsy and inefficient means for ensuring proper treatment. Most patients accept recommendations that are necessary for health. But treatment programs that involve a lot of hands-on effort by parents or the minor himself over a long period of time are almost impossible to carry out effectively unless the family is willing to collaborate in treatment. Courts are more effective at compelling one-shot interventions such as surgery for appendicitis than in imposing long-term treatment on a reluctant patient and family. Even when empowered by a court to override family wishes, a conscientious, ethical physician will attempt to satisfy patients 'and families' desires to the extent compatible with the patient's health (Bester et al. 2017).

A classic recurring example of the problems with long-term involuntary treatment is compelled treatment of anorexia nervosa, which predominantly affects adolescents and young adults. Overall recovery is 50%, but mortality is 5% (Steinhausen 2002). In severe, enduring disease, the mortality is about 20%. Many, but not all, who undergo compelled inpatient treatment of refractory anorexia nervosa relapse after discharge (Yager et al. 2016). The Direct Effects Basis of the State Intervention Test would support involuntary treatment directed toward weight gain and, secondarily, toward the psychological condition, if it often were effective. Such treatment may indeed be effective (Ayton et al. 2009).

Compelled inpatient treatment is controversial because those with anorexia appear to be in full control of their faculties except for their perception of body image. Some believe that self-starvation is not sufficiently indicative of diminished capacity to justify overriding a patient's decision not to eat (Boyle 2019). Finally, what is construed as delusional in an isolated individual may be tolerable if it is part of an ongoing tradition. Consider a hypothetical ancient religious culture, the Neo-Essenes, whose members prize education, asceticism, and non-violence, not unlike Quakers or Jains. They are vegetarian, and minimize injuring or killing any animals. An extreme denomination of this group is called the Anaxagorans, after a philosopher said to have starved himself. Anaxagorans sometimes practice self-starvation as a holy way to die, recognizing that plants as well as animals are living beings. Although most self-starvation is practiced by people with terminal illnesses, occasionally an adolescent female resorts to the practice. Such young women have a psychological profile similar to Western females with anorexia nervosa. They differ mostly in their motivation. Anaxagorans consider them holy. Other Neo-Essenes are conflicted, recognizing that the practice has a long tradition, but considering it extreme and somewhat sad.[4]

We may ask whether self-starvation based on religious explanations of reality is compatible with attribution of capacity. If so, one difference between Annaxagoran

---

[4] See Phillips and Schaefer (2019) for description of a similar practice.

starvation and anorexia nervosa is that the former is part of an established tradition to which millions of people adhere. Another is that Anaxagoran starvation is based on a noumenal theory incommensurate with naturalism, while anorexia nervosa appears to be based on delusion. Most people in Western society undoubtedly feel uncomfortable with the idea of Anaxagoran starvation. They might invoke the Direct Effects Basis to prevent self-starvation, even if it is voluntarily performed by someone who otherwise appears to have capacity. Certainly, we give lip service to the courage and faith of people who accepted martyrdom in the name of religion, as occurred during the Spanish Inquisition. We often regard as heroes people who fight for a cause, and die facing long odds. The Alamo defenders come to mind. The State Intervention Test as an ethical guide is intended to allow states to intervene against parents under certain circumstances, and not to direct them to do so. I regard intervention to prevent Anaxagoran self-starvation as a borderline case. Whether the state should respond proactively should depend on multiple factors, such as the age of the minor, the minor's mental state, and the apparent degree of undue influence, including social pressure, from peers and cybermedia. Certainly, the state should not interfere with parental efforts to stop self-starvation, up to and including forced treatment.

This obviously raises the question of whether parents should be able to interfere with an adolescent minor's joining a cult such as the Waco Branch Davidians (Newport 2006), converting to a different mainstream religion than his parents, making decisions regarding his or her (Hutchinson et al. 2020) gender that appear to be socially influenced, and similar drastic decisions, some of which have implications for health and safety.

11.6.3 End of Life Care

A related question is how to make decisions about or for adolescents who will soon die. Howe (2019) finds that dying adolescents can experience anguish over disagreement with parents and doctors regarding end-of-life treatment. Loss or impending loss of their child can lead parents to overwhelming sadness and feelings of guilt. Parents may not grasp their adolescent children's wishes regarding termination of active care (Friebert et al. 2020). It is best, therefore, to initiate discussions regarding advanced care directives at as early point in the illness if possible, so that communication can be open, and disputes can be resolved (Needle et al. 2018). That being said, it is common for parents of seriously ill children to change their priorities over time from obtaining the best medical care to making sure the child feels loved and comfortable (Hill et al. 2019). Clinicians themselves may feel moral distress not only in the face of disagreement with parents and patients themselves, but in the face of their inability to reverse a tragic situation (Prentice and Gillam 2018). Howe (2019) states that parents' decisions-making capacity often will be affected by their own strong emotions. Sensitivity to patients' and families' emotions and wishes, and ability to work with them, is a difficult skill that must be learned and practiced. If resolution of differences between patients and family is important, then the needs of family members is important, and reconciliation of views must be sought. Clinical ethicists, chaplains, and behavioral health professionals may be able to mediate solutions. It is a tragedy when such cases end in litigation.

The question of physician-assisted death (PAD) in adolescents requires mention. Belgium and the Netherlands are the only jurisdictions that explicitly permit PAD in terminally ill minors (Brouwer et al. 2018). Canada has constitutionalized PAD as a right for people who are "condemned to a life of severe and intolerable suffering" (*Carter v. Canada (AG)*, SCC 5, [2015] 1 SCR 331, note 1 at ¶1). Guichon et al. (2017) would apply this legislation to minors with understanding equivalent to *Gillick* capacity. Canadians should seek legal consultation before agreeing to assist in a minor's death. PAD in general is a sensitive and highly politicized issue. It involves issues that concern the state, but that go well beyond parental authority. My advice to a physician in any nation is that she should not participate in PAD of a minor except under the umbrella of an institution with an ongoing program defined by institutional policies and protected by sound legal support. Assuming that PAD itself does not invoke issues more important than parental choice, then I would support parental choice in this matter, provided that medical staff agree and the decision passes state review. An older adolescent should be in accord, and should not be under undue pressure. Sufficient professional counseling of parents and supervision by the state (to prevent abuse) are critical; death is irreversible. I have discussed state-compelled termination of care, knowingly leading to death, as related to Charlie Gard and Alfie Evans.

We have seen that cognitive understanding precedes emotional maturity by at least a decade. Furthermore, there are no widely accepted test tests to determine whether a person's emotional immaturity negates his cognitive capacity. Also, both by virtue of their social and economic dependency (which makes them susceptible to parental influence) and their high susceptibility to peer pressure, even older adolescents are highly susceptible to undue influence. Finally, some of the interesting and important considerations include the circumstances under which PAD generally should be acceptable—an issue on which I am ambivalent.[5] What seems reasonable to me is that, outside exceptional circumstances, active action that leads to a child's death should require consensus among parent, physician, government, and the minor himself.

[5] The decision to agree to active termination of another's life can cause dissention in the family and guilt among its members. In the era before medical ethics became prominent, before the establishment of the hospice movement, and when people frequently died in hospital, I often saw physicians give suffering terminal patients an infusion of glucose water. This would lead to electrolyte imbalance that would induce death by coma—often aided by narcotics. Logical analysis would declare this to be paternalistic, but death came easily, and patients appreciated the care. Perhaps some things that are intuitively right are difficult to justify philosophically.

11.6.4 Genetic Testing and Disclosure

This is an area in which early disclosure might actually empower the maturing minor. This vast topic, which I must treat superficially, encompasses issues pertinent both to adolescents and to younger children. The standard approach to genetic counseling, attributed to Joan Marks, has been based on value neutrality and non-directive counseling (Bosk 1993). Radical non-directiveness has been questioned and leaders in the field increasingly advocate a shared decision-making model (Benkendorf 2014). Non-directiveness is impossible to achieve in any event, as language without evaluative connotations is a mirage (Michie et al. 1997). Autonomy as completely uncoerced decision is, itself, a mirage. Robinson Crusoe (Defoe 1719/2014) may have enjoyed autonomy without influence or constraint from others, at least until Friday showed up. Most of us are affected by the needs and opinions of those around us, and many of us are happy to have the support and advice of friends, family, and, perhaps, others around us. Some scholars advocate a relational autonomy approach (Shepherd et al. 2017) in shared decision making (Elwyn et al. 2012) in making medical decisions regarding genetic information, and in disclosing genetic information to family members. Exploring issues related to genetic disorders may be more autonomy-enhancing than mere presentation of scientific and clinical data (Wachbroit and Wasserman 1995).

These considerations apply to minors as well, but the application is tricky. Normally, parents are surrogates who make medical decisions on behalf of children, based on the child's interests and needs, and on competing interests of other family members. Dena Davis (1997, 2010), though, applied the open future doctrine to genetic testing of children. She states that the priority in deciding whether to obtain or disclose genetic information is to maximize the child's adult choices. She uses the example of Huntington's disease, a condition that produces a severe movement disorder and dementia in by age 50 in half of children of affected individuals.[6] Davis asks whether parents should be allowed to test their minor children for presence of the genetic defect. She says this should not be done. Because there is no effective medical intervention, and the psychosocial effects of testing and disclosure are uncertain, the choice should be left to the child at the age of legal maturity. Davis' work has influenced many organizational guidelines (Garrett et al. 2019).

I believe Davis's open future argument has it backwards, even if one accepts the priority of an open future (which I do not). Depriving a person of the ability to decide on a test until the age of 18 is not as important to a person's range of future choices as is giving that person the ability to plan his or her life choices realistically, in the context of intrinsic health constraints.

Consider the following hypothetical case. Tulevik disease is caused by transplacental passage of a parasite to the fetus. It causes distinctive, but mild and reversible, symptoms in the mother, and is generally diagnosed prenatally. It causes blindness in half the children of infected mothers. Those affected show no symptoms until they are between ages 30 and 50, at which time they completely lose their eyesight

[6] Not, as Davis (1997) states, in their 50's.

over the course of a week. Tulevik disease otherwise can be only diagnosed by a blood test during the infant's first year of life. His and his family's knowledge of his Tulevik status from infancy might provide at least two advantages over learning of the condition only upon losing eyesight. First, knowing that he will develop Tulevik disease would be an integral part of his life. Onset of Tulevik blindness would not be as socially disruptive, or as psychologically damaging, as unexpected midlife blindness. A child who knows he will become blind might flourish more than one who always wonders whether this will happen. Second, the child would be able to make plans that would best provide for his needs and the needs of those close to him. If affected, he might not pursue a career as an artist or an airplane pilot. He could develop romantic and other relationships based on ability to plan for the inevitable loss of sight, with less chance of disruption that would occur if he suddenly became blind. He might make different financial choices than he would if he anticipated good vision throughout adulthood. On the other hand, if the child is unaffected, he need not fear loss of vision. For affected children, the number of total choices is reduced, but the number of choices that would contribute to maximal flourishing would be increased.

I constructed this hypothetical to block out the genetic etiology, and to enable diagnosis only in childhood. Obtaining and disclosing information that allows the child to maximize his capabilities, though these are constrained by physical factors, seems to be appropriate.

Another reason given for routine non-testing of children for adult-onset genetic disorders is that the majority of adults who may be affected, never having been offered childhood testing, will decline testing (Bennett et al. 2003). But, learning about an inevitable illness while one is an asymptomatic adult is not the same as living one's whole life with the knowledge. This is true of psychological implications as well as implications for life choices, and for effects on ongoing relationships. An analogy is that growing up with economic or other poverty is not the same as growing up with wealth and becoming poor.

Realization during adulthood that one has a 50% chance of developing Huntington's disease can be unsettling and development of symptoms can be depressing. A superb novel by Jennifer duBois (2012) describes the attempt of one such person attempts to find meaning. I accept, though, that, like the arguments against testing and disclosure, my intuition that children would do better with disclosure is not well enough supported to become general policy. It cannot be stated definitively how many carriers of genetic traits such as that associated with Huntington's disease will flourish better (1) knowing about it from early childhood; (2) learning about it in youth or early adulthood; (3) learning about the possibility that they may carry the genetic marker, but not being tested; or (4) being kept in the dark. These questions must be settled empirically. Mood disorders may be a manifestation of preclinical

Huntington's disease,[7] in which case Huntington's disease is an inappropriate model for other genetic conditions.

Can minors understand clinical genetic information, though, and do they want this information? A review article by McGill et al. (2019) suggests that children can grasp the notion of inherited causes of disease and testing for these diseases. Many adolescents have a positive attitude toward testing, though this varies according to the disease and the options for prevention or modification of the adverse effects (Myers et al. 2020). McGowan et al. (2019) found that many adolescents would desire information regarding their genetic predisposition to disease. Attitudes of both children and adults may be context-dependent, unstable, and confused (Strohmaier et al. 2019). The concerns expressed by children, adolescents, and adults overlap greatly, and are summarized in Table 11.1.

Delaying a decision to test for adult-onset diseases until the age of consent denies people the opportunity to learn about genetically-determined conditions while they have an opportunity to have it be part of their self-image, and to avoid the shock of learning of their limitations after formation of their personality, important relationships, and goals. The near unanimity of professional organizations in opposing testing children for adult-onset genetic conditions (Garrett et al. 2019) is based on autonomy considerations.

But interests have priority in decisions for children. What is appropriate, then, is an analysis of the weight of the various implicated interests, including interest in preserving the choice for testing. Other harm objections have been raised regarding childhood testing. Misattributed paternity can be revealed (Li and Liao 2008), which can disrupt families. The incidence of misattributed paternity in the Western world is 1–3% (Larmuseau et al. 2013). Other potential harms include stigma, insurance and employment discrimination, and misunderstanding a carrier state (e.g., sickle cell trait), or even misunderstanding the meaning of carrying a recessive trait for an adult-onset genetic disease (Ross et al. 2013). Insurance discrimination can be resolved through legislation that prevents inquiry into an individual's genomic information, or accession of such information. Employment discrimination cannot take place without a breach of confidentiality and can also be resolved by legislation. Stigma is a greater problem, especially in medically sophisticated populations with a great deal of inbreeding, a high incidence of certain deleterious genetic traits, and arranged marriages, such as certain highly traditional Jewish communities (Rose et al. 2016). But stigma attaches when a parent displays a dominant genetic disorder, regardless of genetic testing. Indeed, testing will remove the stigma in half the children. To the extent that people desire healthy mates and companions, there will always be stigmatization of people who are subject to poor health, for whatever reason. I doubt

[7] Depression and anxiety are frequently found in preclinical carriers (Martinez-Horta et al. 2016). It is not clear whether mood disorders prior to the onset of motor symptoms and dementia are part of the disease process, a reaction of carriers to their situation, or both (Pla et al. 2014), and psychological symptoms may precede disease by many years. Psychological manifestations are reportedly more common in those who have the genetic defect than in genetically normal children of parents with Huntington's disease (Marshall et al. 2007). It is not known whether preclinical psychological mood disorders are influenced by disclosure of carrier status.

Table 11.1 Attitudes of young people and adults towards clinical genetic testing: (After McGill et al. 2019; Frankel et al. 2016; Pereira et al. 2019)

Concern or benefit	Reported by children/adolescents	Reported by parents/clinicians
Benefits		
Informed future reproductive decision-making	√	
Knowledge of risk status	√	
Early lifestyle modification for anticipation or management of the condition	√	√
Inform family members and allow them to act accordingly	√	
Lifestyle changes; screening, breast augmentation (BRCA)		√
Inform reproductive choices		√
Sense of control over situation		√
Strengthening of relationships through the testing experience		√
Positive psychological impact—relief from uncertainty		√
Value of information for its own sake		√
Concerns		
False positives and negatives		√
Difficulties in interpretation: variable penetrance; alleles of uncertain significance		√
Poor understanding of implications if tested too young	√	√
Effect on family		√
Privacy, stigma and discrimination	√	√
Negative psychological impact (e.g., worry, low mood, regret)	√	√
May regret knowledge	√	√
Interference with school and other important activities	√	
Disease prevention may not be possible	√	

(continued)

Table 11.1 (continued)

Concern or benefit	Reported by children/adolescents	Reported by parents/clinicians
Psychological distress for patient and family Parents exaggerate child's vulnerability Impaired bonding with child Blame of self and partner	✓	

that having a 50% chance of a serious adult-onset genetic condition is much less stigmatizing than a certainty of such a condition. Suppose Abelard is dating Heloise, whose father has Huntington's disease. Would Abelard really be more likely to break off the relationship if he knew that Heloise would definitely develop Huntington's disease than if he knew that the odds of her developing Huntington's disease were 50%?

That leaves the question of psychological harm. There is surprisingly little empiric data on this subject, considering the unanimity of organizational policy against childhood testing (Wakefield et al. 2016). The suggestions that there might be anxiety, depression, survivor guilt (for those who test negative), and preoccupation with developing disease have mostly not been demonstrated. This is not surprising, considering that children appear to accommodate to knowledge of existing childhood illnesses that narrow their potential for adult achievement. Indeed, several authors (Dalby 1995; Duncan et al. 2005; Aatre and Day 2011; Wakefield et al. 2016) note that children accommodate well to knowledge that they possess a deleterious gene which may impair their health in the future. The limited amount of knowledge on this subject is due to the early adoption of policies against childhood testing based on hypothetical concerns. It seems intuitive that people who grow up with limitations accept them better than if they suddenly are confronted with them as adults.

What should doctors disclose? Consider two possibilities. First, an adolescent wants testing or sequencing, and his parent refuses. The adolescent should prevail if disclosure is more beneficial than non-disclosure, and if non-disclosure is likely to cause an objectively severe harmful effect. Otherwise, the Direct Effects Basis allows the parent to prevail, even if this is not the best decision. But inability to plan his life may be sufficient harm to override parental wishes. The ability to plan one's future knowing one's limitations may foreseeably avoid severe psychological harm and financial need.

A second possibility is that the parent wants testing, the adolescent assents, but the physician declines to provide it. Here, the parents should prevail. A physician's decision against testing is paternalistic and undermines trust (Vayena and Tasioulas 2013), despite the underpinning of such policies by professional societies (e.g., American Academy of Pediatricians 2013, reaffirmed 2018). According to the Bases in the State Intervention Test parents are the default deciders regarding what is best for children, unless their decision is harmful, overall. More research is necessary to allow confident determination of the effects of disclosure in various clinical contexts. However, if it is not clear whether the net benefit of testing or disclosure is harmful or beneficial, the Test would give parents have the power to make the decision.

To summarize, adolescents have sufficient stake in knowing about characteristics regarding their genomes that might affect their health that their wishes on disclosure should ordinarily be respected, though the final decision for an adolescent without legal decisional competence rests with parents. Parents should make these decisions for younger children. My opinion is based on the premise that testing and disclosure per se are unlikely to cause serious harm to minors. Thus, my conclusion is tentative, and would change if evidence were to refute my empiric assumption. My position does not conform with most organizational recommendations. Physicians involved in these clinical situations should follow local laws and institutional policies.

11.7 Conclusion

Adolescents are likely to have good intellectual understanding of their medical situations. On the other hand, they are likely to exercise poor judgment, and to be unduly susceptible both to peer and parental influence. If both parents and patient refuse treatment that is deemed necessary for an existing or potential grave condition, legal action may be appropriate. However, parents are likely to resist prolonged treatment regimens requiring a lot of parental effort, even if such treatment is that are ordered by a court. In non-urgent situations, when parents and physician disagree, or when parents lose confidence in the physician, the adolescent and family should be allowed to obtain additional opinions or to change physicians on the same basis as an adult would.

This chapter has deferred discussion in one area in which parental opinion often differs from the opinions of *bien pensant* physicians, academicians, and legal authorities—adolescent choices regarding sexuality and reproduction. These issues will be addressed in the next chapter.

References

Aatre, Rajani D., and Sharlene Day. 2011. "Psychological Issues in Genetic Testing for Inherited Cardiovascular Diseases." *Circulation: Cardiovascular Genetics* 4 (1): 81–90. https://doi.org/10.1161/CIRCGENETICS.110.957365.

Alderson, Priscilla. 2017. Children's Consent and the Zone of Parental Discretion. *Clinical Ethics* 12 (2): 55–62. https://doi.org/10.1177/1477750917691887.

Alvarez, Julie A., and Eugene Emory. 2006. Executive Function and the Frontal Lobes: A Meta-analytic Review. *Neuropsychology Review* 16 (1): 17–42. https://doi.org/10.1007/s11065-006-9002-x.

American Academy of Pediatrics Committee on Bioethics, Committee on Genetics, and The American College of Medical Genetics and Genomics Social, Ethical, and Legal Issues Committee.

2013, reaffirmed 2018. Ethical and Policy Issues in Genetic Testing and Screening of Children. *Pediatrics* 131 (3): 620–622. https://doi.org/10.1542/peds.2012-3680 (Reaffirmed. (2018). *Pediatrics* September 142 (3): e20181836. https://doi.org/10.1542/peds.2018-1836.

Ayton, Agnes, Catherine Keen, and Bryan Lask. 2009. Pros and Cons of Using the Mental Health Act for Severe Eating Disorders in Adolescents. *European Eating Disorders Review* 17 (1): 14–23. https://doi.org/10.1002/erv.887.

Badarau, Domnita O., Katharina Ruhe, Thomas Kühne, Eva De Clercq, Anca Colita, Bernice S. Elger, and Tenzin Wangmo. 2017. Decision Making in Pediatric Oncology: Views of Parents and Physicians in Two European Countries. *American Journal of Bioethics Empirical Bioethics* 8 (1): 21–31. https://doi.org/10.1080/23294515.2016.1234519.

Benkendorf, Judith. 2014. Genetic Legacy and the Genomic Future. *Genetics in Medicine* 16 (6): 862–863. https://doi.org/10.1038/gim.2014.36.

Bennett, Robin L., Heather L. Hampel, Jessica B. Mandell, and Joan H. Marks. 2003. Genetic Counselors: Translating Genomic Science into Clinical Practice. *Journal of Clinical Investigation* 112 (9): 1274–1279. https://doi.org/10.1172/JCI20113.

Benston, Shawna. 2016. Not of Minor Consequence?: Medical Decision-Making Autonomy and the Mature Minor Doctrine. *Indiana Health Law Review.* 13 (1): 1–16.

Bester, Johan Christiaan, Martin Smith, and Cynthia Groggins. 2017. A Jehovah's Witness Adolescent in the Labor and Delivery Unit: Should Patient and Parental Refusals of Blood Transfusions for Adolescents Be Honored? *Narrative Inquiry in Bioethics* 7 (1): 97–106. https://doi.org/10.1353/nib.2017.0022.

Binato, Giulia. 2019. Mature Minors and Self-determination in Medical Consent Law: A Comparison Between the Italian Legal System and the English Legal System. *Interdisciplinary Journal of Family Studies* 24 (1): 72–88.

Bosk, Charles L. 1993. The Workplace Ideology of Genetic Counselors. In *Prescribing Our Future: Ethical Challenges in Genetic Counseling*, 25–38, ed. Diane M. Bartels, Bonnie S. LeRoy, and Arthur L. Caplan. London: Taylor & Frances.

Boyle, Sam. 2019. How should the law determine capacity to refuse treatment for anorexia? *International Journal of Law and Psychiatry* 6: 250–259. https://doi.org/10.1016/j.ijlp.2019.05.001.

Brouwer, Marije, Christopher Kaczor, Margaret P. Battin, Els Maeckelberghe, John D. Lantos, and Eduard Verhagen. 2018. Should Pediatric Euthanasia be Legalized? *Pediatrics* 141 (2): e20171343.

Brown, Caruso, E. Amy, and Amy R. Slutzky. 2017. Refusal of Treatment of Childhood Cancer: A Systematic Review. *Pediatrics* 140 (6): e20171951. https://doi.org/10.1542/peds.2017-1951.

Cherry, Mark J. 2013. Ignoring the Data and Endangering Children: Why the Mature Minor Standard for Medical Decision Making Must Be Abandoned. *Journal of Medicine and Philosophy* 38 (3): 315–331. https://doi.org/10.1093/jmp/jht014.

Coleman, Doriane Lambelet, and Philip M. Rosoff. 2015. The Legal Authority of Mature Minors to Consent to General Medical Treatment. *Pediatrics* 131 (4): 786–793.

Coughlan, Kevin W. 2018. Medical Decision-Making in Paediatrics: Infancy to Adolescence. *Paediatrics and Child Health* 23 (2): 138–146. https://doi.org/10.1093/pch/pxx127.

Dalby, Shirley. 1995. GIG Response to the UK Clinical Genetics Society Report "The Genetic Testing of Children. *Journal of Medical Genetics* 32 (6): 490–494.

Davis, Dena S. 1997. Genetic Dilemmas and the Child's Right to an Open Future. *Rutgers Law Review* 28 (2): 549–592.

Davis, Dena S. 2010. *Genetic Dilemmas: Reproductive Technology, Parental Choices, and Children's Futures*, 2nd ed. New York: Oxford University Press.

Defoe, Daniel. 1719. *Robinson Crusoe.* Garden City, NY: Black and White Classics.

Department of Health and Human Services. 2020. *Summary of the HIPAA Privacy Rule.* https://www.hhs.gov/hipaa/for-professionals/privacy/laws-regulations/index.html. Text of rule is recorded in 45 C.F.R. Part 160 and Part 164, Subparts A and E.

Diamond, Adele. 2013. Executive Functions. *Annual Review of Psychology* 64: 135–168. https://doi.org/10.1146/annurev-psych-113011-143750.

Dickens, Bernard M., and Rebecca J. Cook. 2015. Patients' refusal of recommended treatment. *International Journal of Gynecology and Obstetrics* 131 (1): 105–108.

Diekema, Douglas S. 2020. Adolescent Brain Development and Medical Decision-making. *Pediatrics* 146 (Supplement 1): S18–S24. https://doi.org/10.1542/peds.2020-0818F.

duBois, Jennifer. 2012. *A Partial History of Lost Ca uses.* New York: Dial Press.

Duncan, Rony E., Julian Savulescu, Lynn Gillam, Robert Williamson, and Martin B. Delatycki. 2005. An International Survey of Predictive Genetic Testing in Children for Adult-Onset Conditions. *Genetics in Medicine* 7 (6): 390–396. https://doi.org/10.1097/01.GIM.0000170775.39092.44.

Elwyn, Glyn, Dominick Frosch, Richard Thomson, Natalie Joseph-Williams, Amy Lloyd, Paul Kinnersley, Emma Cording, Dave Tomson, Carole Dodd, Stephen Rollnick, Adrian Edwards, and Michael Barry. 2012. *Journal of General Internal Medicine* 27 (10): 1361–1367. https://doi.org/10.1007/s11606-012-2077-6.

Frankel, Leslie Ann, Stacey Pereira, and Amy L. McGuire. 2016. Potential Psychosocial Risks of Sequencing Newborns. *Pediatrics* 137 (Supplement 1): S24–S29. https://doi.org/10.1542/peds.2015-3731F.

Friebert, Sarah, Daniel H. Grossoehme, Justin N. Baker, Jennifer Needle, Jessica D. Thompson, Yao L. Cheng, Jiehuan Wang, and Maureen E. Lyon. 2020. Congruence Gaps Between Adolescents with Cancer and Their Families Regarding Values, Goals, and Beliefs About End-of-Life Care. *JAMA Network Open* 3 (5): e205424. https://doi.org/10.1001/jamanetworkopen.2020.5424.

Garrett, Jeremy R., John D. Lantos, Leslie G. Biesecker, Janet E. Childerhose, Wendy K. Chung, Ingrid A. Holm, Barbara A. Koenig, Jean E. McEwen, Benjamin S. Wilfond, MD, and Kyle Brothers, Clinical Sequencing Exploratory Research (CSER) Consortium Pediatrics Working Group. 2019. Rethinking the 'Open Future' Argument Against Predictive Genetic Testing of Children. *Genetic Medicine* 21 (10): 2190–2198.https://doi.org/10.1038/s41436-019-0483-4

Grootens-Wiegers, Petronella, Irma M. Hein, Jos M. van den Broek, and Martine C. de Vries. 2017. Medical Decision-Making in Children and Adolescents: Developmental and Neuroscientific Aspects. *BMC Pediatrics* 17: 120. https://doi.org/10.1186/s12887-017-0869-x.

Guichon, Juliet, Farah Mohamed, Kim Clarke, and Ian Mitchell. 2017. Autonomy and Beneficence in Assisted Dying in Canada: The Eligibility of Mature Minors. *Alberta Law Review* 54 (3): 775–802.

Hill, Douglas L., Jennifer A. Faerber, Yimei Li, Victoria A. Miller, Karen W. Carroll, Wynne Morrison, Pamela S. Hinds, and Chris Feudtner. 2019. Changes Over Time in Good-Parent Beliefs Among Parents of Children with Serious Illness: A Two-Year Cohort Study. *Journal of Pain Symptom Management* 58 (2): 190–197. https://doi.org/10.1016/j.jpainsymman.2019.04.018.

Howe, Edmund G. 2019. When Adolescents May Die. *Journal of Clinical Ethics*. 30 (2): 77–88.

Hutchinson, Anna, Melissa Midgen, and Anastassis Spiliadis. 2020. In Support of Research into Rapid-Onset Gender Dysphoria. *Archives of Sexual Behavior* 49 (1): 79–80. https://doi.org/10.1007/s10508-019-01517-9.

Ibsen, Henrik. 1882. *An Enemy of the People.* Translated by R. Farquharson Sharp. https://www.gutenberg.org/files/2446/2446-h/2446-h.htm.

Katz, Aviva L., Sally A. Webb, and Committee on Bioethics, American Academy of Pediatrics. 2016. Informed Consent in Decision-Making in Pediatric Practice. *Pediatrics* 138 (2): e20161485.

Kon, Alexander and Wynne Morrison. 2018. Shared decision-making in pediatric practice: A broad view. *Peidatrics* 42 (Suppl 3): S129-S132. https://doi.org/10.1542/peds.2018-0516B.

Lane, Susan H., and Eileen Kohlenberg. 2012. Emancipated Minors: Health Policy and Implications for Nursing. *Journal of Pediatric Nursing* 27 (5): 533–548.

Larmuseau, M.H.D., J. Vanoverbeke, A. Van Geystelen, G. Defraene, N. Vanderheyden, K. Matthys, T. Wenseleers, and R. Decorte. 2013. Low Historical Rates of Cuckoldry in a Western European

Human Population Traced by Y-Chromosome and Genealogical Data. *Proceedings of the Royal Society B* 280 (1772): 20132400. https://doi.org/10.1098/rspb.2013.2400.

Lee, Benjamin, Paul Ishimine, Madeline Joseph, and Sanjay Mehta. 2018. Evaluation and Treatment of Minors. *Annals of Emergency Medicine* 71 (2): 225–232. https://doi.org/10.1016/j.annemergmed.2017.06.039.

Lehto, Juhani E., Petri Juujärvi, Libbe Kooistra, and Lea Pulkkinen. 2010. Dimensions of Executive Functioning: Evidence from Children. *British Journal of Developmental Psychology* 21 (1): 59–80. https://doi.org/10.1348/026151003321164627.

Li, D., and C. Liao. 2008. Incidental Discovery of Nonpaternity During Prenatal Testing of Genetic Disease. *Fetal Diagnosis and Therapy* 24 (1): 39–41.

Marsh, Howard, and John Reynard. 2009. Patient Confidentiality: Ethical, Legal and Regulatory Responsibilities. *BJU International* 104 (2): 164–167.

Martinez-Horta, Saul, Jesus Perez-Perez, Erik van Duijn, Ramon Fernandez-Bobadilla, Mar Carceller, Javier Pagonabarraga, Berta Pascual-Sedano, Antonia Campolongo, Jesus Ruiz- Idiago, Frederic Sampedro, et al. 2016. Neuropsychiatric Symptoms Are Very Common in Premanifest and Early-Stage Huntington's Disease. *Parkinsonism and Related Disorders* 25 (1): 58–64.

Marshall, Jeanine, Kerry White, Marjorie Weaver, Leah Flury Wetherill, Siu Hui, Julie C. Stout, A. Johnson, M.D. Xabier Beristain, Jacqueline Gray, Joanne Wojcieszek, et al. 2007. Specific Psychiatric Manifestations Among Preclinical Huntington Disease Mutation Carriers. *Archives of Neurology* 64 (1): 116–121. https://doi.org/10.1001/archneur.64.1.116.

McCarthy, Claire. 2018. Why Teenagers Eat Tide Pods. *Harvard Health Blog*. https://www.health.harvard.edu/blog/why-teenagers-eat-tide-pods-2018013013241. Accessed 18 Jan 2008.

McGill, B.C., C.E. Wakefield, J. Vetsch, K. Barlow-Stewart, N.A. Kasparian, A.F. Patenaude, M.-A. Young, R.J. Cohn, and M. Tucker. 2019. Children and Young People's Understanding of Inherited Conditions and Their Attitudes Towards Genetic Testing: A Systematic Review. *Clinical Genetics* 95 (1): 10–22. https://doi.org/10.1111/cge.13253.

McGowan, Michelle L., Cynthia A. Prows, Melissa DeJonckheere, William B. Brinkman, Lisa Vaughn, and Melanie F. Myers. 2018. Adolescent and Parental Attitudes About Return of Genomic Research Results: Focus Group Findings Regarding Decisional Preferences. *Journal of Empirical Research in Human Research Ethics* 13 (4): 371–382. https://doi.org/10.1016/j.ajhg.2015.05.022.

Michie, Susan, Faye Bron, Martin Bobrow, and Theresa M. Marteau. 1997. Nondirectiveness in Genetic Counseling: An Empirical Study. *American Journal of Human Genetics* 60 (1): 40–47.

Myers, Melanie F., Lisa J. Martin, and Cynthia A. Prows. 2020. Adolescents' and Parents' Genomic Testing Decisions: Associations with Age, Race, and Sex. *Journal of Adolescent Health* 66 (3): 288–295.

NDAA. 2013. Minor Consent to Medical Treatment Laws. *National District Attorney's Association*. https://ndaa.org/wp-content/uploads/Minor-Consent-to-Medical-Treatment-2.pdf.

Needle, Jenifer S., Cynthia J. Peden-McAlpine, and Joan Liaschenko. 2018. Physicians' Perspectives on Adolescent and Young Adult Advance Care Planning the Fallacy of Informed Decision Making. *Journal of Clinical Ethics* 30 (2): 131–142.

Newport, Kenneth G. C. 2006. *The Branch Davidians of Waco: The History and Beliefs of an Apocalyptic Sect*. Oxford: Oxford University Press.

Pathak, Priya R., and Adriana Chou. 2019. Confidential Care for Adolescents in the U.S. Health Care System. *Journal of Patient Centered Research and Reviews* 6 (1): 46–50. https://doi.org/10.17294/2330-0698.1656.

Pereira, Stacey, Jill Oliver Robinson, Amanda M. Gutierrez, Devan K. Petersen, Rebecca L. Hsu, Caroline H. Lee, Talia S. Schwartz, et al. 2019. Perceived Benefits, Risks, and Utility of Newborn Genomic Sequencing in the BabySeq Project. *Pediatrics* 143 (Supplement 1): S6–S13. https://doi.org/10.1542/peds.2018-1099C.

Phillips, Kathryn and Katherine L. Schaefer. 2019. Annihilation of Desire in Jain Ethics as a Challenge to Western, Subjectivist Notions of Well-Being. *Science, Religion and Culture* 6 (1): 67–76. https://doi.org/10.17582/journal.src/2019.6.1.67.76.

Pla, Patrick, Sophie Orvoen, Frédéric Saudou, Denis J. David· and Sandrine Humbert. 2014. Mood Disorders in Huntington's Disease: From Behavior to Cellular and Molecular Mechanisms. *Frontiers in Behavioral Neuroscience* 8: Article 133. https://doi.org/10.3389/fnbeh.2014.00135.

Prentice, Tricia M., and Lynn Gillam. 2018. Can the Ethical Best Practice of Shared Decision-Making Lead to Moral Distress? *Journal of Bioethical Inquiry* 15 (2): 259–268.

Reddy, Diane M., Raymond Fleming, and Carolyne Swain. 2002. Effect of Mandatory Parental Notification on Adolescent Girls' Use of Sexual Health Care Services. *JAMA* 288 (6): 710–714. https://doi.org/10.1001/jama.288.6.710.

Rose, E., N. Schreiber-Agus, K. Bajaj, S. Klugman, and T. Goldwasser. 2016. Challenges of Pre- and Post-Test Counseling for Orthodox Jewish Individuals in the Premarital Phase. *Journal of Genetic Counseling* 25 (1): 18–24. https://doi.org/10.1007/s10897-015-9880-2.

Ross, Lainie Friedman, Howard M. Saal, Karen L. David, Rebecca R. Anderson, and The American Academy of Pediatrics; American College of Medical Genetics and Genomics. 2013. Technical Report: Ethical and Policy Issues in Genetic Testing and Screening of Children. *Genetics in Medicine* 15 (3): 234–245. https://doi.org/10.1038/gim.2012.176.

Salter, Erica. 2017. Conflating Capacity with Authority: Why We're Asking the Wrong Question in the Adolescent Decision-making Debate. *Hastings Center Report* 37 (1): 32–41.

Shepherd, Rowan Forbes, Tamara Kayali Browne, and Linda Warwick. 2017. A Relational Approach to Genetic Counseling for Hereditary Breast and Ovarian Cancer. *Journal of Genetic Counseling* 26 (2): 283–299.

Silber, Tomas J. 2011. Adolescent Brain Development and the Mature Minor Doctrine. *Adolescent Medicine* 22 (2): 207–212.

Steinberg, Laurence. 2013. Does Recent Research on Adolescent Brain Development Inform the Mature Minor Doctrine? *Journal of Medicine and Philosophy* 38 (3): 256–267. https://doi.org/10.1093/jmp/jht017.

Steinhausen, Hans-Christoph. 2002. The Outcome of Anorexia Nervosa in the 20th Century. *American Journal of Psychiatry* 159 (8): 1284–1293. https://doi.org/10.1176/appi.ajp.159.8.1284.

Strohmaier, Jana, Stephanie H. Witt, Josef Frank, Noemi Lemme, Laura Flatau, Fabian Streit, Jerome C. Foo, et al. 2019. Attitudes Toward the Right to Autonomous Decision-Making in Psychiatric Genetic Testing: Controversial and Context-Dependent. *American Journal of Human Genetics B Neuropsychiatric Genetics* 180 (8): 555–565. https://doi.org/10.1002/ajmg.b.32724.

Ungaru, Yoram. 2011. Making Sense of Adolescent Decision-Making: Challenge and Reality. *Adolescent Medicine* 22 (2): 195–206.

Vayena, Effy, and John Tasioulas. 2013. Genetic Incidental Findings: Autonomy Regained? *Genetics in Medicine* 15 (11): 868–870.

Wachbroit, Robert, and David Wasserman. 1995. Patient Autonomy and Value-Neutrality in Nondirective Genetic Counseling. *Stanford Law and Policy Review* 6 (2): 103–121.

Wakefield, Claire E., Lucy V. Hanlol, Katherine M. Tucker, Andrea F. Patenaude, Christina Signorelli, Jordana K. McLoone, and Richard J. Cohn. 2016. The Psychological Impact of Genetic Information on Children: A Systematic Review. *Genetics in Medicine* 18 (8): 755–762. https://doi.org/10.1038/gim.2015.181.

Warren, Samuel D., and Louis D. Brandeis. 1890. The Right to Privacy. *Harvard Law Review* 4 (5): 193–220.

Weithorn, Lois A. 2020. When Does a Minor's Legal Competence to Make Health Care Decisions Matter? *Pediatrics* 146 (Supplement 1): S25–S32. https://doi.org/10.1542/peds.2020-0818G.

Yager, Joel, Terry Carney, and Stephen Touyz. 2016. "Is Involuntary (Compulsory) Treatment Ever Justified in Patients with Severe and Enduring Anorexia Nervosa?" In *Managing Severe and Enduring Anorexia Nervosa: A Clinician's Guide*, 185–201, ed. Stephen Touyz, Daniel Le Grange, J. Hubert Lacey, and Phillipa Hay. New York: Routledge.

Chapter 12
Sexual and Reproductive Issues I: Education; Reproductive Choices

Abstract It is not necessary to invoke concepts such as reproductive rights or reproductive justice to address the needs of reproductive health. A modus vivendi based on personal and public health needs and sufficiencies will protect the needs of all in a more parsimonious way, while probably generating less conflict than do controversial assertions of reproductive right and justice. Some controversy is inevitable, as traditional pronatal views clash with an apparent need for more antinatal mores generated by adverse Anthropocene changes resulting from rapid population growth and resource consumption over several centuries. The chapter proposes a body of information that all children need to know to protect their safety. It also suggests that, for public health reasons alone (as suggested by Douglas Diekema), reproductively capable minors should be entitled to private and confidential access to prevention of conception and childbirth on the same basis as adults. The chapter discusses, but does not resolve, whether a parent should be permitted to compel the abortion of a fetus carried by a minor who is incompetent to make decisions. It also discusses the prerogative of a minor to place her child for adoption.

Western mores regarding reproduction and sexuality have drastically changed in recent years and will continue to do so. Decreased necessity and desirability of having children, combined with recent technologies that enable us to separate sexual behavior from reproduction, made changes in sexual and reproductive mores possible and attractive. Many people and groups continue to adhere to traditional beliefs. The ability to engage in sexual behavior without fear of pregnancy has expanded the possibilities for adolescent sexual behavior. I have divided the topic into two chapters because of the length of the discussion.

A. J. Jacobs, *Assigning Responsibility for Children's Health When Parents and Authorities Disagree: Whose Child?*, The International Library of Bioethics 90,
https://doi.org/10.1007/978-3-030-87698-2_12

12.1 Theoretical Considerations

Issues of reproductive rights and reproductive justice must be mentioned because of their prevalence, though I am skeptical of the existence of any deontic claims based on non-religious arguments, and I consider law to be based on *modus vivendi* constrained by constitutional limits primarily designed to protect people against the state.

The concept of reproductive rights was initially promoted in opposition to viewpoints that upheld natural law concepts of marriage (Noonan 1965), traditional roles for women and protection of embryos and fetuses from induced abortion (Marquis 1989). Initial battles looked at formal rights. Some later advocates have insisted that formal rights, leading to legal guarantees of contraceptive use and termination of pregnancy, are insufficient (Petchesky 1995). These 'reproductive justice' advocates want all reproductive services to be readily available to all. This involves a panoply of issues, including education in sexuality and control of fertility; actual access to contraception, pregnancy termination, and prenatal care (Macleod et al. 2017). Barriers to access to some services may be present even when there are no legal obstacles (Macleod et al. 2017). For example, when adolescents are covered under parental insurance, parents are notified of claims for payment, including claims for contraceptives; this may preclude minors from seeking oral contraceptives (Fuentes et al. 2018). Some would address these issues of availability in a reformist manner. Others see these issues as one of many intimately connected items in the progressive agenda, linked to as welfare, environment, violence, family structure, and prisoners' rights. The SisterSong Women of Color Reproductive Health Project is generally credited with spearheading this reproductive justice approach (Ross et al. 2001). These writers use the term reproductive justice to define what they consider a state obligation to provide universal availability of services related to the enhancement, care, and prevention of reproduction, going beyond seeking formal rights. Starrs et al. (2018), have reviewed the current status of the reproductive freedom of women.

I will not recapitulate non-consequentialist arguments for or against abortion and contraception. Diekema (2020) credibly asserts that reproductive care exemptions from parental consent requirements exist primarily for public health reasons, implying that reproductive autonomy rights discovered by judges in the course of litigation are pretextual. Federal courts have little jurisdiction over public health, but may define constitutional rights that supersede state legislation based on the *parens patriae* and police power doctrines.

What are the public health considerations? First, public health is concerned with minors at risk. Teens who engage in sexual activity without protection can acquire sexually transmitted infections. If pregnancy is a possibility (or exists), a pregnant adolescent is most tangibly affected. If a confidential and legal option is not available, pregnant teens may obtain unsafe abortions outside the medical care system, especially if they believe their parents would disapprove of either the pregnancy or an abortion. If an adolescent has a child, this will affect the prospects of the adolescent mother (and often the father) for education, livelihood, and future family life whether or not the adolescent is married. Women who give birth as teenagers are more likely than other women to be socio-economically disadvantaged (Gselamu et al. 2019) Pregnant teens are prone to be victims of domestic violence during and following pregnancy (Quinlivan and Evans 2001). The direction of causality of these adverse effects has not been determined. Children of teens are more likely to spend part of their childhood in 1-parent homes, to become teenage parents themselves, and to have intellectual deficits (Baldwin and Cain 1980). The mother's parents may have to assume many of the financial and physical burdens of raising their daughter's child. Teen pregnancy has intergenerational effects. The infant's grandparents are likely to play a major role in caring for the baby. Chen et al. (2007) in an American population-based study, reported that infants born to teenage mothers have increased risk of prematurity, low birth weight, low Apgar scores, and neonatal death. The children have worse behavioral, health, and academic outcomes than children of older mothers (Pogarsky et al. 2006), and these poor outcomes may extend to their grandchildren (Wall-Wieler et al. 2019). Such children are more likely to be involved with the criminal justice system or to be dependent on state support. Thus, there is a negative impact on an adolescent's own parents and to society at large when that adolescent gives birth.

The Indirect Effects Basis of the State Intervention test supports the minor's prerogative in seeking pregnancy prevention and limitation. To the extent that supporting the capabilities of the adolescent is important to society, parents should neither compel a pregnant daughter to give birth nor discourage her from placing the infant for adoption. Sexually mature minors should be permitted to make contraceptive choices. An exception is that minors should not be allowed to elect to have irreversible sterilization. Arguably, the Direct Effect Basis of the Test would allow a parent to authorize abortion because of the socioeconomic and possible physical harm to the adolescent in allowing a pregnancy to continue. In any event, adolescents have the prerogative to abort a pregnancy on the same basis as adults. A segment of academicians supports adult levels of sexual and reproductive freedom for adolescents (Starrs et al. 2018; Buller and Schulte 2018) I suspect, though, that most people in the Western world consider teenage childbirth to be undesirable. I would even guess that many of the scholars who promote an expansive view of adolescent rights would be quite unhappy if their 14-year old daughters gave birth. Furthermore, for actual young teens, sexual debut is likely to be involuntary. The age of sexual initiation is two years younger when initiation is forced than when it is voluntary (Hawks et al. 2019). Childhood sexual abuse or forced sexual intercourse is associated with early menarche (Zabin et al. 2005) and dating older people of the opposite sex (Marín et al. 2000) The CDC recently reported that about half of rapes of both males and females occurred under 18 years of age, with about 11 million female victims and 2 million male victims reporting involuntary sexual experiences (Smith et al. 2018). Those with involuntary sexual encounters under age 11 amounted to 1,232,000 females and 738,000 males. These undoubtedly represent gross underestimates, as a sense of shame is likely to deter young adolescents from frankness about involuntary sexual experiences (Hlavka 2017).[1]

[1] Anecdotal data suggest that at least the first episode of sexual intercourse in newly sexually mature females is forced. Women of my age raised in affluent environments have reported to me discussions

Public health authorities would generally favor programs of education and readily available services to prevent teenage motherhood, while at the same time, supporting teens who become pregnant and choose to carry the pregnancy. As for treating physicians, they should engage with adolescents (and with parents when appropriate and possible) to maximize the health of those adolescents who are pregnant—no matter what the pregnant young women choose to do. This needs to be done in the context of community norms, and in the context of the values of the patient and the patient's family, In Hohfeldian terms, pregnancy is a mixed relationship involving prerogatives of the mother, claims of the mother on resources, powers to change behavior of family members and others, and duties to the fetus and, eventually, the infant.

Reproduction is, among other things, a claim on society's resources, which we now recognize are limited. This claim cannot be categorical. This is not to say that coercive policies such as China's One Child (now Two Child) program are necessary to attain a sustainable ecosphere; that is an open question. However, we no longer can accept unsupported claims that Malthusian ideas have been discredited (Petchesky 1995).

12.2 The Physical Environment and Its Consequences

Let us try to understand the reasons for differences in views regarding sexuality and reproduction, rather than trying to label and blame those who disagree with us. Our sensibilities are not more advanced than are the sensibilities of our forebears. Rather, they probably result from recent changes in our physical environment. These changes have resulted in developed nations' seeking new norms of sexual and reproductive behavior for at least the past century.

Consider the changes in the world since my paternal grandparents were compelled by their families and custom to marry in 1886. My grandfather, Aron, was born in 1862 in a poor, remote town in the Carpathian Mountains. He married Pearl in 1879. Pearl died in 1885, shortly after the birth of her fifth child. Aron married Pearl's sister, Ethel, who was 16. This followed an inescapable local norm requiring marriage of a widower to his deceased wife's oldest unmarried sister. Ethel was only four years older than her oldest niece, who became her new stepdaughter. Ethel had to leave her secondary school and forego plans to go to university, in order to marry Aron.

Norms such as sororate marriage had important survival value at a time when families were the source of support and security for its members. A stepmother who

---

with their peers in junior high school (generally age 11–14) revealing forced sexual encounters those classmates had experienced. My informants believed that such experiences were not rare. It should be presumed that girls' sexual activity below age 15 is not voluntary. The situation with boys is murkier. Boys are unlikely to admit to anyone that they have had an involuntary sexual encounter. For some recent work on the involuntary sex that women, as well as men, inflict on young males, see Curry and Utley (2018), Depraetere et al. (2020), Ohlert et al. (2020).

also was an aunt likely would be better disposed toward her stepchildren than an unrelated stepmother would be. Throughout most of the nineteenth century most economic production depended on muscle power. Food was produced by men and by draft animals driven by men. Much cloth was handspun, and clothing was hand sewn. Death from infection, occupational accidents, and childbirth was frequent. If someone lived past the age at which she could work, she probably often depended for support on her children (Laslett 1988). Understandably, family stability and large families were desirable. Children—an economic necessity—could be conceived only through sexual intercourse. Childbirth was dangerous, with a mortality in England of 5–7 maternal deaths per 1000 live births (Chamberlain 2006). Deaths from ectopic gestations and miscarriages increased that risk. If women had to spend much of their lives and energy reproducing and nursing their children, men, who were generally larger and stronger, had to fill most economically productive jobs. Farming, mining, logging, soldiering, etc., required great strength. Epidemics, wars, and famines threatened survival[2] and reinforced the need for pronatal social arrangements. Conditions of life did not improve much through the nineteenth century. Factory labor was added to the other forms of heavy, dangerous work in which people engaged. And the crowding of urbanization increased the chances of contracting communicable disease.

Because of high childhood mortality, pronatal mores were important to survival of families and society throughout most of history. World population grew slowly until modern times (Roser et al. 2013). Norms and rules favored stable marital arrangements between a man[3] and a woman. The man ideally could father children and perform hard physical work. The woman ideally could bear and raise a sufficient number of children that some would survive to adulthood. She also performed most household chores, which were more difficult and time-consuming than they are now. The privileges of men in such a society were unquestionable, but these social arrangements had survival value at the time.

Longman (2006) describes patriarchy as a system in which marriage is normative, and men, though dominant, are invested in their children. Patriarchy arose in agricultural societies which depended on property that needed protection. Patriarchy was a powerful engine for fertility. More populous societies were able to defend themselves against, and conquer, less populous societies. Patriarchy penalizes men and women who do not marry, and disfavors children born outside marriage. It relies on norms of men marrying and caring for their families. Without such norms, patriarchy degenerates into misogyny. But when men take an interest in their children, and women devote themselves to their children, the result is creation of successive generations of many children. This perpetuated a stable society (Longman 2006).

[2] Examples of disasters that reduced national populations by at least 1/3 include the Irish famine of the 1840s (Boyle and Ó'Gráda 1986), the Thirty Years' War (1618–1648) in Germany (Outram 2001), and the plague epidemic of the 1340s (Kelly 2005).

[3] In this chapter, the terms 'man' and 'woman' refer to biological sex unless the context suggests otherwise. The terms 'male' and 'female,' used as nouns, refer to lived gender roles. The meaning of these latter two words, when used as adjectives, should be inferred from the context.

Patriarchy was not universal, and its absence weakened societies. The utility of norms of reproductive behavior can change with altered circumstances. Sparta was not patriarchal. Its ruling warrior class, the Spartiates, raised children communally and allowed women a high degree of equality. Women managed household economics without interference and owned property (Doran 2011). Impregnation of married women by Spartiates other than their husbands, was open and accepted. Spartiate economic activity was confined to waging war and managing estates worked by slaves. This system worked as long as there were not too many wars and there was land to distribute. When natural disasters and almost constant war reduced the number of Spartiate men, Spartiate mores did not foster repopulation of the Spartiate class, leading to depopulation and Sparta's ultimate decisive military defeat. Spartan society was oriented to produce elite warriors as a priority over reproduction. Antinatal norms can promote damaging population decline. So can cultural preferences for using resources for individual- or couple-oriented goals instead of for family or communal goals (Johansson 1987). The importance of demographic trends for security and for prosperity would seem to justify non-coercive policies to obtain optimal populations. Population goals and policies need to be reevaluated periodically in light of changing conditions. Present worldwide conditions may make pronatal policies inappropriate.

The biosphere may not be able to accommodate humans at a comfortable level of material well-being without marked reduction in the Earth's population. Stress on the biosphere in unquestionable (United Nations 2020). Ecological stress that threatens human survival is caused not only by greenhouse gasses, but by acidification of oceans, widespread extinction of species, depletion of fresh water supplies and of land suitable for agriculture, and loss of forest cover (Ripple et al. 2020). Chemistry Nobelist Paul Crutzen (2002) held that these human-made changes have created a new geologic era that he calls the Anthropocene. Dasgupta and Dasgupta (2017) have calculated on the basis of an economic model that the biosphere can sustain no more than 3.5 billion people if the mean individual income were to be 20,000 $US equivalents. In fact, current world population is over 7 billion, and is expected to reach 10 billion by the end of the century. The adverse effects of population growth on human and other life may pose a challenge to the current consensus regarding reproductive freedom if there is not a marked voluntary reduction in fertility in the near future.

Pronatal norms are obsolete. Globally, the population of the world in 1800 was just under a billion people (Census Bureau 2020). World population had doubled over the previous 300 years, and would double again over the next 130 years. It took 1300 years for world human population to increase an order of magnitude from 100 million, but population will have increased by another order of magnitude, to about 10 billion by 2050, four times as rapidly as it took to reach 1 billion (United Nations 2019). Some self-isolating groups, such as Chasidic Jews, Hutterite Anabaptists, and Old Amish Mennonites, have a population growth exceeding 4%. Even Mormon and conservative Protestant women now have a fertility rate no greater than 2 ½ children per woman. Almost all European nations have fertility rates below replacement.

12.3 Parents, State, Sex, and Reproduction

In the remainder of this chapter I will discuss education in sexuality and reproduction, as well as some sexual and reproductive issues. I will make some assumptions for the sake of argument, not all of which I necessarily agree with. These assumptions reflect what I believe to be the political consensus in developed nations.

I assume in this chapter that the legal consensus of developed nations reflects public opinion, except when I explicitly say otherwise. I assume that commonly used forms of contraceptive are legal and widely available, with no restrictions on non-medical grounds. I further assume that fetuses without self-consciousness or viability are not entitled to legal protection against abortion, and that women are entitled to undergo abortion without medical indication at least in the first trimester. I take it as axiomatic that termination of a previable pregnancy should be legally acceptable when continued pregnancy is significantly more dangerous to a woman than termination of that pregnancy. Finally, I assume that the state should not interfere with sexual expression unless it is non-consensual or provokes harms of the sort that invoke the Bases of the State Intervention Test.

12.3.1 Reproductive Education

It all begins with education. Minors cannot exercise their reproductive options unless they know them. The content of education in reproduction has cognitive and behavioral aspects (Duncan et al. 2008). The need for education on sex and reproduction is widely appreciated throughout the world (Leung et al. 2019; Ivanova et al. 2000) The appropriate scope of reproductive education is controversial. It is likely that progressive, educated parents would agree that education should include not just 'the birds and the bees,' but liberal attitudes toward sexual orientation, gender identity, and special needs (Breuner et al. 2016) as the American Academy of Pediatrics (AAP) recommends. However, a significant number of parents believe in *gender essentialism*—that individuals' social roles should to some degree be determined by their biological sex. This view also is inherent in traditional forms of all three of the principal Abrahamic religions, as well as in Hinduism. It is difficult to find scholarship quantitatively describing the views of the public on the validity of essentialist versus progressive ideas. Questions of whether bathrooms should be segregated by genital anatomy or by gender self-identification (Samar 2017), and whether biological males should be allowed to compete in athletics as women (Pitsiladis et al. 2016) are prominent occupants of the American political agenda.

Gender performativity—the idea that gender is socially and personally determined—dominates American intellectual life. Some facts to the contrary are patent; some people produce ova, while others produce sperm. Sperm producers tend to be larger and stronger than ovum producers. In order to reproduce, ovum producers (who, uniquely, possess uteri) must carry a fetus for nine months, and then must nurse the child (or else administer a synthetic substitute for human milk). The only biological investment of the sperm producer, however, is copulation. This does not negate the fact that women have shown themselves to be the equal of men in most economic and intellectual arenas, and have exceeded men in some; such differences in performance may be partially biologically based (Kurth et al. 2017).[4] But investigating the possibility of other biological differences that might affect social roles is not a good way to advance one's academic career. Even speculating that differences in cognitive capacities might exist is dangerous; Lawrence Summers was forced out of the Harvard presidency (Finder et al. 2006), in part for such speculation (Bloom 2005; Women in Math 2005).

Gender essentialism, like critical gender studies, can consider biological realities irrelevant. There can be moral components to gender essentialism. Some traditionalists divorce roles from capacity. They believe that women should be confined to private spaces regardless of their ability to succeed in public spheres. But Saudi Arabian or Old Amish societies are a far cry from someone like Summers, who would ask if empirical data about differences in cognitive and behavioral capacities of men and women *as groups* might result in differences in success in some areas of endeavor, differences that could favor women as well as favoring men.

Gender essentialism as a moral issue now is commonly confined to the sphere of sexual relations. Traditionalists believe that cis-heterosexuality should be the norm. But secular academicians almost universally accept homosexuality and gender incongruity (gender identification that differs from biological sex) as normal behavior. Religiously conservative parents also are likely to believe that people should confine sexual relations to marriage.

This obviously creates tension with those who believe that the only moral parameters in sexual behavior are the presence of mutual consent. Educators may want to present sexual options in a neutral manner, but may be opposed by parents who do not want certain options presented as acceptable. An extreme example of this is found in strict Jewish groups in which males and females do not interact with each other until the wedding night, and in which many have no idea regarding the sex act before marriage (Estrin 2013). Such people take exception to introducing sex education into their schools (Sherwood 2019). One American appellate court ruled that public school districts may present ideas that are offensive to students' religion, noting that public schools have an assimilative function (*Mozert v. Hawkins County Bd. Of Educ. 827* F. 2d 1058, 6th Circuit Court of Appeals, 1987). School districts have wide discretion in choosing curricula. Parents cannot opt out of a history or biology program either on grounds of dissatisfaction with their content. The *Mozert*

---

[4] Essentialism frequently is countered by destroying straw men. Phillips (2010) described essentialism as attribution of characteristics to *everyone* within a particular category. Except for characteristics that define differences (i.e., lactation and reproductive functions), almost all essentialists would say that differences apply to group averages rather than to everyone in the group. Some authors refer to speculative cringeworthy statements over a century old (Heyman and Giles 2006). Authors may also reject essentialism explicitly because it might lead to conclusions different from those the authors wish to adopt—a form of argument that reasons backwards.

judges would accept private alternatives to public education.[5] They probably would not demand, as UK government officials did (Sherwood 2019), that private schools provide sex education incompatible with the religion's beliefs. Some secular democracies provide state funding for religious schools (Department of Education 2000), but that is currently unconstitutional in the US.

I have discussed the problems related to adolescent sexual activity, including sexually transmitted diseases and pregnancy. But it is not only adolescents who are at risk of, and from, sexual activity. A literature review encompassing data from 24 nations suggests that sexual solicitation of minors, and physical abuse, are common (Barth et al. 2013). Many of these children are sexually immature. There have been numerous media reports of child grooming, sex trafficking of adolescents, and molestation by clergy, scout leaders, and teachers.

Children lacking relevant information about sexuality are especially vulnerable to dangerous consequences. For their own safety children need to understand, at an age-appropriate level, sexuality and the mechanism of reproduction. They need to acquire an appreciation of community norms regarding physical and verbal contact. Minors must learn to recognize sexual advances, and must learn and internalize strategies to deal with inappropriate or unwanted sexual advances. They need to understand that advances are not necessarily heterosexual in nature, and are not sex-or gender-specific. Many people in the area of child behavior maintain that it is important for pre-adolescents and adolescents to be taught about their own developing sexual feelings so that they will understand these feelings, and make better decisions. They should understand, in an age-appropriate manner, the possibility and consequences of sexual transmission of communicable disease. Failure to provide any of this education places children in physical danger, Failure to allow one's children to receive appropriate sex education can therefore trigger state intervention under the Direct Effects Basis of the State Intervention Test. Even Chasidic or Hutterite children can be molested, and can acquire sexually transmitted infections. Acquisition of skills for negotiating the terrain of the contemporary sexual scene is necessary for adolescents. I believe that requiring this scope of information is justified by the Direct Effects Basis. Minors capable of insemination or pregnancy should understand options for prevention of childbirth, including abortion (where abortion is legal).

Such curricula run into the problem that many parents oppose abortion, contraception, and premarital sexual relations on moral grounds. Education in sexuality must be sensitive to these viewpoints. The link between sexual intercourse and reproduction is now weak. Childbirth is preventable through contraception and pregnancy termination as well as through abstinence. Conversely, it is possible for women to become pregnant without performing a sex act. However, the availability of ways to prevent childbirth does not imply their moral acceptability. Sexual and reproduction education should not be a tool for cultural imperialism. It is possible to teach about contraception and pregnancy termination while suggesting that they may not be

[5] These assertions are based on *dicta* in the *Mozert* opinion. *Obiter dicta* are statements in judicial opinions that do not directly address the subject of the controversy at issue. They do not have precedential force, because courts are only permitted to rule on the legal issues in dispute.

appropriate alternatives. Similarly, the reality that an adolescent may receive sexual advances that are not cis-heterosexual need not be accompanied by indoctrination in a particular view of the scope of appropriate sexual activity. The ubiquity of sexual content in the media makes education all the more important. Even prepubertal children have access to pornography on the internet, which may not be accurate or psychologically healthy. They are exposed to information regarding homosexuality and gender incongruence, regardless of what their parents might wish. Schools have a role in helping children acquire accurate information and put this information into perspective.

In the US, with its decentralized education system, communities in most states have leeway in dealing with sexual issues. Districts can tailor sexual and reproductive education to community norms. Those who take exception to these norms have the option of private education or home schooling for their children, if family finances and parent availability permit. Perhaps European nations that finance religious education have the best approach to the conundrum of reconciling general beliefs with parental norms that find those beliefs objectionable.

12.3.2 Adolescent Prerogatives

What begins with education must translate into action. It is not enough to educate adolescents regarding sexuality and reproduction. Public health considerations require that all people with sufficient capacity have the options to take the same steps to control the reproductive consequences of their sexual behavior. All individuals capable of sexual activity, including minors, should have the same legal rights to control sexual expression and use of methods to prevent conception or to terminate pregnancy. In Canada this may mean pregnancy termination for all, on demand (Shaw and Norman 2020), while in Malta it may mean that there will be no elective pregnancy termination for anyone (Caruana-Finkel 2020). This position is justified by both the Indirect Effects Basis of the State Intervention Test and by the direct Effects Basis. Reproductive policy may be sufficiently important to expect less capacity as a basis for decisional competence in this area than in other areas of health care. Furthermore, the welfare of minor mothers is of interest to the state. Even in a subculture fiercely observant of traditional sexual norms, a minor can be raped by an outsider (or even an insider). The minor must be able to obtain diagnosis and treatment of sexually transmitted infections, and must have the prerogative to deal with an accidental pregnancy as she sees fit, though within legal constraints applicable to adults as well. This is an area in which the state will almost always prevail over parents.[6]

The legal systems of most Western nations have a very broad view of adolescent reproductive liberty. Pregnancy termination is legal in the United States, Canada, and in all European nations except Poland, Malta, and some microstates (Library of Congress 2020). Most European nations restrict elective pregnancy termination

[6] The extent to which the government should actively make services available is a political matter, and should be governed by *modus vivendi* and sufficientarian considerations.

to the first trimester. In the US reproductive liberty was guaranteed by *Griswold v. Connecticut*, 381 US 479, Supreme Court, 1965) and subsequent cases, and termed a right to privacy. Freedom to limit childbearing was extended to elective pregnancy termination in 1973 (*Roe v. Wade*, 410 US 113, Supreme Court, 1973). This freedom was grounded in the Due Process clause of the 14th Amendment. Federal courts relied on privacy rather than sex or gender equality as a basis for reproductive freedom.

The Supreme Court, in *Bellotti v. Baird* (443 U.S. 622, 1979, 642), observed that

> the potentially severe detriment facing a pregnant woman is not mitigated by her minority. Indeed, considering her probable education, employment skills, financial resources, and emotional maturity, unwanted motherhood may be exceptionally burdensome for a minor. In addition, the fact of having a child brings with it adult legal responsibility, for parenthood, like attainment of the age of majority, is one of the traditional criteria for the termination of the legal disabilities of minority. In sum, there are few situations in which denying a minor the right to make an important decision will have consequences so grave and indelible.

The Court permitted pregnant minors to bypass parental consent for abortion by application to a court (*Planned Parenthood v. Casey*, 505 U.S. 833, Supreme Court, 1992). This is known as *judicial bypass*.

The right to privacy in connection with decisions affecting procreation thus extends to minors as well as to adults, and should extend beyond pregnancy termination to measures to prevent conception and to treatment for sexually transmitted infections. Paradoxically, even though this care is less invasive than pregnancy termination, protection of the American adolescent seeking contraception is not as robust as with abortion.

Mechanical and hormonal contraception is legal in the United States, Canada, and all European nations. The right of a minor to obtain contraception is affirmed in *Carey v. Population Services Int'l*, 431 US 678, Supreme Court, 1977. This opinion applies to non-prescription contraceptives, but *dicta* imply that it would apply to prescription contraceptives as well. To my knowledge, the question of insertion of implanted long-acting contraceptive devices such as intrauterine devices without parental permission has not been litigated in any state. *Carey* declares that "the [Constitutional]right to privacy in connection with decisions affecting procreation extends to minors as well as to adults." (*Carey*, 693; internal citations and ellipses omitted). Thus, as Hansen and Arora (2018) suggest, implantable long-acting contraceptives should be available to minors on the same basis as they are available to adults. Furthermore, a minor who can consent to insertion should be able to consent to removal. Despite *Carey*, though, only 23 states and the District of Columbia categorically allow minors to consent to contraceptive services (Guttmacher Institute 2020). Four states have no explicit policies, and the remaining states have limitations on when minors may receive contraceptive services.

All states allow minors to seek treatment of sexually transmitted infections, but 19 of them permit the physician to inform the minor's parents if they believe this to be in the child's best interests (Guttmacher Institute 2020). States vary regarding the legal competence of minors to seek prenatal care or place their children for adoption; some of these allow physicians to notify the minor's parents. 27 states require parental notification or consent before a minor places her infant for adoption, but all have a judicial bypass procedure (Guttmacher Institute 2016). It would seem that if a woman has a categorical right to choose abortion, she certainly should have a categorical right to place an infant for adoption.

Even if they can obtain treatment without parental consent, many adolescents (Pathak and Chou 2019) obtain payment coverage from parents' insurance plans. These plans report itemized services to the policyholder (usually a parent), who often pays a share of the expense. This destroys confidentiality vis-à-vis parents for young patients whose care is financially covered by their parents' insurance plans. This may decrease utilization of services (Fuentes et al. 2018) in addition to interfering with the privacy of the young patient.[7] In nations in which all medical costs for minors bypass parents, patients may be able to maintain confidentiality regarding reproductive services. Another challenge to confidentiality is that parents generally have access to medical records. The exceptions under HIPAA are (1) if states allow minors to consent to a procedure (English and Ford 2004), (2) if the procedure is ordered by a judge; and (3) if the parent waives the right to see the medical record (Marcell et al. 2017).

Laws may vary, and may change after publication of this book, so physicians should familiarize themselves with relevant law.

Another possible challenge to privacy of a minor living at home is the occurrence of complications. The complication rate is low from abortions (Raymond and Grimes 2012), from oral contraceptives (Peragallo Urrutia et al. 2013), and from long-acting implantable contraceptives (Peterson and Curtis 2005). Nonetheless, occasional complications will occur, and parents will become aware of the circumstances if the patient is a minor for whom they are responsible.

Interestingly, *dicta* in *Carey*[8] appear to imply a right of minor girls to conceive and bear children. But philosophical and legal support for the notion that the decision to have a baby is the minor's does not acknowledge the reality of the effect that the decision has on others in a family. There is a widespread sentiment in the US that carrying a pregnancy is a more moral choice than terminating a pregnancy since abortion involves killing a unique life (whether or not that fetus is to be considered a person). Deontic reasoning would seem to dictate that if a minor may make the decision to abort a fetus then she should, a fortiori, be able to decide to continue the pregnancy. Judith Jarvis Thompson (1971) famously argued that even if a fetus is a person, there is no obligation to keep another person attached to your body in order to sustain that person's life. But Thompson's argument also implies that if you can decide to unyoke the stranger and kill him, then you also can leave the stranger attached—*if you and the stranger are the only two people whose concerns are relevant*. This argues that the minor may opt to carry her pregnancy. But other people, especially parents, have important interests in whether or not the teen carries

[7] Under the American Affordable Care Act, a child may remain on a parent's policy until age 26, so those affected may be above the age of adolescence.

[8] Readers are reminded that *dicta*, or statements in legal rulings that address issues that are not relevant to deciding the case at hand. They are not precedential, as courts rightly can rule only on matters brought before them. If courts could establish precedent on issues not brought before them, they would not be adjudicating cases—they would be legislating (Abramowicz and Stearns 2005).

the pregnancy. A decision to abort will tangibly affect the parents less than will a decision to carry the pregnancy. I am not prepared to say that parents should be able to compel an adolescent to abort a pregnancy. What of an extreme case—a pregnant 10-year-old?[9] Perhaps there are circumstances in which pregnancy is so deleterious to a child's well-being that the state should at least be permitted to order an abortion over the objection of a pregnant minor and her mother. High odds of death or blindness might be one such situation, and a very young minor mother might be another. Certainly, one who believes in clinical ethics based on resolution of conflicting prima facie principles should be reluctant to have women's (or men's) reproductive freedom prevail over any other rights in all circumstances. If a pregnant child has little or no capacity for rational reflection, then the parent should make the decision based on principles enumerated in this book. The existence of a fetus that is viable *extra utero* should receive much more deference than a pre-viable fetus.

The choice to have a baby is influenced by those around the prospective mother. There is great social influence on family size (Goldstein et al. 2003; Bornstein et al. 2017) and spacing (Duclos et al. 2019). Consider how most Western readers of this chapter would react if their daughter in university became pregnant at age 19 and decided to discontinue her education and raise the child. Most of their highly educated colleagues would regard this as odd and inappropriate. In contrast, a majority of females in sub-Saharan Africa marry before age 18 (Walker 2012).

I am not prepared to call for abortion of a minor's pregnancy against her will if that minor is fairly rational. However, unless the pregnant minor is emancipated, those who will be responsible for the care of her baby must be part of the discussion regarding whether to continue the pregnancy. There is no role for judicial bypass for a child living at home who wants to have a baby. Teen pregnancy is more than a medical issue. A team composed of the appropriate helping professions, such as psychologists and social workers, should be involved with the pregnant adolescent, the father of the fetus (if available) and the adolescent's parents (if they are willing). Ultimately, though, parents can take over as surrogates for the pregnant child only if that child is incapable of rationally evaluating the situation with *Gillick*-level competence.

12.4 Conclusion

Adolescents need to have sufficient education to be able to make reproductive choices appropriate to their age and cultural milieu, and to be able to protect themselves from sexual aggression.

Adolescents who have a rational understanding of reproductive options should be legally competent to make these decisions for themselves. Family involvement is optimal, but if the minor is afraid of repercussions from her family, she should not be required to involve them. If the minor lacks decisional capacity and is likely

[9] I have seen this several times as a physician and administrator.

to be harmed physically or otherwise by her parents, a court should make decisions with appropriate consultation. Absent an informed preference by the minor, it should be rebuttably presumed that contraception is preferable to risk of pregnancy, and that early termination of pregnancy is preferable to giving birth. This enhanced decision-making competence is based on public health considerations. Teen pregnancy substantially disadvantages the teen and it harms society overall, at least in developed societies. A pregnant minor who wants to carry a pregnancy but who is physically or emotionally unable to care for her infant may be an exception to a rule that minors should be allowed to carry a pregnancy against parental opposition.

References

Abramowicz, Michael, and Maxwell Stearns. 2005. Defining Dicta. *Stanford Law Review* 57 (4): 953–1094.

Baldwin, Wendy, and Virginia S. Cain. 1980. The Children of Teenage Parents. *Family Planning Perspectives* 12 (1): 34–43.

Barth, J., L. Bermetz, E. Heim, S. Trelle, and T. Tonia. 2013. The Current Prevalence of Child Sexual Abuse Worldwide: A Systematic Review and Meta-Analysis. *International Journal of Public Health* 58 (3): 469–483. https://doi.org/10.1007/s00038-012-0426-1.

Bloom, Stacie. 2005. In the Debate of Sex and Science, Summers, Hopkins, and the X Chromosome Battle It Out. *Journal of Clinical Investigation* 115 (5): 1107–1108. https://doi.org/10.1172/JCI25238. Accessed 30 Jan 2021.

Bornstein, Brian H., David K. DiLillo, and Hannah Dietrich. 2017. Family Size Preferences in a College Student Sample. *Open Families Studies Journal* 9 (1): 31–36. https://doi.org/10.2174/1874922401709010031.

Boyle, Phelim P., and Cormac Ó'Gráda. 1986. Fertility Trends, Excess Mortality, and the Great Irish Famine. *Demography* 23 (4): 543–562.

Breuner, Cora C., Gerri Mattson, Committee on Adolescence, and Committee on Psychosocial Aspects of Child and Family Health. 2016. Sexuality Education for Children and Adolescents. *Pediatrics* 138 (2): e20161348. https://doi.org/10.1542/peds.2016-1348.

Buller, Ana Maria, and Marie Celine Schulte. 2018. Aligning Human Rights and Social Norms for Adolescent Sexual and Reproductive Health and Rights. *Reproductive Health Matters* 26 (52): 38–45. https://doi.org/10.1080/09688080.2018.1542914.

Caruana-Finkel, Liza. 2020. Abortion in the Time of COVID-19: Perspectives from Malta. *Sexual and Reproductive Health Matters* 28 (1): 1780679. https://doi.org/10.1080/26410397.2020.1780679.

Census Bureau. 2020. Historical Estimates of World Population. United States Census Bureau. https://www.census.gov/data/tables/time-series/demo/international-programs/historical-est-worldpop.html.

Chamberlain, Geoffrey. 2006. British Maternal Mortality in the 19th and Early 20th Centuries. *Journal of the Royal Society of Medicine* 99 (1): 559–563. https://doi.org/10.1177/014107680609901113.

Chen, Xi-Kuan., Shi Wu Wen, Nathalie Fleming, Kitaw Demissie, George G. Rhoads, and Mark Walker. 2007. Teenage Pregnancy and Adverse Birth Outcomes: A Large Population Based Retrospective Cohort Study. *International Journal of Epidemiology* 36 (2): 368–373. https://doi.org/10.1093/ije/dyl284.

Crutzen, Paul J. 2002. Geology of Mankind. *Nature* 415 (6867): 23. https://doi.org/10.1038/415023a.

Curry, Tommy J., and Ebony A. Utley. 2018. She Touched Me: Five Snapshots of Adult Sexual Violations of Black Boys. *Kennedy Institute of Ethics Journal* 28 (2): 205–241. https://doi.org/10.1353/ken.2018.0014.

Dasgupta, Aisha, and Partha Dasgupta. 2017. Socially Embedded Preferences, Environmental Externalities, and Reproductive Rights. *Population and Development Review* 43 (3): 405–441.

Department of Education. 2000. Education Indicator: An International Perspective. Indicator 45: Source of Funds for Education. US Department of Education, Institute of Education Sciences, National Center for Education Statistics. https://nces.ed.gov/pubs/eiip/eiip45s1.asp. Accessed 7 Jan 2021.

Depraetere, Joke, Christophe Vandeviver, Tom Vander Beken, and Ines Keygnaert. 2020. Big Boys Don't Cry: A Critical Interpretive Synthesis of Male Sexual Victimization. *Trauma, Violence, and Abuse* 21 (5): 991–1010. https://doi.org/10.1177%2F1524838018816979

Diekema, Douglas S. 2020. Adolescent Brain Development and Medical Decision-Making. *Pediatrics* 146 (Suppl 1): S18–S24. https://doi.org/10.1542/peds.2020-0818F.

Doran, Timothy Donald. 2011. Demographic Fluctuation and Institutional Response in Sparta. Doctoral Dissertation, University of California, Berkeley, 2011. https://escholarship.org/uc/item/3pk467b6.

Duclos, Diane, Francesca L. Cavallaro, Tidiane Ndoye, Sylvain L. Faye, Issakha Diallo, Caroline A. Lynch, Mareme Diallo, Adama Faye, and Loveday Penn-Kekan. 2019. Critical Insights on the Demographic Concept of "Birth Spacing": Locating *Nef* in Family Well-Being, Bodies, and Relationships in Senegal. *Sexual and Reproductive Health Matters* 27 (1): 136–145. https://doi.org/10.1080/26410397.2019.1581533.

Duncan, Paula, Joseph F. Hagar Jr., and Judith S. Shaw. 2008. Promoting Healthy Sexual Development and Sexuality. In *Bright Futures: Guidelines for Health Supervision of Infants, Children, and Adolescents* compiled by the American Academy of Pediatrics, 169–176. Elk Grove Village, IL: American Academy of Pediatrics. https://brightfutures.aap.org/Bright%20Futures%20Documents/9-Sexuality.pdf.

English, Abagail, and Carol A. Ford. 2004. The HIPAA Privacy Rule and Adolescents: Legal Questions and Clinical Challenges. *Perspectives of Sexual and Reproductive Health* 15 (2): 80–86. https://doi.org/10.1111/j.1931-2393.2004.tb00012.x.

Estrin, Daniel. 2013. The Sex Manual for Ultra-Orthodox Jews. *BBC News*, April 21, 2013. https://www.bbc.com/news/magazine-22152700.

Finder, Alan, Patrick D. Healy, and Kate Zernike, 2006. President of Harvard Resigns, Ending Stormy 5-Year Tenure. *New York Times*, February 22, 2006. https://www.nytimes.com/2006/02/22/education/22harvard.html.

Fuentes, Liza, Megan Ingerick, Rachel Jones, and Laura Lundberg. 2018. Adolescents' and Young Adults' Reports of Barriers to Confidential Health Care and Receipt of Contraceptive Services. *Journal of Adolescent Health* 62 (1): 36–43. https://doi.org/10.1016/j.jadohealth.2017.10.011.

Goldstein, Joshua, Wolfgang Lutz, and Maria Rita Testa. 2003. The Emergence of Sub-Replacement Family Size Ideals in Europe. *Population Research and Policy Review* 22 (5): 479–496.

Gselamu, Liranso, Yoseph Dagne, Martha Gebreyohannes, and Andualem Kelebe. 2019. Psychosocial Effects of Teenage Pregnancy: Systematic Analysis. *Psychology and Behavioral Sciences* 8 (5): 115–118. https://doi.org/10.11648/j.pbs.20190805.12.

Guttmacher Institute. 2016. An Overview of Consent to Reproductive Health Services by Young People. *Guttmacher Institute*, March 14, 2016. https://www.guttmacher.org/state-policy/explore/overview-minors-consent-law.

Guttmacher Institute. 2020. Minors' Access to Contraceptive Services, December, 2020. https://www.guttmacher.org/state-policy/explore/minors-access-contraceptive-services. Accessed 9 Jan 2021.

Hansen, Rosemary T. B., and Kavita Shah Arora. 2018. Consenting to Invasive Contraceptives: An Ethical Analysis of Adolescent Decision-Making Authority for Long-Acting Reversible Contraception. *Journal of Medical Ethics* 44 (9): 585–588. https://doi.org/10.1136/medethics-2018-104855.

Hawks, Laura, Steffie Woolhandler, David U. Himmelstein, David H. Bor, Adam Gaffney, and Danny McCormick. 2019. Association Between Forced Sexual Initiation and Health Outcomes Among US Women. *AMA Internal Medicine* 179 (11): 1551–1558. https://doi.org/10.1001/jamainternmed.2019.3500.

Heyman, Gail D., and Jessica W. Giles. 2006. Gender and Psychological Essentialism. *Enfance; Psychologie, Pedagogie, Neuropsychiatrie, Sociologie* 58 (3): 293–310.

Hlavka, Heather R. 2017. Speaking of Stigma and the Silence of Shame: Young Men and Sexual Victimization. *Men and Masculinities* 20 (4): 482–505. https://doi.org/10.1177%2F1097184X16652656.

Ivanova, Olena, Masna Rai, Kristien Michielsen, and Sónia. Dias. 2000. How Sexuality Education Programs Have Been Evaluated in Low- and Lower-Middle-Income Countries? A Systematic Review. *International Journal of Environmental Research and Public Health* 17: 21. https://doi.org/10.3390/ijerph17218183.

Johansson, S. Ryan. 1987. Status Anxiety and Demographic Contraction of Privileged Populations. *Population and Development Review* 13 (3): 439–470. https://doi.org/10.2307/1973134.

Kelly, John. 2005. *The Great Mortality: An Intimate History of the Black Death, the Most Devastating Plague of All Time*. New York: Harper Collins.

Kurth, Florian, Lutz Jancke, and Eileen Luders. 2017. The Sexual Dimorphism of Broca's Region: More Gray Matter in Female Brains in Brodmann Areas 44 and 45. *Journal of Neuroscience Research* 95 (1/2): 626–632. https://doi.org/10.1002/jnr.23898.

Laslett, Peter. 1988. Family, Kinship and Collectivity as Systems of Support in Pre-Industrial Europe: A Consideration of the 'Nuclear-Hardship' Hypothesis. *Continuity and Change* 3 (2): 153–175. https://doi.org/10.1017/S026841600000093X.

Leung, Hildie, Daniel T. L. Shek, Edvina Leung, and Esther Y. W. Shek. 2019. Development of Contextually-relevant Sexuality Education: Lessons from a Comprehensive Review of Adolescent Sexuality Education Across Cultures. *International Journal of Environmental Research and Public Health* 16: 21. https://doi.org/10.3390/ijerph16040621.

Library of Congress. 2020. Abortion Legislation in Europe. https://www.loc.gov/law/help/abortion-legislation/europe.php.

Longman, Phillip. 2006. The Return of Patriarchy. *Foreign Policy* 153: 56–65.

Macleod, Catriona Ida, Sian Beynon-Jones, and Merran Toerien. 2017. Articulating Reproductive Justice through Reparative Justice: Case Studies of Abortion in Great Britain and South Africa. Culture, Health, and Sexuality 19 (5): 601–615. https://doi.org/10.1080/13691058.2016.1257738.

Marcell, Arik V., Gail R. Burstein, and American Academy of Pediatrics Committee on Adolescence. 2017. Sexual and Reproductive Health Care Services in the Pediatric Setting. *Pediatrics* 140 (5): e20172858. https://doi.org/10.1542/peds.2017-2858.

Marín, Barbara Vanoss, Karin K. Coyle, Cynthia A. Gomez, Scott C. Carvajal, and Douglas B. Kirby. 2000. Older Boyfriends and Girlfriends Increase Risk of Sexual Initiation in Young Adolescents. *Journal of Adolescent Health* 27 (6): 409–418.

Marquis, Don. 1989. Why Abortion is Immoral. *Journal of Philosophy* 86 (4): 183–202. https://doi.org/10.2307/2026961.

Noonan, John T. Jr. 1965. *Tokos* and *Atokion*: An Examination of Natural Law Reasoning against Usury and against Contraception; Note. Natural Law Forum. Paper 109. http://scholarship.law.nd.edu/nd_naturallaw_forum/109. Accessed 15 Dec 2020.

Ohlert, Jeaninne, Thea Rau, Bettina Rulofs, and Marc Allroggen. 2020. Comparison of Elite Athletes' Sexual Violence Experiences in and Outside Sport. *German Journal of Exercise and Sport Research* 50 (4): 435–443. https://doi.org/10.1007/s12662-020-00678-3.

Outram, Quentin. 2001. The Socio-Economic Relations of Warfare and the Military Mortality Crises of the Thirty Years' War. *Medical History* 45 (2): 151–184.

Pathak, Priya R., and Adriana Chou. 2019. Confidential Care for Adolescents in the U.S. Health Care System. *Journal of Patient-Centered Research and Reviews* 6 (1): 46–50. https://doi.org/10.17294/2330-0698.1656.

Peragallo Urrutia, Rachel, Remy R. Coeytaux, Amanda J. McBroom, Jennifer M. Gierisch, Laura J. Havrilesky, Patricia G. Moorman, William J. Lowery, et al. 2013. Risk of Acute Thromboembolic Events with Oral Contraceptive Use: A Systematic Review and Meta-analysis. *Obstetrics and Gynecology* 122 (2, Part 1): 380–389. https://doi.org/10.1097/AOG.0b013e3182994c43

Petchesky, Rosalind Pollack. 1995. From Population Control to Reproductive Rights: Feminist Fault Lines. *Reproductive Health Matters* 3 (6): 152–161. https://doi.org/10.1016/0968-8080(95)90172-8.

Peterson, Herbert B., and Kathryn M. Curtis. 2005. Long-Acting Methods of Contraception. *New England Journal of Medicine* 353 (20): 2169–2175. https://doi.org/10.1056/NEJMcp044148.

Phillips, Anne. 2010. What's Wrong with Essentialism? *Distinktion: Journal of Social Theory* 11 (1): 47–60. https://doi.org/10.1080/1600910X.2010.9672755.

Pitsiladis, Yannis, Joanna Harper, Jonathan Ospina Betancurt, Maria-Jose. Martinez-Patino, Attilio Parisi, Guan Wang, and Fabio Pigozzi. 2016. Beyond Fairness: The Biology of Inclusion for Transgender and Intersex Athletes. *Current Sports Medicine Reports* 15 (6): 386–388. https://doi.org/10.1249/JSR.0000000000000314.

Pogarsky, Greg, Terence P. Thornberry, and Alan J. Lizotte. 2006. Developmental Outcomes for Children of Young Mothers. *Journal of Marriage and Family* 68 (2): 332–344.

Quinlivan, Julie A., and Sharon F. Evans. 2001. A Prospective Cohort Study of the Impact of Domestic Violence on Young Teenage Pregnancy Outcomes. *Journal of Pediatric and Adolescent Gynecology* 14 (1): 17–23.

Raymond, Elizabeth G., and David A. Grimes. 2012. The Comparative Safety of Legal Induced Abortion and Childbirth in the United States. *Obstetrics & Gynecology* 119 (2 Part 1): 215–219. https://doi.org/10.1097/AOG.0b013e31823fe923.

Ripple, William J., Christopher Wolf, Thomas M. Newsome, Phoebe Barnard, and William R. Moomaw. 2020. World Scientists' Warning of a Climate Emergency. *BioScience* 70 (1): 8–12. https://doi.org/10.1093/biosci/biz088.

Roser, Max, Hannah Ritchie, and Esteban Ortiz-Ospina. 2013. World Population Growth. Published online at OurWorldInData.org. https://ourworldindata.org/world-population-growth.

Ross, Loretta J., Sarah L. Brownlee, Dázon Dixon Diallo, Luz Rodriguez, and Latina Roundtable. 2001. The SisterSong Collective: Women of Color, Reproductive Health, and Human Rights. *American Journal of Health Studies* 17 (2): 79–88.

Samar, Vincent J. 2017. The Right to Privacy and the Right to Use the Bathroom Consistent with One's Gender Identity. *Duke Journal of Gender Law and Policy* 24 (1): 33–59.

Shaw, Dorothy, and Wendy V. Norman. 2020. When There Are No Abortion Laws: A Case Study of Canada. *Best Practice and Research: Clinical Obstetrics and Gynaecology* 62 (1): 49–62. https://doi.org/10.1016/j.bpobgyn.2019.05.010.

Sherwood, Harriet. 2019. Sex Education Rules Could Force Haredi Jews into Home Schooling. *The Guardian*, January 20, 2019. http://www.theguardian.com/education/2019/jan/20/ultra-orthodox-haredi-jews-resist-new-sex-education-guidance.

Smith, Sharon G., Xinjian Zhang, Kathleen C. Basile, Melissa T. Merrick, Jing Wang, Marcie-jo Kresnow, and Jieru Chen. 2018. The National Intimate Partner and Sexual Violence Survey: 2015 Data Brief—Updated Release. National Center for Injury Prevention and Control, Centers for Disease Control and Prevention. https://www.cdc.gov/violenceprevention/datasources/nisvs/2015NISVSdatabrief.html?CDC_AA_refVal=https://www.cdc.gov/violenceprevention/nisvs/2015NISVSdatabrief.html.

Starrs, Ann M., Alex C. Ezeh, Gary Barker, Alaka Basu, Jane T. Bertrand, Robert Blum, Awa M. Coll-Seck, et al. 2018. Accelerate Progress—Sexual and Reproductive Health and Rights for All: Report of the Guttmacher—Lancet Commission. *Lancet* 391 (10140): 2642–2692. Accessed 29 June 2021.

Thompson, Judith Jarvis. 1971. A Defense of Abortion. *Philosophy and Public Affairs* 1 (1): 47–66.

United Nations. 2019. World Population Prospects 2019, Online Edition. Revision 1. United Nations, Department of Economic and Social Affairs, Population Division. http://creativecommons.org/licenses/by/3.0/igo/. See also World Population Prospects: The 2019 Revision (XLS).

Population Division of the Department of Economic and Social Affairs of the United Nations Secretariat. June 2019. Accessed 8 July 2019

United Nations. 2020. Climate Change. Peace, Dignity, and Equality on a Healthy Planet. January 11, 2016. https://www.un.org/en/sections/issues-depth/climate-change/.

Walker, Judith Ann. 2012. Early Marriage in Africa: Trends, Harmful Effects and Interventions. *African Journal of Reproductive Health* 16 (2): 231–240.

Wall-Wieler, Elizabeth, Janelle Boram Lee, Nathan Nickel, and Leslie Leon Roos. 2019. The Multigenerational Effects of Adolescent Motherhood on School Readiness: A Population-Based Retrospective Cohort Study. *PLoS ONE* 14: e0211284. https://doi.org/10.1371/journal.pone.0211284.

Women in Math. 2005. Aftermath of Gender Gap Remarks by Harvard President Summers. Blog: Women in Math. https://pages.uoregon.edu/wmnmath/Summers/index.html.

Zabin, Laurie Schwab, Mark R. Emerson, and David L. Rowland. 2005. Childhood Sexual Abuse and Early Menarche: The Direction of Their Relationship and Its Implications. *Journal of Adolescent Health* 36 (5): 393–400. https://doi.org/10.1016/j.jadohealth.2004.07.013.

Chapter 13
Sexual and Reproductive Issues II: Departures from Binary Sexual and Gender Viewpoints

Abstract This chapter addresses phenomena seen in children that represent departure from a gender essentialist viewpoint. This is the idea that normal people can be categorized as male or female, and that social behavior should ordinarily follow from biological sex. Gender essentialism is integral to most traditional religious and philosophical systems, but is now almost excluded from many academic and professional forums. This chapter discusses gender incongruity, and disorders of sexual differentiation, as examples of challenges to the gender essentialist viewpoint.

This chapter will discuss minors whose physiology or behavior is inconsistent with sexual and gender essentialism. There is controversy as to how to regard these states, and how to treat them. I will first raise some theoretical issues.

13.1 Variation, Disease, or Immorality?

Should a feature such as an enlarged clitoris or the desire of an anatomic male with an XY genotype to be treated as a woman be considered normal, diseased, or immoral? We first must define disease. There are two paradigms and intermediate attempts at definition. Some consider disease to be a natural phenomenon (Boorse 2014). Others regard illness as a social construct (Margolis 1976; Goosens 1980) These positions are called, respectively, *naturalism* and *normativism*.

Christopher Boorse (2014) defines disease in terms of departure from normal function. Normality is defined as *biostatistical* typicality for a class such as species, sex, or developmental status (child, adult, etc.). A disease is a state in which a functional ability of one part of an organism is reduced. A healthy 20-year-old should be able to walk and to run, but is not expected to be able to run a marathon. A healthy 80-year-old may not be able to run, but should be able to walk. And statistical rarity is not necessarily departure from health, such as a person whose eyes each are a different color. Not all disease needs to be remedied.

A. J. Jacobs, *Assigning Responsibility for Children's Health When Parents and Authorities Disagree: Whose Child?*, The International Library of Bioethics 90,
https://doi.org/10.1007/978-3-030-87698-2_13

Defining diseases normatively also has its problems. Consider that political dissidents were often hospitalized for 'sluggish schizophrenia' in the USSR, (van Voren 2010). Hybrid theories considering physiological abnormalities combined with normative elements have been proposed (Wakefield 1992; Powell and Scaiffe 2019). Jerome Wakefield (2007), coined a *harmful dysfunction* definition of disease, stating that both dysfunction and generally perceived harm must be present to characterize a state as a disorder. Disease may be mild, such as colorblindness (Wakefield and Conrad 2020). Furthermore, harm does not mean net harm, as when vaccinia infection prevents subsequent smallpox. I accept Wakefield's view, with the stipulation that a harm which defines a disease can affect either the person with the condition or someone else—consider sociopathy or Typhoid Mary (Brooks 1996). This is also consistent with the Indirect Effects Basis of the State Intervention Test. Disease, then, can be contextual, sometimes based on perception of harm or possibility of actual harm. Inability to synthesize a molecule vital to life is a disease when the nutrient is not found in the available diet, but it is not a disease when that nutrient is present. It is not too much of a leap to consider that the way in which a society regards gender incongruence likely will depend on the importance to that society of reproduction. A society that depends on high levels of reproduction for its success will adopt norms that promote conception and childbirth. If perceived as involuntary, sexual behavior not directed toward reproduction may be categorized as a disease. The behavior may be considered immoral if the deviation is attributed to voluntary behavior.

The medical profession has conflicting norms in this regard. When someone who desires children is involuntarily infertile, the affected individual often seeks medical care. Those who treat infertile individuals who voluntarily seek fertility are inclined to view it as a disease (Dupree 2018). This position is endorsed by the American Medical Association and the World Health Organization. One of the reasons for arguing that infertility is a disease is rhetorical—to justify its coverage by payors. But if infertility is a disease, then does one create a disease by performing surgery or giving hormones that destroy fertility? Provided the preferences of the recipient of gender-affirming medical treatment are stable—i.e., that the recipient will not rue the choice later—that person will not experience harm. On the other hand, someone involuntarily incapable of reproduction does experience harm from her condition.

Behavior that is voluntary, and that many people disapprove of, is often categorized as immoral. Most contemporary religions arose in an era when a pronatal stance was important enough for survival of individuals and groups to have moral implications. The Hebrew Bible (Leviticus 20:13), New Testament (1 Timothy 1:10), and Koran (7 [Surat Al-A'rāf]: 80–81) explicitly proscribe male same-sex copulation. Catholicism, conservative Protestantism, Eastern Orthodoxy, Islam, and Judaism consider male homosexual behavior immoral (Hildebrandt 2015). Liberals in Abrahamic traditions have modified their views regarding the immorality of homosexuality (Greenberg 2004; van den Akker et al. 2013; Alipour 2017).

Until 1973, American psychiatry was divided by three competing theories regarding male homosexuality: pathology, immaturity, and normal variation (Drescher 2015). Spurred by homosexual activists within and outside the organization, the American Psychiatric Association voted to remove homosexuality from the DSM as a mental disorder. This episode clearly shows that that characterization of a phenomenon as a disease has a normative component. People must consider a phenomenon to be a disease for it to be characterized as such. Homosexuality met the Boorse criteria of a state shared by a minority of people with a functional deficit in reproductive capacity. However, the normative criteria changed.

The remainder of this chapter will consider two conditions whose status has been in play. *Gender incongruence*, the adoption of public sex roles that differ from biological sex, has been designated in various times and places as normal, diseased, immoral, and even criminal. Ambiguous genital anatomy has variously been called disease, disability, and simple variant.

13.2 Gender Incongruence

As early as 1993, Fausto-Sterling (1993) called for an end to binary classification of people as either male or female. *Transgender*, as used here, is social identification as a member of the opposite sex, while *gender nonconforming* denotes gender expression that is not unambiguously male or female. *Gender dysphoria* is distress or impairment in functioning resulting from gender incongruence. Although a majority of those with gender incongruence are transsexual, many are non-binary, and the number of such individuals appears to be increasing (Richards et al. 2016; Koehler et al. 2018). Gender nonconformity has not been as well-studied as transgender states, and there is no consensus regarding medical treatment (Richards et al. 2016).

A prominent academic obstetrician posted this dialog on Twitter:

> Pt – Is this the ultrasound where I find out #gender? We are having a #GenderRevealParty
>
> Me – "well you will need to wait a few years for that. But you will find out the sex and whether the heart, brain, and other organs are structurally normal."

Two questions: First, is it obligatory for physicians to adopt, for professional purposes, the notions of gender as being fluid, divorced from biological sex, and possibly neither male nor female? Second, how should physicians deal with parents and families that have a traditional binary view of sexuality, and who espouse *gender essentialism* (the idea that social roles should align with a classification of people as biologically male or female)?

All mainstream Western medical organizations of which I am aware whose members engage in treatment of sexuality and reproduction have taken positions averring that gender is divorced from sexuality, that gender need not be binary, and that gender incongruence should not be regarded as pathological. (e.g., Rafferty et al. 2018). Physicians in the Western world who disagree with this characterization probably would be well-advised to either refer gender dysphoric patients elsewhere for care, or to separate their personal beliefs from their medical practice.

13.2.1 Natural History

Gender incongruity is inversely correlated with age. One advocacy organization calculates that 0.7% of Americans from ages 13–17 identify as gender incongruent, compared to 0.5% of those over 65 years old (Herman et al. 2017). These figures are comparable to statistics reported from other Western nations (Arcelus et al. 2015).

There is little question that gender incongruent persons are stigmatized. Gender incongruent individuals are more likely than the general US population to have experienced domestic and sexual violence, depression, suicide attempts, expulsion from their home (or leaving home because of hostility), and problems in school. They are more likely to have attempted suicide, used illegal drugs, or dropped out of school before completing a diploma or degree (Kaltiala-Heino et al. 2018). Though most parents are supportive of their gender incongruent children and their choices (James et al. 2016), those parents who are not supportive can have a profound negative impact on the physical and mental well-being of their gender incongruent child (Kaltiala-Heino et al. 2018). Siblings' attitudes tend to echo those of the parents.

Peer groups are another story. Competition for friends and a place in social hierarchy is a constant feature of adolescence (Redhead et al. 2021). Competition is based on prestige and intimidation. Any sort of non-conformity can place adolescents at a disadvantage. Physical and verbal bullying directed against gender incongruent youth is common (Clark et al. 2014, Kaltiala-Heino et al. 2018).

Gender non-conforming youth are likely to have fewer friends and fewer opportunities for sexual expression. If they are taking puberty-blocking hormones their physical immaturity is likely to affect their peer relationships in myriad ways (Schulz and Sisk 2016; Cardoos et al. 2017). Much child and adolescent behavior is directed toward a struggle for resource control (Hawley 2015).[1] Strategies for social dominance consist of prosocial and coercive strategies. The simultaneous use of both is the most successful among both males and females (Vermande et al. 2018). Aggression is associated with popularity and social dominance (Pellegrini et al. 2011). Being relegated to a submissive role can lead to unhappiness, stress, and long-term habits of submission (Hawley 2015). High levels of testosterone and size have been associated with social dominance in boys, with cortisol (associated with stress and anxiety) likely blunting these effects (Knight et al. 2020). People with atypical sexual presentation or behavior are at a disadvantage in the fierce world of adolescent status competition and group formation. Requirements that teens act civilly in school and other organized activities are gratifying, but they will not change the constant battle for social status that (as we all should recall) is a dominant feature of life as an adolescent.

Serious psychiatric diagnoses appear to be more common among gender incongruent children and adolescents than among cisgender individuals. There is higher prevalence of autism spectrum disorders among gender-non-conforming individuals

---

[1] That is also true of child and adult behavior, of course. Evolving sexuality adds a new dimension and a sense of urgency to this, however.

than is present in the general population (Strang et al. 2014). There is a high incidence of both affective disorders and of personality disorders in patients with gender incongruence (Hepp et al. 2005), as well as a higher frequency of self-harm in gender incongruent minors (Peterson et al. 2017). The directionality of the relationship between gender incongruence and psychiatric illness has not been established.

The etiology and natural history of gender incongruence are poorly understood. It has been proposed, for example, that there are at least two variants of male-to female transgenderism (Lawrence 2017). One variant is androphilic, or being exclusively attracted to males. The other variant results in a variety of kinds of gender preference. These people are said to manifest autogynephilia, which is the disposition of a biologic man to be sexually aroused by thinking of himself as a female (Blanchard 1989). The concept of autogynephilia is controversial. Furthermore, there have been recent reports of female-to-male transgenderism in teenagers arising with no prior signs, often occurring in multiple members of a social circle, perhaps mutually reinforcing and further reinforced by cybermedia (Marchiano 2017; Littman 2018; Hutchinson et al. 2020). These authors postulate social contagion. This is contemporaneous with a rapid change in sex ratio of adolescents presenting for care of gender dysphoria. The evidence for rapid-onset gender dysphoria with social contagion as an etiological factor has been challenged (Restar 2020). If such rapid-onset gender incongruence exists, it may arise from multiple etiologies. The understanding of the etiology of gender incongruence is in its infancy.

The natural history of childhood gender incongruence is not well understood either. Available evidence strongly suggests that the large majority of children expressing transgender identification eventually will 'desist' to identification with their natal sex (Drescher et al. 2016). It is not possible to tell conclusively which children will persist in transgender behavior and which will desist. However, the intensity of transgender identification in childhood seems to be correlated with persistence (Steensma et al. 2013). It is possible that parental reinforcement of gender incongruity is associated with persistence (Fast and Olson 2018). Many desisters appear to revert to cisgender presentation with a homosexual sexual orientation (Priest 2019).

13.2.2 Treatment

Drescher et al. (2016) characterize three possible treatment strategies for gender incongruity in children. One, called *gender affirmation* (Rafferty et al. 2018) encourages children to affirm the incongruent gender identity. The child's transgender identity is accepted and reinforced with early social transition to the gender opposite natal sex. Social transition means overt identification with gender identity, such as name changes, wearing clothing associated with perceived gender, etc. Gender affirmation is based on the presumption that this is associated with better mental health. Some evidence has been published to support this hypothesis (Olson et al. 2016). The concern is that many of these children will desist anyway—perhaps 80% of boys. The preferability of gender affirmation is based on two assumptions. First, that transgender persistence to adulthood is not inferior to desistence in terms of flourishing. Second, it assumes that children who socially transition but later revert to gender identification congruent with their biological sex will not be worse off than if they had not socially transitioned as children (Drescher et al. 2016). There is no decisive empirical evidence to support or refute either of these contentions. Furthermore, gender affirmation is based on an assumption, or at least a hope, that being a member of a gender minority will not lead to permanent setbacks in various facets of flourishing unrelated to sexual and social, and occupational adjustment.

The second treatment strategy is called *watchful waiting*. Formal social transitioning is delayed past childhood. This option is an acceptable option to gender affirmation, at least in Europe (van de Grift et al. 2020). It differs from gender affirmation in that social transitioning is discouraged in pre-pubescent children, and possibly in early adolescence. Children are not discouraged in their gender-incongruent behavior, though, and therapists encourage parents to facilitate their children's either continuing their incongruous gender identification or assuming a gender compatible with their assigned sex at birth. The watchful waiting approach is intended to allow the child easily to persist or desist, while minimizing stress arising from differences between a child's feelings about him or herself and how that child is expected to behave.

The last approach, *promotion of gender identification with natal sex* is discouraged in the US and Western Europe.

As a child approaches adolescence, endogenous hormones will stimulate development of primary and secondary sex characteristics consistent with natal sex. Strong transgender identification in childhood is likely to be associated with gender persistence, as are gender dysphoria persistent in adolescence, and social transition in childhood (Shumer et al. 2016). Minors are psychosocially supported using a strategy of either gender affirmation (as supported by the American Academy of Pediatrics; see Rafferty et al. 2018) or of watchful waiting (as currently recommended by the World Professional Association for Transgender Health (Coleman et al. 2012) and the Endocrine Society (Hembree et al. 2009). Medical adjunctive treatment may be appropriate with either of these approaches as a child enters adolescence. Puberty blockers (GnRH agonists) should be considered—certainly if dysphoria is present or if the child seems confident in his or her gender identification. Hormone therapy should be given only in the context of a program of holistic medical and psychosocial care. Transgender children should be counseled regarding future fertility before hormone treatment is given, and perhaps encouraged to bank gametes. Few adolescents do this, unfortunately (Chen et al. 2017). The main concerns of treatment with GnRH agonists are osteoporosis, possible infertility, and the social stigma of sexual immaturity. Such treatment is said to be psychologically beneficial overall (de Vries et al. 2014). When the minor reaches the age of legal competence, puberty-inducing hormones compatible with the child's gender identification are a therapeutic option. Surgery should ordinarily be deferred until adulthood.

Legal affirmation should take place only when gender stability is probable, and in accordance with local law. Clinicians should be aware of local law that might limit their therapeutic options. Legal changes are not necessarily in the direction of liberalization. A recent English case, *Bell v Tavistock*, [2020] EWHC 3274 (Admin),[2] held that minors under age 16 are unlikely to be *Gillick*-competent to consent to puberty blocking treatment, and all but required clinicians to obtain a court order before initiating such treatment. The court held (¶137) that a child cannot adequately understand the consequences of gender affirmation without having undergone puberty, whose changes are part of understanding one's gender identity. Also, informed consent would require an understanding of the risks, benefits, and alternatives of cross-sex hormones, since most of these minors eventually take them (¶138). The court concluded that, because of the uncertain effects of hormonal management of gender incongruity, even minors 16 years and older must have a court hearing before receiving puberty blockers (¶146–147, 152). This opinion has been appealed.

Adolescence is a time of turmoil and experimentation (Evans 2020). Furthermore, many gender-incongruent youth have other significant psychological issues, which may precede their gender incongruence rather than arise from it. All adolescents are anxious and confused about their sexuality. Gender issues have become highly politicized. It is not only religious conservatives who are active in the political arena. Progressive advocacy groups also attempt to control the gender agenda. Neither they nor religious conservatives seek to be objective, and there have been attacks on opponents' livelihoods. The removal of Kenneth Zucker as head of the Toronto Center for Addiction and Mental Health under pressure from activists is a case in point.[3] Those who practice in this area or who offer opinions are aware that it is a minefield in which activists seek to discredit their opponents and, at times, seek to destroy their careers (Pilgrim and Entwhistle 2020). In this context, I discuss situations in which vulnerable adolescents with gender incongruence must deal with unaccepting parents.

13.2.3 When the Patient Is from an Unaccepting Family or Milieu

The rationale for a gender affirmation approach, as opposed to a watchful waiting approach, is that its psychological results are said to be superior in young people, especially if the family is accepting of the gender transition (de Vries et al. 2014). It is not clear, however, whether the serious reported problems, including a high rate of suicidal ideation and attempts (Aitken et al. 2016; Peterson et al. 2017) and depression is due to intrinsic factors, a general dissatisfaction with one's body and

---

[2] The text of the opinion is available at https://www.judiciary.uk/wp-content/uploads/2020/12/Bell-v-Tavistock-Judgment.pdf (accessed 13 January, 2021).

[3] Zucker sued over his firing. Ontario settled the lawsuit, issuing an apology, correcting untrue statements it used, in part, as a basis for firing Zucker, and paying Zucker a settlement CA, $ 586.000. After his firing, Zucker continued to collaborate with prominent people in the field, and remains editor of the Archives of Sexual Behavior. The Ontario government had closed the service after firing Zucker, thereby avoiding a decision as to whether to rehire Zucker.

self (Peterson et al. 2017), or to an unfriendly and unsupportive environment (de Vries et al. 2014; Shiffman et al. 2016). Most clinicians employ watchful waiting, gender affirmation, or a combination of the two, as a psychosocial basis for their practice. Use of puberty blockers is theoretically compatible with either approach, though the blocked teen must negotiate the social aspects of adolescence as one who is not sexually mature.

Parents, for a variety of reasons, may not accept treatment that envisions their children assuming an adult gender incongruity. Many parents, with appropriate counseling, come to support, or at least accept, their children's gender journey. Many parents have beliefs that make it difficult for them to accept gender behavior discordant from natal sex.

In other cases, the matter will come to the attention of health care professionals because of harm or incipient harm to a minor. The legal systems of Western nations do not consider gender incongruity to be harmful to society, so the Indirect Effects Basis of the State intervention Test is irrelevant. The stigma of gender incongruence, and the limitation in the number of available sexual partners,[4] are insufficient to invoke the Direct Effects Basis. Treatments available to minors do not include surgery, it has not been firmly established whether puberty blocking drugs permanently affect physiologic reproductive capacity. Medical standards have accepted psychosocial treatment that might cause or promote irreversible gender identification in a manner that impairs or destroys fertility.[5] That leaves possible physical harm as the only issue relevant to the Direct Effects Basis. Possible complications of puberty arrest include hypothyroidism (Naderi et al. 2019), osteoporosis, and arrest of fertility, genital development, capacity for full sexual function and brain development (Laidlaw et al. 2019). Long-term follow-up of the Dutch cohort and other populations of people treated with hormones from pubescence probably will educe the long-term effects of prolonged puberty delay.

Dubin et al. (2020) would seek court intervention when there is domestic violence as a result of gender issues, or when a child engages in self-harm, or is likely to, as a result of gender dysphoria. This seems appropriate. All children with gender dysphoria require in-depth psychological evaluation and treatment, in which parents often should be involved. In dealing with families, clinical judgment requires sensitivity and flexibility. Child behavior that would be managed by gender affirmation in a family that treasured gender variety might better be treated with watchful waiting in a family committed to gender essentialism, in order to preserve the child's relationship with his family in the long run. Whatever the beliefs of the physician, the family and its beliefs should be treated with respect. The clinician's concern is the safety of the child.

Unrelated to clinical decisions, physicians and other citizens should be committed to programs of clinical and basic investigations aimed at elucidating the causes and

---

[4] I have argued earlier in other contexts that maximization of present or future choice is not a sufficient reason for interfering with parents' decisions regarding their children.

[5] Paradoxically, many of the same professionals who support gender-affirming treatment vehemently oppose genital modification for ritual reasons.

natural history of the various facets of gender variation, and to finding ways to promote flourishing of children and adolescents who express gender incongruity. As a thorough understanding of the biology (Hilton and Lundberg 2021) and neurophysiology (e.g., Skorska et al. 2021) of gender incongruence emerges, we can anticipate that treatment options will broaden and that flourishing of youth with gender incongruity will be enhanced.

13.3 Children with Differences (or Disorders) of Sexual Differentiation (DSD)

I will conclude this chapter with a discussion of children whose bodies do not fully conform to male or female anatomy and physiology. The term *disorders of sexual development or differences of sexual development* (DSD) is preferable to 'intersex'.

Men presumptively have the ability to produce sperm, transfer it to women via their urethras, and fertilize their ova. Women presumptively have the ability to produce ova, copulate with men, and carry fertilized ova in their uteri to give birth to a child. A defining characteristic of DSD is that it is present at birth, though it might not be identified at birth. Frequency of DSD has been estimated at 1 in 5,000 that can be identified at birth (Shteyler et al. 2020), to 2% (Blackless et al. 2000) based on all detectable abnormalities, clinically significant or otherwise.

Sexual assignment has been of primary importance in almost all societies, most likely because of the supreme importance of reproduction. The frequent presence of physiologically unimportant variations from a complete male or female phenotype and genotype (Ainsworth 2015), such as with a vestigial uterus located in the inguinal canal of a 70-year-old father of four (Sherwani et al. 2014) is minimally important. The ability to present oneself as a desirable member of one's sex is important to social, mating (Walter et al. 2020), and occupational (Elkins 2020) success. An attractive physique is an important determinant in human mating choice (Kordsmeyer et al. 2018; Perilloux and Cloud 2019; Zhang et al. 2019).

There are multiple reasons why parents might have a strong preference for children whose physical appearance is characteristically male or female. One is an innate or strongly conditioned human response to physical cues associated with masculinity or femininity. Another is the desire of parents to see children achieve social, economic, sexual, and reproductive success. Parents may believe, with reason, that a child with DSD would be happier, more fulfilled, and generally flourish more with typical anatomy and physiology. This has led to the frequent use of surgery to change the intersex child's anatomy to conform to an appearance more typical of a paradigmatic sex. There are several forms of surgery, each adapted to a specific condition, and most having several alternative technical approaches. Congenital adrenal hyperplasia, a syndrome in genetic females that results in androgen production and clitoral enlargement, (Speiser and White 2003), often is treated by surgically reducing clitoral size by excising corpora cavernosa important in sexual arousal. Another approach is to spare the cavernosa, separating it from the glans and the rest of the shaft, and anchoring it beneath the labial skin (Creighton et al. 2012). Vaginoplasty may be performed as required to construct or expand a vagina to allow coitus, and is best deferred until maturity when anatomic conditions are more favorable and the patient is more likely to practice the vaginal dilatation that is initially required. Both vaginoplasty and vaginal dilatation appear to be successful in creating a coital vagina (Callens et al. 2014). Hypospadias repair in males should be performed, if at all, by 18 months for the best surgical success and the lowest complication rate (Creighton et al. 2012). Gonadal removal for undescended testes is warranted in those conditions in which the rate of gonadal cancer is high (Gardner and Sandberg 2018) as in some forms of gonadal dysgenesis (McCann-Crosby et al. 2014). Orchiopexy—transposing undescended testes into the scrotum—is reasonably performed in childhood to maximize the chances of sperm production at puberty (Creighton et al. 2012).

I take it for granted that that most people with congenital adrenal hyperplasia would benefit from typical genital morphology, provided that sexual satisfaction and reproductive capacity were satisfactory. Activists have questioned the appropriateness of at least some such surgery. First, they claim that a high proportion of these operations are unsuccessful, leading to complications, and failing to achieve their objective of creating a child able to function sexually or reproductively. They frequently cite cosmetic clitoral surgery in congenital adrenal hyperplasia as a condition in which early surgery has often led to poor clinical results. Though there are few immediate complications, long-term success is less certain. Minto et al. (2003) found in a retrospective study in the UK that those who had undergone clitoral surgery had markedly worse sexual function than those with an intact clitoris. However, it was not stated how many had clitoridectomy and how many had nerve-sparing clitoral reduction, which began replacing clitoridectomy toward the end of the time Minto's cohort had surgery. Nor is it known whether the surgical group had more marked anatomical abnormalities to begin with. Also, even the group with an intact clitoris reported poor sexual function. A French group also found poor results with regard to sexual sensitivity, satisfaction, and reproduction (Gastaud et al. 2007) But a Swedish study of comparable size with almost all patients undergoing clitoroplasty, reported much higher levels of sexual satisfaction (Nordenskjöld et al. 2008). Also, the specific genotype may be important in determining sexual function in people with congenital adrenal hyperplasia, regardless of whether surgery is performed (Schernthaner-Reiter et al. 2019). The 2006 Consensus Statement (Lee et al. 2006) was drafted in the context of availability only of now-obsolete surgical techniques. Improving surgical techniques and better choice of patients may make it possible to achieve typical anatomy with good function. Meanwhile, a decision to operate should be up to the parents, supported by expert counseling.

But much of the opposition to correction is not based on concerns about bad results. Some is based on deontic autonomy considerations (Brussels Collaboration 2019). Other objections are based on disability theory, seeking not to pathologize anatomical differences (Crocetti et al. 2020). Still others are based on critical gender theory (Jones 2018), feminism (Dreger and Herndon 2009), and other theoretical approaches that seek to normalize non-binary differences. Deferring surgery until an age beyond which body image, sexual identity, and status self-perception are formed is, itself, a parental choice, and not a neutral one. Also, the use of a stringent definition of necessity that allows surgery only to deal with urgent physical danger (Brussels Collaboration 2019; Earp 2021) would seem to bar removal of gonads for cancer prevention, moving testes into the scrotum to allow future fertility, and vaginal creation or dilatation in minors, as there is no immediate danger in these circumstances. Parents and physicians might find this position irrelevant to determining the best way to care for the children they are responsible for. They may prefer that their children not be cannon fodder in ideological warfare. Removing streak gonads that will never produce hormones or germ cells, but will develop cancer up to half the time clearly is justifiable on the basis of beneficence. It also is compatible with respect for autonomy. Based on presumed substituted judgment; reasonable people competent to consent would consent to such an operation. Even open choice supports this surgery; people who die of cancer have no further choices. The Brussels Collaboration would bypass the standard decision-making process between doctor and parent—shared decision-making (Sandberg et al. 2019). This is based on a controversial construction of non-emergency surgery as a physical assault. Less extreme scholars who approach the subject from a human rights perspective accept that operation with clear medical benefit is indicated, even if hypospadias repair and clitoral reduction are not (Hegarty et al. 2020). The question of the risks and benefits in clitoral surgery for congenital adrenal hyperplasia is ultimately empiric, and decisions should be based on the best evidence. However, human rights arguments can be impervious to empiric considerations.

13.4 What Do Children And Parents Want?

The concept of sex as a binary phenomenon, as well as of gender as a binary, has come under attack (Blackless et al. 2000; DuBois et al. 2020). Others have a bias towards promoting certain viewpoints regarding gender and sex—specifically, in trying to break down binary identification (Garland and Travis 2018; Cannoot 2021). It is not clear that living as neither man nor woman will best promote flourishing in children capable of such characterization with appropriate treatment. The 2016 update of the 2006 Consensus Statement takes note of all these ethical concerns (Lee et al. 2016) At any rate, quality of life of people with disorders of sexual differentiation has been poorly studied, both qualitatively and quantitatively (Machado et al. 2016; Lee et al. 2016). This is difficult to study because of the heterogeneity of the conditions, their rarity, their wide range of severity, the variations of presentation within each syndrome, differences in treatment, and the wide variety in surgical procedures and the quality with which they are performed.

Some of the literature is tendentious in its criticisms of surgery. Much of this surgery is elective, but characterizing it as cosmetic (Diamond and Garland 2014; Cannoot 2021) is inaccurate (Gardner and Sandberg 2018). Authors also portray an inaccurate, stereotyped narrative of distraught parents, subject to undue influence from bigoted physicians pushing a binary gender agenda on vulnerable parents

(Garland and Travis 2018). Autonomy is described as extremely important for children. Paraphrasing Jones (2017), Cannoot (2021) opines that there is no matter more central to the child than bodily integrity. When I was a child, I did not think of bodily integrity as central, or think much about medical autonomy at all, except that I was afraid of doctors and dentists. Perhaps I was unusual, but the literature suggests otherwise. A classic paper suggested that primary school children worry most about school, health, and personal harm (Silverman et al. 1995). Family instability is a subject of concern when parents are not getting along (Coe et al. 2017). Adolescents are most concerned with personal competence (Fisher et al. 2017) and with social functioning (La Greca and Lopez 1998). Intolerance of uncertainty is a major issue for many children and adolescents (Osmanağaoğlu et al. 2018). If we are most concerned with flourishing, this seems to be related to good relationships with parents and with economic and social stability and security (Bethell et al. 2019; Murray and Lebrun-Harris 2020). It does not appear that autonomy is a high priority for school-age children and adolescents, and bodily integrity ordinarily is not on their minds at all.

Parents should have wide discretion in setting priorities in raising their children. Professionals should encourage them to think of their children's flourishing. Flourishing involves many factors, and bodily integrity is hardly crucial if changing a bodily contour has benefits that a reasonable person would say compensate for the bodily alteration in question (Mazor 2019). Not many people would object to operating on a patient with a disorder of sexual differentiation if failure to operate was likely to be fatal or seriously injurious. Thus, gonads likely to develop malignancies should be removed. Other necessary treatments include mineralocorticoid administration for salt-wasting congenital adrenal hyperplasia. I would consider fertility-preserving surgery to be indicated at any age.

The guidepost for what parents should be allowed to choose, and for what physicians should be allowed to offer, is the Direct Effects Basis of the State Intervention Test. Parents should have wide discretion to choose, with the aid of their physician, a treatment plan that does not markedly increase the risk of sexual or reproductive dysfunction. They should be allowed to raise their children in a manner that they reasonably believe enhances the chances of their children's social, sexual, and reproductive success. Patients with disorders of sexual differentiation should be should be evaluated, and treated in an appropriate way, in a center that cares for many such patients, and that has a full panoply of resources to deal with medical, surgical, social, and psychological issues.[6]

[6] It is to be expected that, at times, the medical consensus will be incorrect. It is a certainty that current treatments for every illness known to humanity will be superseded by better treatments.

13.5 Conclusion

The brain may be a fruitful place to look for intersex and intergender differences as a guide to exploring their biology. Morphologic sex differences between brains are well-established, and genetic influences may be more critical than hormonal influences (Lentini et al. 2013). Rodent models show that immunological and epigenetic factors may contribute to sex differentiation in the brain (McCarthy et al. 2017). Sex differences in brain biology govern complex behavioral patterns such as empathy, in both humans and in other mammals (Christov-Moore et al. 2014).

Some work on biology of transgender brain has recently begun. One study suggests that adolescent brains may resemble those of their experienced gender more than those of their genetic sex (Nota et al. 2017). Another morphologic study shows that models that distinguish cis-males from cis-females does not distinguish between trans-males and trans-females (Baldinger-Melich et al. 2020). The limited work on this subject is reviewed by Frigerio et al. (2021). An appreciation of the neurobiology of sex and gender will help to reveal degree of plasticity of sex and of gendered behavior. The current necessary reliance on our intuitions, and on our conceptualization of these phenomena has resulted in controversies not susceptible to immediate empiric resolution.

As with any decision whose basis is not well understood, parents should be allowed to set standards and boundaries for their minor children, subject to the two Bases of the State Intervention Test.

References

Ainsworth, Claire. 2015. Sex Redefined. *Nature* 518 (7539): 288–291. https://doi.org/10.1038/518288a.

Aitken, Madison, Doug P. VanderLaan, Lori Wasserman, Sonja Stojanovski, and Kenneth J. Zucker. 2016. Self-Harm and Suicidality in Children Referred for Gender Dysphoria. *Journal of the American Academy of Child & Adolescent Psychiatry* 55 (6): 513–520. https://doi.org/10.1016/j.jaac.2016.04.001.

Alipour, Mehrdad. 2017. Essentialism and Islamic Theology of Homosexuality: A Critical Reflection on an Essentialist Epistemology Toward Same-Sex Desires and Acts in Islam. *Journal of Homosexuality* 64 (14): 1930–1942. https://doi.org/10.1080/00918369.2017.1289001.

Arcelus, J., W.P. Bouman, W. Van Den Noortgate, L. Claes, G. Witcomb, and F. Fernandez-Aranda. 2015. Systematic Review and Meta-Analysis of Prevalence Studies in Transsexualism. *European Psychiatry* 30 (6): 807–815. https://doi.org/10.1016/j.eurpsy.2015.04.005.

Baldinger-Melich, Pia, Maria F. Urquijo Castro, René Seiger, Anne Ruef, Dominic B. Dwyer, Georg S. Kranz, Manfred Klöbl, et al. 2020. Sex Matters: A Multivariate Pattern Analysis of Sex- and Gender-Related Neuroanatomical Differences in Cis- and Transgender Individuals Using Structural Magnetic Resonance Imaging. *Cerebral Cortex* 30 (3): 1345–1356. https://doi.org/10.1093/cercor/bhz170.

Bethell, Christina, Jennifer Jones, Narangerel Gombojav, Jeff Linkenbach, and Robert Sege. 2019. Positive Childhood Experiences and Adult Mental and Relational Health in a Statewide Sample: Associations Across Adverse Childhood Experiences Levels. *JAMA Pediatrics* 173 (11): e193007. https://doi.org/10.1001/jamapediatrics.2019.3007.

Blackless, Melanie, Anthony Charuvastra, Amanda Derryck, Anne Fausto-Sterling, Karl Lauzanne, and Ellen Lee. 2000. How Sexually Dimorphic Are We? Review and Synthesis. *American Journal of Human Biology* 12 (2): 151–166. https://doi.org/10.1002/(SICI)1520-6300(200003/04)12:2%3c151::AID-AJHB1%3e3.0.CO;2-F.

Blanchard, Ray. 1989. The Concept of Autogynephilia and the Typology of Male Gender Dysphoria. *Journal of Nervous and Mental Disease* 177 (10): 616–623. https://doi.org/10.1097/00005053-198910000-00004.

Boorse, Christopher. 2014. A Second Rebuttal on Health. *Journal of Medicine and Philosophy* 39 (6): 683–724. https://doi.org/10.1093/jmp/jhu035.

Brooks, Janet. 1996. The Sad and Tragic Life of Typhoid Mary. *CMAJ* 154 (6): 915–916.

Brussels Collaboration. 2019. Medically Unnecessary Genital Cutting and the Rights of the Child: Moving Toward Consensus. *American Journal of Bioethics* 19 (10): 17–28. https://doi.org/10.1080/15265161.2019.1643945.

Byne, William, Susan J. Bradley, A. Eli Coleman, Evan Eyler, Richard Green, Edgardo J. Menvielle, Heino F. L. Meyer-Bahlburg, Richard R. Pleak, and D. Andrew Tompkins. 2012. Report of the American Psychiatric Association Task Force on Treatment of Gender Identity Disorder. *Archives of Sexual Behavior* 41 (4): 759–796. https://doi.org/10.1007/s10508-012-9975-x.

Callens, Nina, Griet De Cuypere, Petra De Sutter, Stan Monstrey, Steven Weyers, Piet Hoebeke, and Martine Cools. 2014. An Update on Surgical and Non-Surgical Treatments for Vaginal Hypoplasia. *Human Reproduction Update* 20 (5): 775–801. https://doi.org/10.1093/humupd/dmu024.

Cannoot, Pieter. 2021. Do parents really know best? Informed consent to sex assigning and 'normalising' treatment of minors with variations of sex characteristics. *Culture, Health, and Sexuality* 23(4): 564-578.

Cardoos, Stephanie L., Ahna Ballonoff Suleiman, Megan Johnson, Wouter van den Bos, Stephen P. Hinshaw, and Ronald E. Dahl. 2017. Social Status Strategy in Early Adolescent Girls: Testosterone and Value-Based Decision Making. *Psychoneuroendocrinology* 81: 14–21. https://doi.org/10.1016/j.psyneuen.2017.03.013.

Chen, Diane, Lisa Simons, Emilie K. Johnson, Barbara A. Lockart, and Courtney Finlayson. 2017. Fertility Preservation for Transgender Adolescents. *Journal of Adolescent Health* 61 (1): 120–123. https://doi.org/10.1016/j.jadohealth.2017.01.022.

Christov-Moore, Leonardo, Elizabeth A. Simpson, Gino Coudé, Kristina Grigaityte, Marco Iacoboni, and Pier Francesco Ferrari. 2014. Empathy: Gender Effects in Brain and Behavior. *Neuroscience and Biobehavioral Reviews* 46 (Pt 4): 604–627. https://doi.org/10.1016/j.neubiorev.2014.09.001.

Clark, Terryann C., Mathijs F.G. Lucassen, Pat Bullen, Simon J. Denny, Theresa M. Fleming, Elizabeth M. Robinson, and Fiona V. Rossen. 2014. The Health and Well-Being of Transgender High School Students: Results from the New Zealand Adolescent Health Survey. *Journal of Adolescent Health* 55 (1): 93–99. https://doi.org/10.1016/j.jadohealth.2013.11.008.

Coe, Jesse L., Patrick T. Davies, and Melissa L. Sturge-Apple. 2017. The Multivariate Roles of Family Instability and Interparental Conflict in Predicting Children's Representations of Insecurity in the Family System and Early School Adjustment Problems. *Journal of Abnormal Child Psychology* 45 (2): 211–224. https://doi.org/10.1007/s10802-016-0164-6.

Coleman, E., W. Bockting, M. Botzer, P. Cohen-Kettenis, G. DeCuypere, J. Feldman, L. Fraser, et al. 2012. Standards of Care for the Health of Transsexual, Transgender, and Gender-Nonconforming People, Version 7. *International Journal of Transgenderism* 13 (4): 165–232. https://doi.org/10.1080/15532739.2011.700873.

Creighton, Sarah, Steven D. Chernausek, Rodrigo Romao, Philip Ransley, and Joao Pippi Salle. 2012. Timing and Nature of Reconstructive Surgery for Disorders of Sex Development—Introduction. *Journal of Pediatric Urology* 8 (6): 602–610. https://doi.org/10.1016/j.jpurol.2012.10.001.

Crocetti, Daniela, Surya Monro, Valentino Vecchietti, and Tray Yeadon-Lee. 2020. Towards an Agency-Based Model of Intersex, Variations of Sex Characteristics (VSC) And DSD/Dsd Health. *Culture, Health and Sexuality* 25: 1–16. https://doi.org/10.1080/13691058.2020.1825815.

de Vries, Annelou L.C., Jenifer K. McGuire, Thomas D. Steensma, Eva C.F. Wagenaar, Theo A.H. Doreleijers, and Peggy T. Cohen-Kettenis. 2014. Young Adult Psychological Outcome After Puberty Suppression and Gender Reassignment. *Pediatrics* 134 (4): 696–704. https://doi.org/10.1542/peds.2013-2958.

Diamond, Milton, and Jameson Garland. 2014. Evidence Regarding Cosmetic and Medically Unnecessary Surgery on Infants. *Journal of Pediatric Urology* 10 (1): 2–6. https://doi.org/10.1016/j.jpurol.2013.10.021.

Dreger, Alice D., and April M. Herndon. 2009. Progress and Politics in the Intersex Rights Movement: Feminist Theory in Action. *GLQ: A Journal of Lesbian and Gay Studies* 15 (2): 199–224. https://muse.jhu.edu/article/261479. https://doi.org/10.1215/10642684-2008-134.

Drescher, Jack. 2015. Out of DSM: Depathologizing Homosexuality. *Behavioral Sciences* 5 (4): 565–575. https://doi.org/10.3390/bs5040565.

Drescher, Jack, Peggy T. Cohen-Kettenis, and Geoffrey M. Reed. 2016. Gender Incongruence of Childhood in the ICD-11: Controversies, Proposal, and Rationale. *Lancet Psychiatry* 3 (3): 297–304. https://doi.org/10.1016/S2215-0366(15)00586-6.

Dubin, Samuel, Megan Lane, Shane Morrison, Asa Radix, Uri Belkind, Christian Vercler, and David Inwards-Breland. 2020. Medically Assisted Gender Affirmation: When Children and Parents Disagree. *Journal of Medical Ethics* 46 (5): 295–299. https://doi.org/10.1136/medethics-2019-1055672019.

DuBois, L. Zachary., James K. Gibb, Robert-Paul. Juster, and Sally I. Powers. 2020. Biocultural Approaches to Transgender and Gender Diverse Experience and Health: Integrating Biomarkers and Advancing Gender/Sex Research. *American Journal of Human Biology* 33 (1): e23555. https://doi.org/10.1002/ajhb.23555.

Dupree, James M. 2018. Insurance Coverage of Male Infertility: What Should the Standard Be? *Translational Andrology and Urology* 7 (Suppl 3): S310–S316. https://doi.org/10.21037/tau.2018.04.25.

Earp, Brian D. 2021. Male or female genital cutting: Why 'health benefits' are morally irrelevant. *Journal of Medical Ethics* Published Online ahead of print: 18 January 2021. https://doi.org/10.1136/medethics-2020-106782.

Elkins, Kathleen. 2020. The Highest Paid Actors and Actresses of 2019, According to Forbes. CNBC, February 9, 2020. https://www.cnbc.com/2020/02/07/the-10-highest-paid-actors-and-actresses-of-2019.html.

Evans, Marcus. 2020. Freedom to Think: The Need for Thorough Assessment and Treatment of Gender Dysphoric Children. *BJPsych Bulletin*, Cambridge University Press, July 21, 2020, 1–5. https://doi.org/10.1192/bjb.2020.72.

Fast, Anne A., and Kristina R. Olson. 2018. Gender Development in Transgender Preschool Children. *Child Development* 89 (2): 620–637. https://doi.org/10.1111/cdev.12758.

Fausto-Sterling, Anne. 1993. The Five Sexes. *The Sciences* 33 (2): 20–24. https://doi.org/10.1002/j.2326-1951.1993.tb03081.x.

Fisher, Emma, Edmund Keogh, and Christopher Eccleston. 2017. Everyday Worry in Adolescents with and Without Chronic Pain: A Diary Study. *Psychology, Health and Medicine* 22 (7): 800–807. https://doi.org/10.1080/13548506.2017.1280175.

Frigerio, A., I. Ballerini, & M. Del C. Valdés Hernández. 2021. Structural, Functional, and Metabolic Brain Differences as a Function of Gender Identity or Sexual Orientation: A Systematic Review of the Human Neuroimaging Literature. *Archives of Sexual Behavior*. Online ahead of print. https://doi.org/10.1007/s10508-021-02005-9

Gardner, Melissa, and David E. Sandberg. 2018. Navigating Surgical Decision Making in Disorders of Sex Development (DSD). *Frontiers in Pediatrics* 19 (6): 339. https://doi.org/10.3389/fped.2018.00339.

Garland, Fae, and Mitchell Travis. 2018. Legislating Intersex Equality: Building the Resilience of Intersex People through Law. *Legal Studies* 38 (4): 587–606. https://doi.org/10.1017/lst.2018.17.

Gastaud, F., C. Bouvattier, L. Duranteau, R. Brauner, E. Thibaud, F. Kutten, and P. Bougnères. 2007. Impaired Sexual and Reproductive Outcomes in Women with Classical Forms of Congenital Adrenal Hyperplasia. *Journal of Clinical Endocrinology and Metabolism* 92 (4): 1391–1396. https://doi.org/10.1210/jc.2006-1757.

Goosens, William K. 1980. Values, Health, and Medicine. *Philosophy of Science* 47 (1): 100–115. https://doi.org/10.1086/288912.

Greenberg, Steven. 2004. *Wrestling with God and Men: Homosexuality in the Jewish Tradition.* Madison: University of Wisconsin Press.

Grift, Tim C. van de, Zosha, J. van Gelder, Margriet G. Mullender, Thomas D. Steensma, Annelou L.C. de Vries, and Mark-Bram Bouman. 2020. Timing of Puberty Suppression and Surgical Options for Transgender Youth. *Pediatrics* 146 (5): e20193653. https://doi.org/10.1542/peds.2019-3653.

Hawley, Patricia H. 2015. Social Dominance in Childhood and Its Evolutionary Underpinnings: Why It Matters and What We Can Do. *Pediatrics* 135 (Suppl 2): S31–S38. https://doi.org/10.1542/peds.2014-3549D.

Hegarty, Peter, Marta Prandelli, Tove Lundberg, Lih-Mei. Liao, Sarah Creighton, and Katrina Roen. 2020. Drawing the Line Between Essential and Nonessential Interventions on Intersex Characteristics with European Health Care Professionals. *Review of General Psychology* 11 (1): 1–14. https://doi.org/10.1177/1089268020963622.

Hembree, Wylie C., Peggy Cohen-Kettenis, A. Henriette, Delemarre-van de Waal, Louis J. Gooren, Walter J. Meyer III, Norman P. Spack, Vin Tangpricha, and Victor M. Montori. 2009. Endocrine Treatment of Transsexual Persons: An Endocrine Society Clinical Practice Guideline. *Journal of Clinical Endocrinology & Metabolism* 94 (9): 3132–3154. https://doi.org/10.1210/jc.2009-0345.

Hepp, U., B. Kraemer, U. Schnyder, N. Miller, and A. Delsignore. 2005. Psychiatric Comorbidity in Gender Identity Disorder. *Journal of Psychosomatic Research* 58 (3): 259–261. https://doi.org/10.1016/j.jpsychores.2004.08.010.

Herman, Jody L., Andrew R. Flores, Taylor N.T. Brown, Bianca D.M. Wilson, and Kerith J. Conron. 2017. Age of Individuals Who Identify as Transgender in the United States. Williams Institute, UCLA School of Law. http://williamsinstitute.law.ucla.edu/wp-content/uploads/Age-Trans-Individuals-Jan-2017.pdf.

Hildebrandt, Achim. 2015. Christianity, Islam and Modernity: Explaining Prohibitions on Homosexuality in UN Member States. *Political Studies* 63 (4): 852–869. https://doi.org/10.1111/1467-9248.12137.

Hilton, Emma N., and Tommy R. Lundberg. 2021. Transgender Women in the Female Category of Sport: Perspectives on Testosterone Suppression and Performance Advantage. *Sports Medicine* 51 (2): 199–214. https://doi.org/10.1007/s40279-020-01389-3.

Hutchinson, Anna, Melissa Midgen, and Anastassis Spiliadis. 2020. In Support of Research into Rapid-Onset Gender Dysphoria. *Archives of Sexual Behavior* 49 (1): 79–80. https://doi.org/10.1007/s10508-019-01517-9.

Jones, Melinda. 2017. Intersex Genital Mutilation—A Western Version of FGM. *International Journal of Children's Rights* 25 (2): 396–411. https://doi.org/10.1163/15718182-02502008.

Jones, Tiffany. 2018. Intersex Studies: A Systematic Review of International Health Literature. *SAGE Open* 8 (2): L 2158244017745577. https://doi.org/10.1177/2158244017745577.

Kaltiala-Heino, Riittakerttu, Hannah Bergman, Marja Työläjärvi, and Louise Frisén. 2018. Gender Dysphoria in Adolescence: Current Perspectives. *Adolescent Health, Medicine and Therapeutics* 9 (March 2, 2018): 31–41. https://doi.org/10.2147/AHMT.S135432.

Knight, Erik L., Amar Sarkar, Smrithi Prasad, and Pranjal H. Mehta. 2020. Beyond the challenge hypothesis: The emergence of the dual-hormone hypothesis and recommendations for future research. *Human Behavior* 123: 104657. https://doi.org/10.1016/j.yhbeh.2019.104657.

Koehler A., Jana Eyssel, and Timo O. Nieder. 2018. Genders and individual treatment progress in (non-)binary trans individuals. *Journal of Sexual Medicine* 15 (2): 102-113.

Kordsmeyer, Tobias L., John Hunt, David A. Puts, Julia Ostner, and Lars Penke. 2018. The Relative Importance of Intra- and Intersexual Selection on Human Male Sexually Dimorphic Traits. *Evolution and Human Behavior* 39 (4): 424–436. https://doi.org/10.1016/j.evolhumbehav.2018.03.008.

La Greca, Annette M., and Nadja Lopez. 1998. Social Anxiety Among Adolescents: Relations and Friendships. *Journal of Abnormal Child Psychology* 26 (2): 83–94. https://doi.org/10.1023/A:1022684520514.

Laidlaw, Michael, Michelle Cretella, and Kevin Donovan. 2019. The Right to Best Care for Children Does Not Include the Right to Medical Transition. *American Journal of Bioethics* 19 (2): 75–77.

Lawrence, Anne A. 2017. Autogynephilia and the Typology of Male-to-Female Transsexualism. *European Psychologist* 22 (1): 39–54. https://doi.org/10.1027/1016-9040/a000276.

Lee, Peter A., Christopher P. Houk, S. Faisal Ahmed, and Ieuan A. Hughes. 2006. Consensus Statement on Management of Intersex Disorders. *Pediatrics* 118 (2): e488–e500. https://doi.org/10.1542/peds.2006-0738.

Lee, Peter A., Anna Nordenström, Christopher P. Houk, S. Faisal Ahmed, Richard Auchus, Arlene Baratz, Katharine Baratz Dalke, et al. 2016. Global Disorders of Sex Development Update since 2006: Perceptions, Approach and Care. *Hormone Research in Paediatrics* 85 (3): 158–180. https://doi.org/10.1159/000442975.

Lentini, E., M. Kasahara, S. Arver, and I. Savic. 2013. Sex Differences in the Human Brain and the Impact of Sex Chromosomes and Sex Hormones. *Cerebral Cortex* 23 (1): 2322–2336. https://doi.org/10.1093/cercor/bhs222.

Littman, Lisa. 2018. Rapid-Onset Gender Dysphoria in Adolescents and Young Adults: A Study of Parental Reports. *PLoS ONE* 13 (8): e0202330–e0202330.

Machado, Paula, Angelo Brandelli Costa, Henrique Nardi, Anna Fontanari, Igor Araujo, and Daniela Knauth. 2016. Follow-up of Psychological Outcomes of Interventions in Patients Diagnosed with Disorders of Sexual Development: A Systematic Review. *Journal of Health Psychology* 21 (10): 2195–2206. https://doi.org/10.1177/1359105315572454.

Marchiano, Lisa. 2017. Outbreak: On Transgender Teens and Psychic Epidemics. *Psychological Perspectives* 60 (3): 345–366. https://doi.org/10.1080/00332925.2017.1350804.

Margolis, Joseph. 1976. The Concept of Disease. *Journal of Medicine and Philosophy* 1 (3): 238–255. https://doi.org/10.1093/jmp/1.3.238.

Mazor, Joseph. 2019. On the Strength of Children's Right to Bodily Integrity: The Case of Circumcision. *Journal of Applied Philosophy* 36 (1): 1–16.

McCann-Crosby, Bonnie, Roshanak Mansouri, Jennifer E. Dietrich, Laurence B. McCullough, V. Reid Sutton, Elise G. Austin, Bruce Schlomer, et al. 2014. State of the Art Review in Gonadal Dysgenesis: Challenges in Diagnosis and Management. *International Journal of Pediatric Endocrinology* 2014 (1): 4. https://doi.org/10.1186/1687-9856-2014-4.

McCarthy, Margaret M., Bridget M. Nugent, and Kathryn M. Lenz. 2017. Neuroimmunology and Neuroepigenetics in the Establishment of Sex Differences in the Brain. *Nature Reviews. Neuroscience* 18 (8): 471–484. https://doi.org/10.1038/nrn.2017.61.

Minto, Catherine L., Lih-Mei. Liao, Christopher R.J. Woodhouse, Phillip G. Ransley, and Sarah M. Creighton. 2003. The Effect of Clitoral Surgery on Sexual Outcome in Individuals Who Have Intersex Conditions with Ambiguous Genitalia: A Cross-Sectional Study. *Lancet* 361 (9365): 1252–1257. https://doi.org/10.1016/S0140-6736(03)12980-7.

Murray, Evva Assing, and Lydie Lebrun-Harris. 2020. Associations Between Parent-Reported Family Economic Hardship and Mental Health Conditions in U.S. Children. *Journal of Children and Poverty* 26 (2): 191–214. https://doi.org/10.1080/10796126.2020.1764188.

Naderi, Fariba, Zahra Soheilirad, and Zahra Haghshenas. 2019. The Influence of Gonadotropin-Releasing Hormone Agonist Treatment on Thyroid Function Tests in Children with Central Idiopathic Precocious Puberty. *Medical Archives* 73 (2): 101–103. https://doi.org/10.5455/medarh.2019.73.101-103.

Nordenskjöld, Agneta, Gundela Holmdahl, Louise Frisén, Henrik Falhammar, Helena Filipsson, Marja Thorén, Per Olof Janson, and Kerstin Hagenfeldt. 2008. Type of Mutation and Surgical

Procedure Affect Long-Term Quality of Life for Women with Congenital Adrenal Hyperplasia. *Journal of Clinical Endocrinology & Metabolism* 93 (2): 380–386. https://doi.org/10.1210/jc.2007-0556.

Nota, Nienke M., Baudewijntje P.C. Kreukels, Martin den Heijer, Dick J. Veltman, Peggy T. Cohen-Kettenis, Sarah M. Burke, and Julie Bakker. 2017. Brain Functional Connectivity Patterns in Children and Adolescents with Gender Dysphoria: Sex-Atypical or Not? *Psychoneuroendocrinology* 86: 187–195. https://doi.org/10.1016/j.psyneuen.2017.09.014.

Olson, Kristina R., Lily Durwood, Madeleine DeMeules, and Katie A. McLaughlin. 2016. Mental Health of Transgender Children Who Are Supported in Their Identities. *Pediatrics* 137 (3): e20153223. https://doi.org/10.1542/peds.2015-3223.

Osmanağaoğlu, Nihan, Cathy Creswell, and Helen F. Dodd. 2018. Intolerance of Uncertainty, Anxiety, and Worry in Children and Adolescents: A Meta-Analysis. *Journal of Affective Disorders* 225 (1): 80–90. https://doi.org/10.1016/j.jad.2017.07.035.

Pellegrini, Anthony D., Cary J. Roseth, Mark J. van Ryzin, & David W. Solberg. 2011 Popularity as a Form of Social Dominance: An Evolutionary Perspective. In *Popularity in the Peer System*, ed. Antonius H. N. Cillessen, David Schwartz, & Lara Mayeux. New York: Guilford Press.

Perilloux, Carin, and Jaime M. Cloud. 2019. Mate-by-Numbers: Budget, Mating Context, and Sex Predict Preferences for Facial and Bodily Traits. *Evolutionary Psychological Science* 5 (3): 294–299. https://doi.org/10.1007/s40806-019-00187-z.

Peterson, Claire M., Abigail Matthews, Emily Copps-Smith, and Lee Ann Conard. 2017. Suicidality, Self-Harm, and Body Dissatisfaction in Transgender Adolescents and Emerging Adults with Gender Dysphoria. *Suicide and Life-Threatening Behavior* 47 (4): 475–482. https://doi.org/10.1111/sltb.12289.

Pilgrim, David, and Kirsty Entwistle. 2020. GnRHa ('Puberty Blockers') and Cross Sex Hormones for Children and Adolescents: Informed Consent, Personhood and Freedom of Expression. *New Bioethics* 26 (3): 224–237. https://doi.org/10.1080/20502877.2020.1796257.

Powell, Russell, and Eric Scarffe. 2019. Rethinking "Disease": A Fresh Diagnosis and a New Philosophical Treatment. *Journal of Medical Ethics* 45 (9): 579–588. https://doi.org/10.1136/medethics-2019-105465.

Priest, Maura. 2019. Transgender Children and the Right to Transition: Medical Ethics When Parents Mean Well but Cause Harm. *American Journal of Bioethics* 19 (2): 45–59. https://doi.org/10.1080/15265161.2018.1557276.

Rafferty, Jason, Committee on Psychosocial Aspects of Child and Family Health, Committee on Adolescence, and Gay Section on Lesbian. 2018. Ensuring Comprehensive Care and Support for Transgender and Gender-Diverse Children and Adolescents. *Pediatrics* 142 (4): e20182162. https://doi.org/10.1542/peds.2018-2162.

Redhead, Daniel, Joey Cheng, and Rick O'Gorman. 2021. Status Competition and Peer Relationships in Childhood. In *Encyclopedia of Evolutionary Psychological Science*, ed. Todd K. Shackelford and Viviana A. Weekes-Shackelford. Cham, Switzerland: Springer. https://doi.org/10.1007/978-3-319-16999-6_3639-1

Restar, Arjee Javellana. 2020. Methodological Critique of Littman's (2018) Parental-Respondents Accounts of 'Rapid-Onset Gender Dysphoria.' *Archives of Sexual Behavior* 49 (1): 61–66. https://doi.org/10.1007/s10508-019-1453-2.

Richards, Christina, Walter Pierre Bouman, Leighton Seal, Meg John Barker, Timo O. Nieder, and Guy T'Sjoen. 2016. Non-Binary or Genderqueer Genders. *International Review of Psychiatry* 28 (1): 95–102. https://doi.org/10.3109/09540261.2015.1106446.

Sandberg, David E., Melissa Gardner, Kristin Kopec, Megan Urbanski, Nina Callens, Catherine E. Keegan, Beverly M. Yashar, et al. 2019. Development of a Decision Support Tool in Pediatric Differences/Disorders of Sex Development. *Seminars in Pediatric Surgery, Reproductive Anomalies and Differences of Sex Development* 28 (5): 150838. https://doi.org/10.1016/j.sempedsurg.2019.150838.

Schernthaner-Reiter, Marie Helene, Sabina Baumgartner-Parzer, Hans Christian Egarter, Michael Krebs, Alexandra Kautzky-Willer, Kathrin Kirchheiner, Anton Luger, and Michaela Bayerle-Eder. 2019. Influence of Genotype and Hyperandrogenism on Sexual Function in Women with Congenital Adrenal Hyperplasia. *Journal of Sexual Medicine* 16 (10): 1529–1540. https://doi.org/10.1016/j.jsxm.2019.07.009.

Schulz, Kalynn M., and Cheryl L. Sisk. 2016. The organizing actions of adolescent gonadal steroid hormones on brain and behavioral development. *Neuroscience and Biobehavioral Reviews* 70: 148-158. https://doi.org/10.1016/j.neubiorev.2016.07.036.

Sherwani, Afak Yusuf, Abdul Qayoom Shah, Abdul Majeed Wani, Ahmad Chalkoo Bashir, Ahmad Khan Bashir, Farooq Ahmad Sofi, Ashfaq Amin Wani, et al. 2014. Hysterectomy in a Male? A Rare Case Report. *International Journal of Surgery Case Reports* 5 (1): 1285–1287. https://doi.org/10.1016/j.ijscr.2014.10.020.

Shiffman, Marc, Margaret M. Lumley, Susan P. Lollis, Doug P. VanderLaan, Hayley Wood, S. Kathleen Hughes, Allison Owen-Anderson, and Kenneth J. Zucker. 2016. Behavioral and emotional problems as a function of peer relationships in adolescents with gender dysphoria: A comparison with clinical and nonclinical controls. *Psychology of Sexual Orientation and Gender Diversity* 3(1): 27–36. http://dx.doi.org/10.1037/sgd0000152.

Shteyler, Vadim M., Jessica A. Clarke, and Eli Y. Adashi. 2020. Failed Assignments—Rethinking Sex Designations on Birth Certificates. *New England Journal of Medicine* 383 (25): 2399–2401. https://doi.org/10.1056/NEJMp2025974.

Shumer, Daniel E., Natalie J. Nokoff, and Norman P. Spack. 2016. Advances in the Care of Transgender Children and Adolescents. *Advances in Pediatrics* 63 (1): 79–102. https://doi.org/10.1016/j.yapd.2016.04.018.

Silverman, Wendy K., Annette M. La Greca, and Shari Wasserstein. 1995. What Do Children Worry About? Worries and Their Relation to Anxiety. *Child Development* 66 (3): 671–686. https://doi.org/10.1111/j.1467-8624.1995.tb00897.x.

Skorska, Malvina N., Sofia Chavez, Gabriel A. Devenyi, Raihaan Patel, Lindsey T. Thurston, Meng-Chuan. Lai, Kenneth J. Zucker, M Mallar Chakravarty, Nancy J. Lobaugh, and Doug P. Vander-Laan. 2021. A Multi-Modal MRI Analysis of Cortical Structure in Relation to Gender Dysphoria, Sexual Orientation, and Age in Adolescents. *Journal of Clinical Medicine* 10 (2): 345. https://doi.org/10.3390/jcm10020345.

Speiser, Phyllis W., and Perrin C. White. 2003. Congenital Adrenal Hyperplasia. *New England Journal of Medicine* 349 (8): 776–788. https://doi.org/10.1056/NEJMra021561.

Steensma, Thomas D., Jenifer K. McGuire, Baudewijntje P.C. Kreukels, Anneke J. Beekman, and Peggy T. Cohen-Kettenis. 2013. Factors Associated with Desistence and Persistence of Childhood Gender Dysphoria: A Quantitative Follow-Up Study. *Journal of the American Academy of Child and Adolescent Psychiatry* 52 (6): 582–590. https://doi.org/10.1016/j.jaac.2013.03.016.

Strang, John F., Lauren Kenworthy, Aleksandra Dominska, Jennifer Sokoloff, Laura E. Kenealy, Madison Berl, Karin Walsh, et al. 2014. Increased Gender Variance in Autism Spectrum Disorders and Attention Deficit Hyperactivity Disorder. *Archives of Sexual Behavior* 43 (8): 1525–1533. https://doi.org/10.1007/s10508-014-0285-3.

Van den Akker, Hanneke, Rozemarijn van der Ploeg, & Peer Scheepers. 2013. Disapproval of Homosexuality: Comparative Research on Individual and National Determinants of Disapproval of Homosexuality in 20 European Countries. *International Journal of Public Opinion Research* 25 (1): 64–86. https://doi.org/10.1093/ijpor/edr058

van Voren, Robert. 2010. Political Abuse of Psychiatry—An Historical Overview. *Schizophrenia Bulletin* 36 (1): 33–35. https://doi.org/10.1093/schbul/sbp119.

Vermande, Marjolijn M., Patricia A. Gilholm, Albert H.A. Reijntjes, Dave J. Hessen, Elisabeth H.M. Sterck, and Anne M. Overduin-de Vries. 2018. Is Inspiring Group Members an Effective Predictor of Social Dominance in Early Adolescence? Direct and Moderated Effects of Behavioral Strategies, Social Skills, and Gender on Resource Control and Popularity. *Journal of Youth and Adolescence* 47 (9): 1813–1829. https://doi.org/10.1007/s10964-018-0830-9.

Wakefield, Jerome C. 1992. Disorder as Harmful Dysfunction: A Conceptual Critique of DSM-III-R's Definition of Mental Disorder. *Psychological Review* 99 (2): 232–247. https://doi.org/10.1037/0033-295X.99.2.232.

Wakefield, Jerome C. 2007. The Concept of Mental Disorder: Diagnostic Implications of the Harmful Dysfunction Analysis. *World Psychiatry* 6 (3): 149–156.

Wakefield, Jerome C., and Jordan A. Conrad. 2020. Harm as a Necessary Component of the Concept of Medical Disorder: Reply to Muckler and Taylor. *Journal of Medicine and Philosophy* 45 (3): 350–370. https://doi.org/10.1093/jmp/jhaa008.

Walter, Kathryn V., Daniel Conroy-Beam, David M. Buss, Kelly Asao, Agnieszka Sorokowska, Piotr Sorokowski, Toivo Aavik, et al. 2020. Sex Differences in Mate Preferences Across 45 Countries: A Large-Scale Replication. *Psychological Science* 31 (4): 408–423. https://doi.org/10.1177/0956797620904154.

Zhang, Lingshan, Anthony J. Lee, Lisa M. DeBruine, and Benedict C. Jones. 2019. Are Sex Differences in Preferences for Physical Attractiveness and Good Earning Capacity in Potential Mates Smaller in Countries with Greater Gender Equality? *Evolutionary Psychology* 17 (2): 1474704919852921. https://doi.org/10.1177/1474704919852921.

Chapter 14
Male Circumcision

Abstract Circumcision consists of removal of the male prepuce (foreskin), leaving the penile glans (head) intact. Over a billion men alive today have undergone circumcision. The procedure has been widely performed for at least four millennia, largely as a religious or cultural rite. Performed on a healthy young boy under reasonably hygienic conditions, circumcision carries minimal risk of severe injury. There is no convincing evidence that it is a significant cause of urinary, reproductive, or sexual dysfunction. This chapter reviews the evidence on both sides of the circumcision debate. The chapter rejects or refutes deontic arguments against circumcision. Finding no strong evidence that childhood circumcision is a health risk, the chapter applies the State Intervention Test and finds that state interference with parental authorization of circumcision falls outside appropriate state scope of action.

This chapter and the next will discuss rituals involving genital alteration. This chapter deals with boys and the next chapter with girls. I ask two questions to frame the issue. First, why might parents who are interested in their children's welfare want to subject their minor children to genital alteration? Motivation for non-medical childhood circumcision might be hygiene, health benefit, cultural practice, aesthetics (which blends with cultural practice), or satisfaction of religious demands. The second question is based on the historical fact that so far as is known, only Antiochus Epiphanes IV, Hadrian, Stalin and Hitler outlawed ritual male circumcision (Freeman 1999). Why would liberals and progressives want to emulate the example of these despots?

Ritual genital cutting of infants is contentious. Ensuring that children are treated for serious diseases evokes little disagreement. Even enhancement procedures are more controversial among academicians than among parents and the general public. There has been no tsunami of opposition to cosmetic cleft lip replacement or orthodontia. By contrast, opposition to infant genital cutting either affirms cultural positions regarding sexual expression or reflects hostility toward cultures which engage in these rituals (Shweder 2009). Legislative bodies in much of Western Europe have considered restricting or abolishing ritual circumcision of children (Aktürk 2019). The level of antipathy often directed at procedures that involve genital alteration, often combined with contempt for groups that practice them, raises questions

A. J. Jacobs, *Assigning Responsibility for Children's Health When Parents and Authorities Disagree: Whose Child?*, The International Library of Bioethics 90,
https://doi.org/10.1007/978-3-030-87698-2_14

regarding the objectivity and motivation of some opponents. I will conclude that childhood male circumcision is permitted by the State Intervention Test.

Many of us have strong loyalty to some community. A *community* is a group of people whom one would succor, support, and uphold. Much current liberal thought sees the state as the appropriate primary community. However, the allegiance of many people is to other institutions. These may include one's ethnic group, region, or co-linguists; consider Kashmir or Quebec. One's primary group also be one's family, business entity, ideological faction, profession, or religion. These alternatives to the state are buttressed either by strongly-binding norms which dictate how members should think or behave, or by strong personal ties that transcend beliefs. It may be in the interest of the state to attenuate the importance of such groups, since they compete with the state for allegiance. However, the state can supervise economic and security affairs without being the primary object of allegiance. Consequently, the state should tolerate groups that do not threaten it or endanger its citizens.

Some groups employ rituals that physically alter the genitalia of children, mostly with religious justifications. This chapter asks when circumcision is appropriate, and the next chapter examines female genital alteration (FGA). Some of the points I make apply to both male circumcision and to female genital alteration. This should be readily apparent to readers, even if I do not repeat the same arguments in both chapters.

14.1 Ritual Childhood Circumcision

Circumcision is removal of the penile prepuce (foreskin), and should not be used to denote any procedure performed on females except for selective removal of the clitoral prepuce. Circumcision has been practiced for millennia. Over a billion living males—one-third of males worldwide—have been circumcised (World Health Organization 2008), many living in areas with extensive programs of biomedical investigation. Therefore, the risks of circumcision should be well-characterized; controversy regarding its physical risks is surprising. Besides ritual applications, circumcision may be performed for reasons of health, cultural conformity, and aesthetics.

14.2 Circumcision and Health

The safety of infant circumcision when performed on healthy infants has been well documented in a large population study (El Bcheraoui 2014). Most infant circumcision (IC) complications were mild. Mortality is probably about 2/1,000,000 in healthy infants (Royal Dutch Medical Society 2010). IC can be performed safely by trained non-physician providers (Ben-Chaim et al. 2005), and by obstetric and pediatric residents (Heras et al. 2018). Adult circumcision has a much higher complication rate than childhood circumcision at any age, with about 1% frequency of serious complications (Friedman et al. 2016). Circumcision of children beyond infancy is intermediate in risk between IC and circumcision of adults (El Bcheraoui et al. 2014). If circumcision of a male is inevitable, it is best performed in infancy (Cohen-Almagor 2021).

Morris et al. (2019) recently published a comprehensive review of the health effects of childhood circumcision. Infant circumcision reduces the incidence of childhood urinary tract infection. Circumcised men have a lower incidence of many sexually transmitted infections, including HPV[1] and HIV. The success of circumcision in reducing heterosexual transmission of HIV has led the World Health Organization (WHO) to endorse circumcision in HPV-prevalent regions, beginning at age 15 (World Health Organization 2008). This recommendation was based on results of three highly powered and well-designed randomized trials 2007, (reviewed by Krieger 2012). The value of these trials has been disputed by authors with a history of fierce opposition to childhood circumcision on ideological grounds (Boyle and Hill 2011; van Howe and Storms 2011). However, the efficacy of circumcision in decreasing heterosexual HIV transmission (Farley et al. 2020), and even homosexual transmission (Yuan et al. 2019) has been confirmed by observational studies in sub-Saharan Africa. A group of opponents of these programs (Fish et al. 2020) condemns these circumcision programs as neo-colonialism and compares them to the notorious Tuskegee study in which effective treatment against syphilis was denied to Black patients. The circumcision programs seem the opposite of this in that they make effective treatment available to Blacks. Problems encountered during rollout of circumcision programs, which Fish et al. characterized as a reckless (if not deliberate) assault on African men, are more convincingly explained as problems frequently associated with institution of a novel large-scale effort (Reed et al. 2018). Morris et al. (2019) summarize evidence suggesting that infant circumcision has a protective effect against other sexually transmitted infections, on meatal stenosis, and on penile and prostate cancer. I am unaware of claims that circumcision interferes with male fertility or overall reproductive capability. Sexual issues will be considered below. The health benefits of circumcision are great enough that infant circumcision should be available at parents' discretion, and should be covered by health care payors (American Academy of Pediatrics 2012).

The effects of circumcision on sexual satisfaction and performance are not as clear-cut as the medical safety of circumcision. In premodern times, the medical, social and economic consequences of unconstrained sexual expression and of pregnancy out of wedlock could be harsh. Maimonides, the Arab–Jewish philosopher writing in the twelfth century, spent his entire life in locales where circumcision was universal. Maimonides stated (1186) without evidence that circumcision had a moderating influence on both male and female sexual drive. He believed that tempering the sex drive allows people to make decisions that are congruent with their best interests instead of their immediate passions. Maimonides is frequently

---

[1] The importance of circumcision in HPV control may be lessened where vaccination against HPV is common.

cited for having had anachronistic opinions (O'Hara and O'Hara 1999). Worse, he has been inappropriately cited as evidence that circumcision actually weakens male libido (Boyle et al. 2000). Boyle et al. (2002) also inaccurately cited Maimonides as stating that weakening the sex drive was the purpose of Jewish circumcision.[2]

Since then, we have learned that the sexual effects of childhood circumcision are difficult to study empirically. Randomized trials on sexuality following childhood circumcision are absent. They would be both unethical and impossible to run. Valid case–control studies are difficult to conduct, as well-constructed control groups are hard to select. Circumcision status is highly correlated with religious, ethnic, and other demographic differences, creating inevitable bias in retrospective studies. Recruitment of subjects for surveys introduces additional unintentional and intentional bias, as those willing to answer questions may differ from the overall population in their demographic and experiential characteristics. Also, members of a circumcised *or* uncircumcised minority may be dissatisfied because of pervasive societal messages that their penile appearance is inappropriate. The best-designed case–control studies of sexual satisfaction in men who had infant circumcision (e.g., Laumann et al. 1997; Homfray et al. 2015) show little difference (See, also, Shabanzadeh et al. 2016; Morris and Krieger 2020). Bossio and Pukall (2018) found that men's attitudes about their circumcision status was a better predictor of sexual functioning than circumcision status itself. Furthermore, sexually dissatisfied men might incorrectly attribute their sexual problems to their circumcision status. Both circumcision and sexual dysfunction are quite common, as is post hoc*ergo propter hoc*[3] reasoning. Also, preferences regarding a partner's circumcision status may be due to cultural expectations and sexual experience. Icelandic women (0.1% circumcision rate) may well have different preferences in a male partner than women in Israel (91% circumcision rate) (percentages obtained from Morris et al. 2016).

Two other possible negative effects of circumcision on sexuality have been suggested. The first is that it has a negative effect on the quality of sexual activity between biological males (Bossio et al. 2015). Earp and Darby (2017, 30) observed that circumcision eliminates the possibility of practices requiring manipulation of the foreskin as may occur in sex between males.

Second, men may be distressed simply by having been circumcised as children Hammond and Carmack (2017). Their study was published in a human rights journal rather than a medical journal, and their methodology was shaky.[4] Earp and Darby (2017) claim without data that there have been widespread attempts to reverse

---

[2] In fact, Maimonides (1186/1904) wrote, "[E]very one that is circumcised enters the covenant of Abraham… This purpose of the circumcision is as important as [modification of sexual desire], and perhaps more important." (Maimonides 1186).

[3] A rough translation is: *It came after this, therefore it happened because of this.*

[4] The idea that the prepuce is more sensitive than the glans is widely reported in the literature. It is based on a chain of citations resting on a few questionable sources, some of which was retracted (Morris et al. 2019).Morris et al. offer refuting data (Bhat et al. 2008), on the other hand, found that the density of Meissner's corpuscles in the prepuce is relatively low. The main conclusion that can be drawn from the literature is that the sensory neuroanatomy of the mature prepuce has not been adequately described. At any rate, arguments from anatomy are a distraction. Histology is an intermediate variable, with the end variable being sexual function. Sexual satisfaction involves

circumcision, but the literature suggests that such attempts are unusual (Özer and Timmermans 2020).

14.3 The Case Against Circumcision

Those who would interfere with families must affirmatively justify this interference. I have suggested earlier in this book that assertions of right should not be used as an intervention principle. This is not because human rights documents preclude circumcision of minors (Jacobs and Arora 2015); rather, it is because assertions of rights lack sufficient foundation and precision to ground an ethical basis for state intervention. The UN structure of declarations and conventions provide for hundreds of rights, many of which are in conflict. They can be construed either to permit or discourage circumcision (Jacobs 2013; Jacobs and Arora 2015) They affirm parental powers, guarantee family and cultural rights, and guarantee children the right to practice their religion. The documents, furthermore, neither have internal attempts at rational justification nor do they constitute national positive law. To the extent that I accept their authority in the ensuing discussion, it is only for the sake of argument.

The dispute over circumcision has deep cultural roots and began long before Paul Cassin and others drafted the United Nations Declaration of the Rights of Man. Ritual childhood circumcision is required by most branches of Judaism (Ganzfried 1961; Klein 1992; Union for Reform Judaism 2011) and Islam (al-Sabbagh 1996). Judaism "affirm[s] male circumcision as an integral part of the divine covenant (*brit milah*) that has existed for five thousand years between God and the Jewish people" (Union for Reform Judaism 2011). In contrast, ritual childhood circumcision is disfavored in Christian and post-Christian Europe. The Christian canon describes ritual childhood circumcision as alternatively unnecessary (Romans 4) or affirmatively sacrilegious (Galatians 5:2–4). Christian doctrine abrogated the Jewish requirement for ritual childhood circumcision (Acts 15:1–32). Physical circumcision was rejected by early theologians such as the heretical Marcion and the orthodox Justin and Origen. Simultaneously, pagan emperors of the Nerva-Antonine dynasty attempted to prevent Jews from circumcising converts and slaves and, in extreme cases, to prevent them from circumcising their children. The theologically-based Christian and culturally-based Roman hostility to ritual childhood circumcision continued in secular guises during the Enlightenment. Voltaire was famously critical of Judaism and Jewish practice, though he was not a racial anti-Semite. Immanuel Kant translated into secular language both the universalistic Christian viewpoint and the Christian emphasis on doctrine as opposed to specific rules for action (Kant, 1793/1960). Kant was palpably hostile to Jewish religion, which he termed not a genuine religion (Kant 1793/1960). To Kant, Judaism was merely a tribal political union whose specific

---

other, and likely more important, factors than density of sensory receptors in the various sites within the penis.

legislation, absence of afterlife, paucity of theological speculation, and belief in collective responsibility distinguished it from true religion. Indeed, Kant (1798) advocated the destruction of the Jewish religion, which he distinguished from physical eradication of Jews.

Not surprisingly, few Europeans are circumcised (Morris et al. 2016), mostly from religious minorities.[5] The notion of a universal, reason-based morality has led to a European constitutional order based on a theory of human rights that is conceptually Eurocentric (Mutua 2007). European constitutional documents such as the European Charter of Human Rights require courts to protect an extensive catalog of rights that individuals hold not only against government, but against all non-state parties. UN rights documents were not considered at the time of adoption to forbid circumcision, as is evidenced by their adoption by Islamic states and Israel. These nations would not have agreed to the abolition of childhood circumcision.

At least six putative rights considerations have been invoked to suggest that governments ought to prohibit non-medical childhood circumcision. First is that circumcision is painful (Rosen 2010). In some parts of Africa, circumcision is publicly performed on pubescent boys as a rite of passage, and both the pain and the public nakedness are essential to the ritual (Niang and Boiro 2007). Some groups consider this to be appropriate to demonstrate that pubescent boys possess the highly desirable trait of fortitude. Conditions in some of these places are harsh, and circumcision, even performed in pubescent boys without pain relief, may not be exceptionally brutal in the context of life in those places. (Brusa and Barilan (2009). Minimization of pain, however, is important in the Western context. Adequate analgesia is available in the West and should be used, so pain should not be an issue (Cohen-Almagor 2021). Shweder (2016) recounts a conversation with an American professor who grew up in Kenya. The professor was circumcised at age 13 and recounted it as the most painful experience in his life. Nonetheless, the physical rite, and the ensuing initiation into the history of his community and its expectations of men, made the experience overwhelmingly positive. He regarded his assimilation into the community and bonding with his peers as a huge boon. There are painful initiation rites in many cultures; playing on American high school football teams comes to mind. Most participants consider the resulting bonding to be worth the pain.

The second rights allegation is that childhood circumcision violates a right to bodily integrity (Svoboda 2013b). Circumcision is a *de minimis* breach of bodily integrity (Jacobs and Arora 2015). Dekkers et al. (2005) characterize ritual childhood circumcision as a prima facie violation. *De minimis* harms should not addressed under the rubric of human rights. Being jostled on a train station platform is not comparable to being thrown under a train (Jacobs 2021). It was a professed concern for bodily integrity, though, that formed the rationale of the non-binding European Parliament (2013) that called for regulation of ritual childhood circumcision. Circumcision is widely practiced outside nations whose culture is European or Hispanic, suggesting that opposition arises from a cultural positionality as much as from a reasoned concern for foreskin integrity. The roster of European academic physicians who characterized

[5] Except in heavily Islamic Albania, Kosovo, North Macedonia, and Bosnia.

as culturally biased the AAP recommendation that infant circumcision be a matter of parental choice (Frisch et al. 2013) should reexamine their claim that their desire to ban childhood circumcision altogether is objective. The history of relations between Jews and the broader population in many of their nations over the last century suggests that deep-seated hostility toward Judaism may be as much of a motivating factor as a reverent concern for the intact body.

The third assertion is that circumcision violates the infant's autonomy (Brussels Collaboration 2019). This issue has been addressed and refuted (Freeman 1999; Brusa and Barilan 2009; Mazor 2013, 2019; Jacobs and Arora 2015). On the one hand, circumcision opponents claim that elective circumcision may be authorized only by the male himself as a consenting adult (Svoboda 2013a). On the other hand, another conception of autonomy holds that parents, as surrogates, may act in their perception of the child's interests and needs. Ritual childhood circumcision conforms to the expectations of their well-established cultures. It addresses both the intrinsic value of circumcision to the parents and their community, and to their desire to see their children accepted. It also involves anticipating what the grown child would retrospectively have wanted his parents to have done. Parents, then, should do what they reasonably believe the child is most likely to desire as an adult (Brusa and Barilan 2009). Also, an infant boy's interest in deferring a decision regarding circumcision must be balanced against the interest in being integrated into his family's religious and cultural milieu, and in the interest of having a maximally safe circumcision if ultimate circumcision is inevitable or highly likely. Opponents argue that men may regret the fact of their circumcision. On the other hand, grown children might well resent the omission of circumcision at an age when it is significantly less painful, risky, and complicated, and disruptive to their lives. One can always resent one's parents' choices. There are many things that adult children regret having done to them. These may not be physically irrevocable, but the effects of decisions that have emotional and social impact extending into adulthood obviously have a permanent effect. Adults may resent their parents having other children or resent having been an only child. They may be angry that their parents compelled them to take music or religion lessons after school, or angry that they did not receive these. We all can be angry at our parents, and there always is someone whose own agenda makes them eager to stoke our anger in the service of their cause. Boys not circumcised during childhood form a body image that includes their foreskin; deferring circumcision is not a neutral act. A Jew or Muslim who is not circumcised is deprived of the experience of maturation and socialization typical to their native culture (Brusa and Barilan 2009).

Mazor (2013, 2019) correctly views childhood circumcision as a matter of balancing interests rather than as a question of right, and sees a boy's integration into a circumcising religious community as outweighing interest arguments against infant circumcision. An influential child rights scholar (Freeman 1999) regards parental power to authorize child circumcision as compatible with the child-friendly British legal principle of paramountcy (*Children Act, 1989, cl. 31(2), Eng, Wales*, I(1)), which prioritizes child interests over all other considerations in all legal proceedings. The alternative to integration into a minority cultural group is not elevation to some sublime state of autonomous judgment and choice. Realistically, the alternative to immersion in a minority culture is integration into the predominant society and adoption of its views. David Brooks (2020) praises such indoctrination as conducive to the happiness and well-being of members of society. This has a sinister ring to survivors (and their descendants) of the many programs of ethnic cleansing and extermination with which we have become familiar in the last century or so.

The fourth argument is that child circumcision is said to limit the child's putative right to an open future (Darby 2013). In fact, most decisions made for children narrow the child's future. Parents and communities shape and narrow a child's passions, activities, beliefs, and aspirations. The focus on circumcision as a major limiting factor seems wildly disproportionate. Childhood circumcision opponents' fifth contention is that circumcision impairs sexual function. This is unlikely, as discussed earlier in this chapter. Finally, circumcision prevents some forms of sexual expression, particularly in the context of sexual acts between two anatomic males. This may be true, but it does not prevent satisfactory overall sexual relationships, including physical relationships with other men. This limitation is not a sufficient reason to abolish infant circumcision.

I now turn to the question of sex and gender. The first question is whether the rite of circumcision express and reinforce a view of gender as binary and biologically determined? Ritual childhood circumcision certainly is compatible with this viewpoint, which is embodied in traditional Judaism and Islam. This is not the entire story, though. Liberal forms of Judaism, such as Conservative and Reform, have retained ritual infant circumcision. Meanwhile, they affirm full religious rights for transgender and gender non-conforming people (Union for Reform Judaism 2003; Rabbinical Assembly 2016).[6] Whatever its original rationale, ritual childhood circumcision is not inextricably linked to a position on gender identity. Furthermore, the experience of circumcision does not deter biologic males from assuming a gender incongruous orientation.

Second, does circumcision reinforce male dominance? This assertion is not convincing. Certainly, only boys are subject to body-altering rituals in Judaism. Furthermore, sexist justifications for this physical ritual were proffered in times when male dominance was taken for granted (Carlin 2016). The traditional criterion for Jewish identity is being born to a Jewish woman; paternity is irrelevant.[7] The egalitarian approach of Reform and Conservative Judaism regarding all aspects of personal status, and the generally favorable attitudes of members of these movements toward gender equality show, however, that there is no necessary connection between ritual childhood circumcision and male superiority.

[6] The Rabbinical Assembly is the organization of rabbis in the Conservative movement, and is as definitive a source of authority as exists within that movement.

[7] Reform Judaism and some other progressive movements consider someone with one Jewish parent, and who affirms Judaism, to be Jewish (Central Conference of American Rabbis 1983). Whether by parental descent or the traditional patrilineal descent, Judaism considers that a person acquires the privileges and responsibilities of being Jewish by birth. Being Jewish does not require a voluntary commitment, except for converts.

It is doubtful that resolution of gender issues would be sufficient to resolve the objections of critics. Consider a hypothetical example of a novel Jewish practice (Jacobs 2021). A liberal Jewish movement is committed to ideals of autonomy, acceptance of all sexual and gender expression, and to the idea that a distinguishing physical mark is essential. It wants, though, to make it easy for Jews to leave Judaism as adults, and to remove a physical stigma. The group substitutes the following rite for circumcision. It tattoos a 2 mm *mogen David* (six-pointed star) in an inconspicuous place in the inner thigh of each newborn Jewish child. The tattoo can easily and safely be removed using a laser if the child later decides to renounce Judaism. All of the arguments I have raised so far against circumcision are countered, except for the autonomy and bodily integrity considerations. Clearly, though, these are *de minimis* and easily reversible physical stigmata, and they should not affect the child's socialization or sexual expression It would seem as though the ceremony would not be worth much attention, as it does not even affect the 'salient' (Munzer 2018) genitalia. I suspect, though, that this rite would still be objectionable to many who oppose circumcision. The particularity of Judaism contradicts the claim to universality of Christianity as expressed by Paul, Marcion, and the church fathers; the claim to the universality of ethics, as expressed by Kant (1793), and the political universality of Marxism, as Svenungsson (2011) identifies in the works of Marxist critics of Judaism such as Žižek and Badiou. This is not just about Judaism; Contemporary European critics are also concerned with a *de minimis* ceremonial vulvar nick as performed by some Muslims, and doubtless would not like it any better if a nick were applied to the small of the backs of both boys and girls (Sarajlic 2020).

14.4 The State Intervention Test and Circumcision

The State Intervention Test does not warrant government interference with childhood circumcision, except to ensure that it is being performed safely and humanely. This is affirmed in the Direct Effects Basis. The physical complications of childhood circumcision are either minor or rare. Ritual childhood circumcision often is performed outside the health care system. It therefore is reasonable for government to ensure the competence of non-medical practitioners. The government also has the authority under the Test to forbid direct oral aspiration of blood from the penis following foreskin removal, known as *Metzitzah B'peh* (Kerlee 2004). This unusual practice, followed by some traditional groups, causes potentially fatal herpes encephalitis in about 1 in 3000 children (Cherpes et al. 2012). However, a government that tries to enforce these measures may encounter resistance, so that governments should consider compromises such as testing *mohalim* (trained religious providers of circumcision) for herpes as a harm-reducing alternative to banning the practice (Jacobs and Arora 2017).

There is insufficient evidence suggesting significant psychological distress to justify proscription of infant circumcision under the State Intervention Test. The inability to engage in a full range of tactile experiences, such as docking (a practice in which a man inserts his erect penis into an orifice created by another man's manually dilating his foreskin) (Harrison 2002) does not seem to reach the severe physiological or psychological harm needed to invoke the Direct Effects Basis. It is possible to have a highly satisfactory sexual relationship without a prepuce. Indeed, there are sufficient health benefits to justify elective infant circumcision (American Academy of Pediatrics 2012). The medical benefits of childhood are reviewed by Morris et al. (2019).

Now let us consider the Indirect Effects Basis. Let us assume for argument's sake that childhood circumcision carries no health benefits, and is being performed only as a ritual. To invoke government power to ban circumcision on the basis of the Indirect Effects Basis it would be necessary to demonstrate a burden to society and its members. Childhood circumcision does not significantly harm third parties. The question, then, is whether childhood circumcision transgresses societal norms to such an extent that it should be banned. In a nation such as the United States or Korea, where non-medical circumcision is common, this is not the case. What about countries in which non-medical circumcision is rare? The question here is whether the social transgression is so great that a religion which regards circumcision as a central tenet cannot be tolerated. Some opponents of circumcision, such as the Royal Dutch Netherlands Association (2010) attempt to finesse this question by declaring that it would not pose much of a problem for Judaism or Islam to simply drop the rite from its requirements. After all, some Jews and Muslims (albeit a small minority) reject circumcision (Kesvani 2017). This condescending view ignores the fact that religious requirements are based on a complex interaction among canonical texts, hermeneutic traditions, and communal practice. Dutch physicians are free to approve or disapprove of Jewish (or Islamic) practice. They cannot, however, determine what is doctrinal or heretical in Judaism or any other religious community to whose membership they do not belong. Participation in a religious tradition is an organic, lived, group experience (Orsi 2003; Stringer 2008). Outsiders cannot tell others what is necessary, optional, or forbidden within the context of their religions or analogous belief systems. It is disingenuous to do this by citing statements or writings of selected Jews (or Muslims), or by their own interpretation of canonical texts. This is akin to telling a Quaker that the existence of Christian military chaplains shows that Christianity sanctions combat. Nor is there a monolithic approach to this question; Jews are subdivided into movements, each with its approach to religious practice, and views about who has the authority to rule in this area. Just as Baptists and Russian Orthodox disagree on the timing of baptism, different Jewish movements determine their own sanctioned practices and beliefs.

A society that seeks to abolish ritual childhood circumcision is at least incidentally committed to exclusion of mainstream Jews and Muslims. If ritual childhood circumcision is outlawed, then its practitioners will either have to abandon this core belief, leave the state, or face the state's legal penalties, much like Jews and Muslims during the Spanish Inquisition. Alternatively, in a society in which circumcised men are merely treated with disfavor and those who circumcise their children are treated with hostility, it is possible that the practice, or the religions that requires it, will be voluntarily abandoned. The Indirect Effects prong is flexible, but using state power to curb childhood circumcision departs drastically from liberalism.

The constraints in the Test overcome suppression of ritual childhood circumcision. Briefly, the Likelihood Constraint applies because severe effects of childhood circumcision either are rare or hypothetical. The Comparability of Effect Constraint applies because the effects of childhood circumcision are not of greater magnitude than many other elective and aesthetic procedures performed on minors. For example, aesthetic orthodontia, which is so common as to be a rite of passage in the affluent West, is more painful and dangerous than childhood circumcision, often involving dental extraction. Finally, the negative effects of punishment of IC exceed any harms of IC itself.

14.5 Conclusion

At least a third of males alive today have undergone circumcision. It is often performed for aesthetic or cultural reasons, or to enhance health. Its safety is well-established, as are certain health benefits. Most often, it has been performed as a religious requirement.

Religion is not only—and generally not primarily—a matter of belief. Gunn (2003) speaks of religion as having three principal attributes, which vary according to the religion and the religionist. These are beliefs, individual connection, and community or social cohesion.[8] Different religions place different emphases on each of these attributes, and approach each of them differently. Them differently. Thus, regarding belief, Christianity is monotheistic, Hinduism polytheistic, and Confucianism non-theistic. Individual Sufis and Pentecostals seek mystical experiences; Unitarians and Reform Jews not so much. As for community, Judaism and Shinto are tied to national communities, while Islam claims universality. American courts, recognizing the protean nature of religion and bound by a written constitution that bars the government from establishing religion, have refused to interpret religious doctrine (*Serbian Eastern Orthodox Diocese v. Milivojevich*, 426 U.S. 696, Supreme Court, 1976). On the other hand, some European courts have interpreted the religions of its citizens. The English Supreme Court ruled that religion was strictly a matter of doctrine (*R (E) v Governing Body of JFS* [2009] UKSC 15, in which the UK Supreme Court stated that a school could not define membership in Judaism using genealogical criteria, though Jewish descent is the traditional defining characteristic of a Jew.[9]

[8] One might add a fourth view, that of religion as a way to muster noumenal forces to alter the physical world. The use of religion to manipulate physical reality is present in traditional religions (Kroesbergen 2019). The prosperity gospel (Bowler 2013) and Wicca (Pearson 2000) are current American examples of using religion to influence physical outcomes.

[9] This is an oversimplification of the issues. The mother professed belief in Judaism but had not been born Jewish, and had undergone a conversion procedure considered invalid by the school authorities. The court held that her profession of Jewish belief made her Jewish. In any event, this court took it upon itself to define Judaism in terms of belief, analogous to Protestantism.

Philosophers such as Kant (1793/1960) have promoted the factual error that religion is principally about theological speculation and affirmation. Doctrine is not of primary importance to most religious adherents, even when it forms the intellectual basis for the religion. The typical Christian is not preoccupied with the nature of the Trinity or with transubstantiation (Stringer 2008). Rather, religion provides community, spirituality, solace, perhaps an opportunity to change one's circumstances through prayer and ritual (Stringer 2008), and, in the case of religions such as traditional Judaism and Islam, the ordering of their lives through comprehensive religious laws.

U.S. v. Seeger, 380 US 163, Supreme Court 1965, 187, adopted Tillich's broad, but doctrinally based, definition of religion as the source of one's being and ultimate concern, so that American laws against religion do not require a belief in transcendental entities such as gods or laws of karma. Some secular beliefs and belief systems have religious overtones. The founding metaphorical myths of Rawls's original position and other contractarian views of pre-state humanity seem comparable in function to the narrative of Genesis 1:1–11:9, when both are construed metaphorically. However, after supplying a founding myth, Rawls (2005) called for elimination of non-public reasons from political discourse and for voting. Among Rawls' basic primary goods is the social basis for self-respect (Rawls 2005), which I have argued is provided by belonging to groups with shared beliefs, relationships, and practices, and to families—one of whose roles is to live and perpetuate these beliefs and practices. Furthermore, in non-ideal societies, people will pursue their own interests. The most a liberal can expect is that we will attempt to use the government as a shield, and not as a sword to unnecessarily restrict others.

Using the law as a sword is what many opponents of circumcision are advocating. They would ban all forms of ritual sexual ceremonies—harmful, *de minimis*, or even beneficial to health—ostensibly on the basis of their beliefs in the overriding importance of autonomy and of maximal sexual expression (Brussels Collaborative 2019; Earp 2021). Earp (2021) describes the Brussels manifesto as an international consensus statement, but this consensus seems limited to activists, many in academics, who are committed abolish clitoral surgery in children with congenital adrenal hyperplasia, circumcision, and all forms of female genital alteration. It is not a consensus outside those who prepared the manifesto. Opponents of genital rituals criticize the objectivity of those who would leave the matter to individual families (Frisch et al. 2013), while implying that their own desire to abolish the practice is objective. Some opponents have stated (Earp 2021) or implied (van Howe 2015)[10] that, since some drafters of the American Academy of Pediatrics policy recommending parent choice are Jewish and favor allowing circumcision of Jews for non-medical reasons, they cannot fairly evaluate medical evidence. This is in contrast to the supposed objectivity of those opposed to circumcision.

[10] van Howe (2015) criticized the preponderance of one ethno/religious group in the composition of the AAP panel without specifically identifying that group. Three of the eight members of the panel that drafted the statement had current or birth surnames that are commonly held by Jews, with no particular cluster of other nationally identifiable birth names. This composition was reflective of the demographics of the upper echelon of academic pediatrics in the US in the early twenty-first century.

I find no convincing reason to believe that secular philosophers stand in a superior moral position to Jewish or religious authorities with regard to making binding demands on other individuals. Parents must decide soon after their sons' births whether to raise them with a circumcised or an uncircumcised body image. There is no compelling ethical or moral reason to favor the ability to be on the receiving end of docking[11] over full integration into a Jewish or Islamic community.

Circumcision usually is safe when performed under hygienic conditions by operators with expertise. Evidence for positive health effects is sufficient to justify elective circumcision outside the ritual setting. There is wide experience in the Western world with circumcision, so that most people know circumcised men. Isolated claims that do not mirror ordinary experience, such as the assertions in the literature that circumcision is associated with autism (Frisch and Simonsen 2015), PTSD (Ramos and Boyle 2000), and enhanced sociosexuality[12] and sensation seeking (Miani et al. 2020) should be viewed with skepticism. I conclude that hygienically-performed circumcisions are permissible in healthy male infants.

Female genital alteration, in contrast to circumcision, comprises a wide range of procedures, the effects of which are not well studied. The extent ranges from a simple needle prick to removal of the entire external genitalia. It is to this range of procedures that I now turn.

References

Aktürk, Şener. 2019. Comparative politics of circumcision bans in Western Europe: A causal narrative. *APSA Preprints*. https://doi.org/10.33774/apsa-2019-d0gw1.

al-Sabbagh, Mohammed Lufti. 1996. *Islamic Ruling on Male and Female Circumcision*. Geneva: World Health Organization. http://apps.who.int/iris/bitstream/handle/10665/119559/dsa54.pdf?sequence=1&isAllowed=y.

American Academy of Pediatrics. 2012. Task force on circumcision. Circumcision policy statement. *Pediatrics* 130 (3): 585–586.

Ben-Chaim, Jacob, Pinhas M. Livne, Joseph Binyamini, Benyamin Harda, David Ben-Meir, and Yoram Mor. 2005. Complications of circumcision in Israel: A one year multicenter survey. *Israel Medical Association Journal IMAJ* 7 (6): 368–370.

Bhat, Ghulam Mohammad, Mohammad Akbar Bhat, Kulbeer Kour, and Bashir Ahmad Shah. 2008. Density and structural variations of Meissner's corpuscle at different sites in human glabrous skin. *Journal of the Anatomic Society of India* 57 (1): 30–33.

Bossio, Jennifer A., Caroline F. Pukall, and Katie Bartley. 2015. You either have it or you don't: The impact of male circumcision on sexual partners. *Canadian Journal of Human Sexuality* 24 (2): 104–119.

[11] A sexual practice in which one man extends his prepuce over the glans of another man's penis, for the purpose of sexual pleasure, especially for the man whose glans is covered by the other man's prepuce. It should be clear that I am using 'docking' as a metonym for any sexual activity that requires a penile prepuce. In this context, I use 'docking' as a metonym for sexual practices requiring a foreskin.

[12] Sociosexuality is the willingness to engage in physical sex outside of a committed relationship (Penke and Asendorpf 2008). A number of studies (e.g., Koladich and Atkinson 2016) link sociosexuality with the Dark Triad of narcissism, Machiavellianism, and psychopathy.

Bossio, Jennifer A., and Caroline F. Pukall. 2018. Attitude toward one's circumcision status is more important than actual circumcision status for men's body image and sexual functioning. *Archives of Sexual Behavior* 47 (3): 771–781.

Bowler, Kate. 2013. *Blessed: A history of the prosperity gospel*. New York: Oxford University Press.

Boyle, Gregory. J., J. Steven Svoboda, Christopher P. Price, and J. Neville Turner. 2000. Circumcision of healthy boys: Criminal assault? *Journal of Law and Medicine* 7 (3): 301–10.

Boyle, Gregory J., Ronald Goldman, J Steven Svoboda, and Ephrem Fernandez. 2002. Male circumcision: Pain, trauma and psychosexual sequelae. *Journal of Health Psychology* 7 (3): 329–343.

Boyle, Gregory J., and George Hill. 2011. Sub-Saharan African randomized clinical trials into male circumcision and HIV transmission: Methodological, ethical and legal concerns. *Journal of Law and Medicine* 19 (2): 316–333.

Brooks, David. 2020. This is how Scandinavia got great. *New York Times* § A: 27. https://www.nytimes.com/2020/02/13/opinion/scandinavia-education.html?action=click&module=Opinion&pgtype=Homepage.

Brusa, Margherita, and Y. Michael Barilan. 2009. Cultural circumcision in EU public hospitals—An ethical discussion. *Bioethics* 23 (8): 470–482.

Brussels Collaboration on Bodily Integrity. 2019. Medically unnecessary genital cutting and the rights of the child: Moving toward consensus. *American Journal of Bioethics* 19 (10): 17–28. https://doi.org/10.1080/15265161.2019.1643945.

Carlin, Na'ama. 2016. *Written Through Blood: The Moral Complexities of Jewish Ritual Circumcision*. Ph.D. Dissertation, University of New South Wales. http://unsworks.unsw.edu.au/fapi/datastream/unsworks:45083/SOURCE02?view=true.

Central Conference of American Rabbis. 1983. *Reform Judaism: Resolution on Patrilineal Descent: The Status of Children of Mixed Marriages*. https://www.jewishvirtuallibrary.org/reform-movement-s-resolution-on-patrilineal-descent-march-1983#:~:text=Committee%20on%20Patrilineal%20Descent%20adopted%20on%20March%2015%2C,is%20mixed%20marriage%2C%20with%20all%20its%20attendant%20implications.

Cherpes, Thomas L., Dean B. Matthews, and Samantha A. Maryak. 2012. Neonatal herpes simplex virus infection. *Clinical Obstetrics and Gynecology* 55 (4): 938–944.

Cohen-Almagor, Raphael. 2021. Should Liberal Government regulate male circumcision performed in the name of Jewish tradition? *SN Social Sciences* 1: 8. https://doi.org/10.1007/s43545-020-00011-7.

Darby, Robert J. L. 2013. The child's right to an open future: Is the principle applicable to non-therapeutic circumcision? *Journal of Medical Ethics* 39 (7): 463–468.

Dekkers, Wim, Cor Hoffer, and Jean-Pierre. Wils. 2005. Bodily integrity and male and female circumcision. *Medicine, Health Care and Philosophy*. 8 (2): 179–191.

Earp, Brian D. (2021). Male or female genital cutting: Why 'Health Benefits' are morally irrelevant. *Journal of Medical Ethics*, online ahead of print [please include Day Month Year]. https://doi.org/10.1136/medethics-2020-106782.

Earp, Brian D., and Robert Darby. 2017. Circumcision, sexual experience, and harm. *University of Pennsylvania Journal of International Law* [Online Symposium, re: Vol. 37, Iss. 2]. https://www.researchgate.net/profile/Brian_Earp/publication/315763686_Circumcision_sexual_experience_and_harm/links/5911160baca272ec9a391cd3/Circumcision-sexual-experience-and-harm.pdf.

El Bcheraoui, Charbel, Xinjian Zhang, Christopher. S. Cooper, Charles E. Rose, Peter H. Kilmarx, and Robert T. Chen. 2014. Rates of adverse events associated with male circumcision in US medical settings, 2001 to 2010. *JAMA Pediatrics* 168 (7): 625–34.

European Parliament. 2013. Resolution 1952: Children's right to physical integrity. Available at http://assembly.coe.int/nw/xml/XRef/Xref-XML2HTML-en.asp?fileid=20174.

Farley, Timothy M.M., Julia Samuelson, M. Kate Grabowski, Wole Ameyaw, Ronald H Gray, and Rachel Baguley. 2020. Impact of male circumcision on risk of HIV infection in men in a changing

epidemic context: Systematic review and meta-analysis. *Journal of the International AIDS Society* 23 (6): e25490. https://doi.org/10.1002/jia2.25490.
Fish, Max, Arianne Shahvisi, Tatenda Gwaambuka, Godfrey B. Tangwa, Daniel Ncayiyana, and Brian D Earp. 2020. A new tuskegee? Unethical human experimentation and western neocolonialism in the mass circumcision of african men. https://doi.org/10.1111/dewb.12285. Online ahead of print.
Freeman, Michael D.A.. 1999. A child's right to circumcision. *BJU International* 83 (Suppl. 1): 74–78.
Friedman, B., J. Khoury, N. Petersen, T. Yahalom, M. Paul, and A. Neuberger. 2016. Pros and cons of circumcision: An evidence-based overview. *Clinical Microbiology and Infection* 22 (9): 768–774.
Frisch, Morten, Yves Agarin, Vidantas Balaskas, Ragnar Bjarnason, Su-Anna Boddy, Piotr Cadorna, Robert P.E. de Giver, et al. 2013. Cultural bias in the AAP's 2012 technical report and policy statement on male circumcision. *Pediatrics* 131 (4): 796–800.
Frisch, Morten, and Jacob Simonsen. 2015. Ritual circumcision and risk of autism spectrum disorder in 0- To 9-year-old boys: National cohort study in Denmark. *Journal of the Royal Society of Medicine* 108 (7): 266–279. https://doi.org/10.1177/0141076814565942.
Ganzfried, Solomon. 1961. *Code of Jewish Law*, translated by Hyman E. Goldin. New York, Hebrew Publishing Company.
Gunn, T. Jeremy. 2003. The complexity of religion and the definition of "religion" in international law. *Harvard Human Rights Journal* 16(1): 189-215.
Hammond, Tim, and Adrienne Carmack. 2017. Long-term adverse outcomes from neonatal circumcision reported in a survey of 1,008 men: An overview of health and human rights implications. *International Journal of Human Rights* 21 (2): 189–218.
Harrison, Daniel M. 2002. Rethinking circumcision and sexuality in the United States. *Sexualities* 5 (3): 300–316.
Heras, Andrea, Victoria Vallejo, Marcela I. Pineda, Allan J. Jacobs, and Lourdes Cohen. 2018. Immediate complications of elective newborn circumcision. *Hospital Pediatrics* 8 (10): 615–619.
Homfray, Virginia, Clare Tanton, Kirstin R. Mitchell, Robert F. Miller, Nigel Field, Wendy Macdowall, Kaye Wellings, Pam Sonnenberg, Anne M. Johnson, and Catherine H. Mercer. 2015. Examining the association between male circumcision and sexual function: Evidence from a British probability survey. *AIDS* 29 (11): 1411–1416.
Jacobs, Allan J. 2013. The ethics of circumcision of male infants. *Israel Medical Association. Journal: IMAJ* 15 (1): 60–64.
Jacobs, Allan J. 2021. Is physical alteration a sufficient reason to prohibit ritual infant circumcision? *Journal of Religion and Health.* 60 (3): 1672–1693. https://doi.org/10.1007/s10943-020-01139-9.
Jacobs, Allan J., and Kavita Shah Arora. 2015. Ritual male infant circumcision and human rights. *American Journal of Bioethics* 15 (2): 30–39.
Jacobs, Allan J., and Kavita Shah Arora. 2017. Punishment of minor female genital ritual procedures: Is the perfect the enemy of the good?. *Developing World Bioethics* 17 (2): 134-140.
Kant, Immanuel. 1793. *Religion Within the Limits of Reason Alone*, translated by Theodore M. Greene & Hoyt H. Hudson. New York: Harper Torchbooks.
Kant, Immanuel. 1798. *The conflict of the faculties*, translated by Mary J. Gregor. Lincoln: University of Nebraska Press.
Kerlee, Jamie Cole. 2004. Too much religious freedom? Infants infected with Herpes after Jewish Mohel applies oral suction to circumcised penises. *Journal of Law and Health* 19 (2): 297–411.
Kesvani, Hussein. 2017. The first generation of Jewish and Muslim Men conflicted about having their sons circumcised. *MEL Magazine*. https://melmagazine.com/en-us/story/the-first-generation-of-jewish-and-muslim-men-conflicted-about-having-their-sons-circumcised-2.
Klein, Isaac. 1992. *A guide to Jewish religious practice*. New York: Jewish Theological Seminary of America.

Koladich, Samantha J., and Breanna E. Atkinson. 2016. The dark triad and relationship preferences: A replication and extension. *Personality and Individual Differences* 94 (3): 253–255. https://doi.org/10.1016/j.paid.2016.01.023.

Krieger, John N. 2012. Male circumcision and HIV infection risk. *World Journal of Urology* 30 (1): 3–13. https://doi.org/10.1007/s00345-011-0696-x.

Kroesbergen, Hermen. 2019. Religion without belief and community in Africa. *Religions* 10(4}: 292-311. https://doi.org/10.3390/rel10040292.

Laumann, Edward O., Christopher M. Masi, and Ezra W. Zuckerman. 1997. Circumcision in the United States: Prevalence, prophylactic effects and sexual practice. *JAMA* 277 (13): 1052–1057.

Maimonides, Moses. 1186. *The guide for the perplexed*, translated by M. Friedländer. New York: E.F. Dutton. https://en.wikisource.org/wiki/The_Guide_for_the_Perplexed_(Friedlander)/Part_III/Chapters.

Mazor, Joseph. 2013. The child's interests and the case for the permissibility of male infant circumcision. *Journal of Medical Ethics* 39 (7): 421–428.

Mazor, Joseph. 2019. On the strength of children's right to bodily integrity: The case of circumcision. *Journal of Applied Philosophy* 36 (1): 1–16.

Miani, Alessandro, Gian Antonio Di Bernardo, Astrid Ditte Højgaard, Brian D. Earp, Paul J. Zak, Anne M. Landau, Jørgen Hoppe, and Michael Winterdahl. 2020. Neonatal male circumcision is associated with altered adult socio-affective processing. *Heliyon Cell Press* 6(11): e05566.

Morris, Brian J., and John N. Krieger. 2020. The contrasting evidence concerning the effect of male circumcision on sexual function, sensation, and pleasure: A systematic review. *Sexual Medicine* 8 (4): 577–598. https://doi.org/10.1016/j.esxm.2020.08.011.

Morris, Brian J., Richard G. Wamai, Esther B. Henebeng, Aaron A. R. Tobian, Jeffrey D. Klausner, J. Banerjee, & Catherine A. Hankins. 2016 estimation of country-specific and global prevalence of male circumcision. *Population Health Metrics* 14 (1): 1–13 [published correction appears in *Population Health Metrics* 2016: 14:11. https://doi.org/10.1186/s12963-016-0073-5.

Morris, Brian J., Catherine A. Hankins, Eugenie R. Lumbers, Adrian Mindel, Jeffrey D. Klausner, John N. Krieger, and Guy Cox. 2019. Sex and male circumcision: women's preferences across different cultures and countries: A systematic review. *Sexual Medicine* 7 (2): 145–161. https://doi.org/10.1016/j.esxm.2019.03.003.

Munzer, Stephen R. 2018. Examining nontherapeutic circumcision. *Health Matrix* 28 (1): 1–77.

Mutua, Makau. 2007. Standard setting in human rights: Critique and progress. *Human Rights Quarterly* 29 (7): 547–629.

Niang, Cheikh Ibrahima, and Hamadou Boiro. 2007. 'You Can Also Cut My Finger!': Social construction of male circumcision in West Africa, a case study of senegal and Guinea-Bissau. *Reproductive Health Matters* 15 (29): 22–32. https://doi.org/10.1016/S0968-8080(07)29312-7.

O'Hara, K. and J. O'Hara. 1999. The effect of male circumcision on the sexual enjoyment of the female partner. *BJU International* 83 (Suppl. 1): 79-84.

Orsi, Robert A. 2003. Is the study of lived religion irrelevant to the world we live in? *Scientific Study of Religion* 42 (2): 169–174.

Özer, Müjde., and Floyd Timmermans. 2020. An Insight into circumcised men seeking foreskin reconstruction: A prospective cohort study. *International Journal of Impotence Research* 32 (6): 611–616. https://doi.org/10.1038/s41443-019-0223-y.

Pearson, Joanne Elizabeth. 2000. *Religion and the return of magic: Wicca as esoteric spirituality*. PhD thesis, Lancaster University.

Penke, Lars, and Jens B. Asendorpf. 2008. Beyond global sociosexual orientations: a more differentiated look at sociosexuality and its effects on courtship and romantic relationships. *Journal of Personality and Social Psychology* 95 (5): 1113–1135. https://doi.org/10.1037/0022-3514.95.5.1113.

Rabbinical Assembly. 2016. Resolution affirming the rights of transgender and gender non-conforming people. http://www.rabbinicalassembly.org/story/resolution-affirming-rights-transgender-and-gender-non-conforming-people.

Rawls, John. 2005. *Political liberalism*. Expanded. New York: Columbia University Press.

Reed, J.B., R. Patel, R. Baggaley. 2018. Lessons from a decade of voluntary medical male circumcision implementation and their application to HIV pre-exposure prophylaxis scale up *International Journal of STD and AIDS* 29 (14): 1432–43. https://doi.org/10.1177/0956462418787896.

Ramos, Samuel and Gregory J. Boyle. 2000. Ritual and medical circumcision among filipino boys: Evidence of post-traumatic stress disorder. *Humanities & Social Sciences papers*. Paper 114. http://epublications.bond.edu.au/hss_pubs/114.

Rosen, Michael. 2010. Anesthesia for ritual circumcision in neonates. *Pediatric Anesthesia* 20 (12): 1124–1127.

Royal Dutch Medical Association. 2010. "Non-Therapeutic Circumcision of Male Minors.

Sarajlic, Eldar. 2020. Children, Culture, and Body Modification." *Kennedy Institute of Ethics Journal*, 30, no. 2: 167–90. *Project MUSE*, doi:https://doi.org/10.1353/ken.2020.0005.

Shabanzadeh Daniel, Signe Düring, and Cai Frimodt-Møller. 2016. Male circumcision does not result in inferior perceived male sexual function—A systematic review. *Danish Medical Journal* 63 (6): A5245.

Shweder, Richard A. 2009. Shouting at the Hebrews: Imperial liberalism v liberal pluralism and the practice of male circumcision. *Law Culture the Humanities* 5 (2): 247–265.

Shweder, Richard A. 2016. Equality now in genital reshaping: brian earp's search for moral consistency. *Kennedy Institute of Ethics Journal* 26 (2): 145–154. https://doi.org/10.1353/ken.2016.0016.

Stringer, Martin D. 2008. *Contemporary Western Ethnography and the Definition of Religion*. London: Continuum.

Svenungsson Jayne. 2011. Enlightened prejudices: Anti-Jewish tropes in modern Philosophy. In *Rethinking Time: Essays on History, Memory and Representation,* Vol. 9, edited by Hans Ruin and Anders Ers. Stockholm: Södertörn Philosophical Studies, 279–90.

Svoboda, J. Steven. 2013a. Tortured bodies, tortured doctrines: informed consent as a legal fiction inapplicable to neonatal male circumcision. In *Genital Cutting: Protecting Children from Medical, Cultural, and Religious Infringements*, edited by George C. Denniston, Frederick M. Hodges, and Marilyn Fayre Milos. Cham, Switzerland: Springer, 1–28.

Svoboda, J. Steven. 2013b. Circumcision of Male Infants as a Human Rights Violation. *Journal of Medical Ethics* 39 (7): 169–174.

Union for Reform Judaism. 2003. Support for the inclusion and acceptance of the transgender and bisexual communities. Commission on Social Action. https://web.archive.org/web/20140103063847/http://urj.org/socialaction/aboutus/reso/?syspage=article&item_id=1872.

Union for Reform Judaism. 2011. Resolution on anti-circumcision initiative. Board of Trustees.. http://urj.org/about/union/governance/reso/?syspage=article&item_id=68500.

van Howe, Robert S. 2015." Presumptions Are Not Data and Data Are Often Not Informative." *American Journal of Bioethics*, 15, no. 2: 40–3. https://doi.org/10.1080/15265161.2014.990761.

van Howe, Robert S., and Michelle R. Storms. 2011. How the circumcision solution in Africa will increase HIV infections. *Journal of Public Health in Africa* 2 (1): 11–15.

World Health Organization. 2008. *Male circumcision: Global Trends and Determinants Of Prevalence, Safety And Acceptability*, 2008. Available at http://apps.who.int/iris/bitstream/handle/10665/43749/97892?sequence=1.

Yuan, Tanwei, Thomas Fitzpatrick, Nai-YingKo, Yong Cai, Yingqing Chen, Jin Zhao, Linghua Li, Junjie Xu, et al. 2019. Circumcision to prevent HIV and other sexually transmitted infections in men who have sex with men: A systematic review and meta-analysis of global data. *Lancet Global Health* 7 (4):, e436-e–447. https://doi.org/10.1016/S2214-109X(18)30567-9.

Chapter 15
Female Genital Alteration

Abstract Female genital alteration (FGA) encompasses a wide range of procedures. Minimal FGA consists of a simple nick with a sharp instrument, leaving no residua. Most Malay and Indonesian girls probably undergo such a vulvar nick. The other extreme of FGA is to remove the entire external genitalia and to surgically narrow the vaginal orifice to render penile penetration difficult or impossible. This procedure, called infibulation, has been prevalent in the Horn of Africa. FGA performance in various places by poorly trained operators under unhygienic conditions increases the risk of all variants of FGA. The frequent absence of analgesia augments likely psychological trauma, though these procedures have become increasing medicalized. All forms of ritual FGA in children are illegal in Western nations, so that outcomes have not been well studied. States in which FGA is indigenous must deal with FGA in the context of their own cultural and legal environment. Where it is tolerated, it is hoped that objective evidence of its effects will be forthcoming, so that policies can be informed by data. In the West, some ritual FGA procedures have acceptable comparable secular procedures. Aesthetic labia minora reduction and clitoral hood retraction (in physically mature women), for example, are legal. Application of the State Intervention Test shows no acceptable application of FGA in physically immature girls except, in some cases, for a vulvar nick. More extensive procedures, performed in physically mature and mentally maturing minors, should be evaluated for acceptability on the basis of individual procedures, in the context of mainstream practices.

Childhood male circumcision might be performed for hygiene, aesthetics, cultural reasons, religious demands or prevention of disease. But no health benefit is claimed for Female Genital Alteration (FGA), an inclusive name for many practices which injure or alter the female external genitalia. Rather, FGA is performed for religious, cultural, and aesthetic purposes. The aesthetic benefits may be to enhance one's personal body image or to make oneself more attractive to potential sexual partners. The chapter on circumcision concentrated on a defense of the practice. This chapter

A. J. Jacobs, *Assigning Responsibility for Children's Health When Parents and Authorities Disagree: Whose Child?*, The International Library of Bioethics 90,
https://doi.org/10.1007/978-3-030-87698-2_15

will discuss why FGA might be performed as a ritual. Many of the arguments in this chapter and the last apply to both circumcision and FGA.[1]

Ritual genital alteration is FGA that is normative practice within a cultural or religious group. Behavioral science provides evolutionary hypotheses that help us to understand rituals.[2] Rituals are procedures that groups adopt to foster solidarity, affiliation, voluntary participation and cooperation among members (Henrich 2016). Examples of rituals include oaths, liturgy, hazing (Salinas and Boettcher 2018), and military behavior such as uniforms and saluting. Rituals engender commitment to the group. The greater the burden group membership places on the individual, the greater will be the personal cost of the group's rituals (Whitehouse 1996). Members' ties to the group are reinforced by the personal investment in the ritual. Someone who has undergone ritual genital alteration has, figuratively as well as literally, 'skin in the game.' High-cost rituals are instrumental in steering individuals to accept the group as a community that supports its members in return for active allegiance, perhaps to the extent of being willing to die for the group (Whitehouse 2018). Some criticize rituals involving the genitalia as prioritizing group interests over individual autonomy. That, of course, is the point. The world in which children live determines and reinforces their values, even in milieus that proclaim allegiance to autonomy. Except in self-isolating communities, these values are the predominant values of society. So even supposedly 'autonomous' decisions are strongly conditioned by socialization and education. Progressive suburban youths may believe themselves to be more autonomous than they perceive Mennonites or Orthodox Jews to be, but this feeling of autonomy may be illusory. They are almost certainly not going to choose careers in farming or diamond cutting over law or banking, and are unlikely to choose to have children before their careers are established. Socialization in different environments makes different values and priorities likely. To counter powerful and ubiquitous socialization by the prevailing society, groups competing with the state for members' loyalty may resort to powerful rituals, including isolation and physical stress. University fraternities may accomplish this through initiation rituals involving branding (Niederwork and Twyman 2015), paddling, or other stressful events (Finkel 2002). Initiation into professions such as medicine or the Catholic priesthood involve years of isolating and all-consuming training.

Intergroup competition is an integral part of human existence (Henrich 2016). Success in intergroup competition occurs through combat, survival under harsh conditions, differential migration, differential reproduction, and transmission of group norms based on a group's prestige and success.[3] Beyond the question of allegiance, it is important to foster prosocial behavior within the group to promote group survival. This is fostered by rituals that encourage solidarity and discourage cheating,

---

[1] I define *female genital alteration* as any physical invasion of external female genitalia performed for non-medical or non-cosmetic reasons. This term 'female genital alteration' was probably proposed by Davis (2001). It is preferable to either 'female genital cutting' or 'female genital mutilation' (Arora and Jacobs 2016).

[2] For an overview of evolutionary psychology, see Buss and von Hippel (2018).

[3] Societies may reject the assimilation of members of some outgroups (Whitman 2017), while the membership status of others may be insecure; (Kremelberg 2016)

defection, or free-riding (Henrich 2004). Even simple, low-cost rituals unattached to substantively unimportant matters can affect both in-group identification and monitoring of out-groups by in-group participants (Wen et al. 2020).

WHO estimates that up to 140 million women have been subjected to some form of FGA (World Health Organization 2014). This is a marked underestimate. WHO data are based largely on African prevalence. In fact, FGA frequently is performed on the Arabian Peninsula (Alsibiani and Rouzi 2010) and the Indian subcontinent (Abrol 2018), and is widespread in Iran (Latham 2016), Iraq (Kizilhan 2011; Shabila et al. 2014), Malaysia (Rashid and Iguchi 2019), and Indonesia (Bočko 2016). Studies from western Asia suggest an incidence of FGA of about 50%, mostly clitoral amputation or vulvar nick. In Southeast Asia, the vulvar nick predominates, and most Indonesian Muslim girls probably receive it (Bočko 2016). Although the procedure is widely associated with Islam, it is practiced in Africa by some Christian denominations (Shay et al. 2012), Ethiopian Jews (Grisaru et al. 1997), and various groups outside Abrahamic traditions (Ahmadu 2017).

The WHO classification system (World Health Organization 1998) of the various FGA procedures is neither comprehensive nor well-correlated with health consequences. Type I is excision of the prepuce and distal clitoris. Type II is excision of part or all of the clitoris and labia minora. Type III, or infibulation, is excision of part or all of the external genitalia and narrowing of the vaginal opening, leaving a narrow orifice to allow menstruation and urination. Type IV is a catchall category of less extensive procedures that includes vulvar nicking, piercing, or scraping. Partial removal of the clitoral prepuce or the labia minora is not explicitly covered by the WHO classification.

Western nations categorically disapprove of all forms of FGA (Earp and Johnsdotter 2021). Europeans and North Americans long have had direct contact with circumcised men, since Jews have lived in Europe for over two millennia. European Christian nations have mostly tolerated ritual infant circumcision to the extent they tolerated the presence of Jews. Europe was unfamiliar with FGA, though, until it colonized Africa and Asia. Immigration from Africa a few decades ago first brought large numbers of women whose had undergone FGA into Europe. At about the same time, Fran Hosken's writings (1979) and advocacy were instrumental in persuading the United Nations to condemn FGA. This advocacy portrayed FGA in a distorted and stereotyped manner. It was implied that infibulation was the norm, and that its purpose was to physically control women's reproductive lives (Hosken 1979). Certainly, infibulation is likely to diminish sexual pleasure and to make intercourse physically impossible until marriage, but it is practiced only in northeast Africa. Stereotypically, this terrifying and excruciatingly painful procedure is performed on children without their consent, prior knowledge, or analgesia (Goodwin and Jones 2008). As late as 2016, Macklin (2016) erroneously wrote that the purpose of FGA is as a tool for men to control women. This view has established a conceptual framework for subsequent scholarship and political action. The WHO is committed to eradicating all female genital cutting, opposing even minimal cutting as a harm reduction measure to prevent more severe cutting (Askew et al. 2016).

Complications of FGA can be immediate, obstetric, or long-term gynecologic (Lurie et al. 2020). I lean towards skepticism regarding published claims regarding complication rates because the poor quality of most studies (Berg et al. 2014, 2017) probably biases them toward overestimating those rates.[4] The nature of the complications are well known, but vary with context and type of cutting; a prick with a sterile lancet is not dangerous, but removal of the entire external genitalia with a dirty razor blade and then sewing the introitus almost closed is likely to cause major short-term and long-term problems. Immediate complications of invasive forms of FGA include pain, bleeding, wound separation, and infection. Chronic problems include pain, scarring, and dyspareunia. Infibulation may result in urinary retention, menstrual difficulties, and infertility. Psychological consequences have been reported (Bendiksen et al. 2021). Obstetrical problems of infibulation include prolonged or obstructed labor leading to cesarean section, hemorrhage, vulvovaginal tears, and fistulas (Berg and Underland 2013). Case-control studies are difficult to execute because social, physical, educational, and cultural differences between cut and uncut women make it difficult to match controls. Publication bias—the tendency to publish only great differences between groups—may be present, especially given the political saliency of FGA. Controls usually are lacking in clinical reports.

The harm done by different kinds of FGA varies with the extent of the procedure. Presumably, complications are minimal for vulvar nicks. Partial labial removal in adults and adolescents is common in Western nations for both functional and cosmetic reasons (Wood 2018). There are few serious complications, and high satisfaction with the aesthetic and sexual outcomes. The most significant minor complication is transient suture line separation (Özer et al. 2018). Sexual dysfunction or chronic pain are rare, and most often due to excessive excision. It is likely that the same operation, performed for ritual reasons in a medical setting, would have similar outcomes, but it is often done in a non-sterile manner outside the global North. Isolated clitoral hood resection in adults is performed in developed nations to enhance clitoral sensitivity and sexual satisfaction (Hunter 2016). Ritual vulvar ablation often involves clitoral hood excision with or without partial clitoral amputation.[5] It is reported that the ability to achieve orgasm is common even following ritual partial clitoral excision (Catania et al. 2007). On the other hand, some women report persistent pain following partial clitoral amputation. Popular media document pain in Bohra girls who have undergone resection of clitoral or periclitoral tissue (Bengali and Parth 2016). But

---

[4] I have never performed an invasive procedure on a woman for religious, cultural, or aesthetic reasons. I have often removed some or all of the vulva for cancer or premalignant conditions, and have performed labia minora reduction on <5 adults who were experiencing pain or chafing from markedly hyperplastic labia minora.

[5] I have practiced gynecology since beginning residency in 1973, and have performed a number of examinations of prepubertal girls for injuries, foreign bodies, and various lesions. Because of the small size of the prepubertal clitoris and the tight adherence of its hood, I believe that separation of the hood from the clitoral head before puberty runs a high risk of injury to the clitoral glans, even when done well. This would be true even with microsurgical techniques. I therefore believe that incision or resection of the clitoral prepuce (though performed commonly in mature women for sexual enhancement) *is unsafe in prepubertal girls.*

one European study did not observe increased prevalence of vulvar pain in women with clitoral amputation (Catania et al. 2007). One case-control study reported no difference in dyspareunia between cut and uncut women (Morison et al. 2001). The obstetrical complications that follow infibulation (Berg and Underland 2013), even in the West, may result in part from substandard obstetric care (Small et al. 2008) or from treatment choices made by infibulated patients (Brown et al. 2010), as well as from the infibulation itself. Obstetrical injuries observed in Sweden are correlated with extent of FGA (Essén et al. 2002, 2005). Studies (e.g., Frega et al. 2013) showing differences in obstetric outcome in type I and II FGA often do not correct for co-morbid conditions, ethnicity, or socioeconomic variables. A recent meta-analysis (Lurie et al. 2020) concluded that individuals with FGA are at higher risk for dyspareunia, dysuria, perineal tears, episiotomy, and prolonged labor, with an odds ratio between 2.0 and 3.0 for each of these variables. This review did not stratify for extent of the FGA procedure. It is difficult to conceive of how vulvar nicks or tattoos could cause chronic physiological dysfunction.

Psychological sequelae have been reported, often without further elaboration as to its nature or severity (Utz-Billing and Kentinich 2008). Some studies have shown greater psychopathology in women who underwent FGA than in uncut women (Piroozi et al. 2020). Psychological complications are especially likely if there were physical complications or if the woman was cut involuntarily (Ahmed et al. 2017) However, one study in Egypt, where most women undergo FGA, showed no differences between cut and uncut women. This was based on psychological test administration rather than on clinical presentation, which was the outcome variable in most studies (Obaid et al. 2019). There are problems with comparing cut and uncut women with regard to psychopathology The processes of subject selection may often have been biased, especially when the studies were conducted in Europe. There may be differences between the groups that accounted both for psychopathology and correlation with cutting, such as success in adaptation to the new culture. Furthermore, women with FGA living in a Europe that is hostile to these ritual practices, may be confronted with the message that they are mutilated, have disgusting external genitalia and are impaired sexually (Johnsdotter 2018). They may develop negative feelings about what happened to them, taught to them by their new society. This phenomenon is termed *psychological mutilation* in a manifesto written by a team of 15 eminent scholars, most of whom are unsympathetic to FGA (Public Policy Advisory Network 2012).

Societies that practice ritual FGA almost always have corresponding male circumcision rituals. All these rituals celebrate division of the population into male and female genders on the basis of biological sex. But, although Western critics often claim that FGA is a tool of male domination, anthropologists report otherwise. Either males or females may set expectations with regard to sexuality in an African society (Johnsdotter 2013). Furthermore, the rationale for FGA can change with cultural changes. Ahmadu (2017) describes a society that changed from a matrilineal society with a dominant goddess to a patriarchal society practicing an Abrahamic religion. The rationale for FGA changed along with the dominant religion. Most of the reasons justifying both FGA performance and abandonment have been enumerated by Berg and Denison (2013). I have modified their analysis slightly. Besides male control and possession of women, reasons for FGA may include: male sexual pleasure, local sexual mores, marriageability, social expectations both within the culture group and vis-à-vis other ethnic groups, religious dictates, aesthetic standards, and perception that the altered external genitalia are cleaner and predisposed to health. Societal factors that may reduce the frequency of FGA, or the radicality or FGA procedures, include male perception of more enjoyable sex with uncut women, changed views of religious requirements, perception that FGA is dangerous or unhealthy, a desire to conform with enlightened or sophisticated global standards, and legal proscription. Whatever the reasons, the prevalence of FGA seems to be declining in some African nations (Engelsma et al. 2020).

Meanwhile, female external genitalia have been modified ever more frequently in the West for aesthetic, sexual, and social reasons. Piercing and tattooing are common in Western society; up to 1% of youths in some locations may have genital tattoos and the same percentage may have a pierced vulva. Various authors have noted two apparent inconsistencies pertaining to FGA. One is that circumcision of male children is treated more favorably in North America and Europe than is even *de minimis* FGA. This may be because of the greater documentation of the safety of circumcision (see previous chapter). It may also be because of the greater familiarity with circumcision. The other inconsistency is that the very same procedures that the West condemns as human rights violations when done for religious reasons, or as a non-Western cultural practice are performed on a large scale in the West for aesthetic reasons—often on adolescents (Boddy 2020; Earp 2021). Earp (2021) calls for regarding all genital alteration—male and female, Western and non-Western—in the same light, and banning it in individuals below the age of consent unless medically urgent. I also regard comparable procedures in males and females as morally equivalent (Arora and Jacobs 2016; Jacobs and Arora 2017). I would, however, apply the State Intervention Test to the question of government interference with any of these procedures.

15.1 Female Genital Alteration and the State Intervention Test

I ask when a state may ethically reverse parental decision to allow their daughters' FGA, or punish the parents for such a decision. I am not giving parents advice regarding whether to have these procedures performed.

A spirit of humility should guide intervention in the laws and customs of other societies. Consider that nations practicing FGA may have harshly critical opinions of North American reproductive policies such as pregnancy outside marriage or late abortion (Nnamuchi 2012), just as we may feel negatively about ritual FGA. Everyone's default position should be respect, toleration, and a commitment to live and let live unless serious tangible consequences are likely to arise. Current concepts of human rights, as expressed in the largely hortatory conventions and declarations of the United Nations, are said to be Eurocentric, and under the domination of Western powers (Mutua 2007). Fewer than a billion of the 7 billion people on Earth reside in North America and Europe. Those of us who live in WEIRD (Western, educated industrialized, rich, and democratic) nations (Henrich 2020) should be aware that we will not indefinitely control the international rights agenda. Western nations should opt for mutual tolerance, if only for prudential reasons. We should consider that FGA may be critical to the fabric of societies in which it is normative. It may provide their members—even women—with the best opportunities for individual and group survival under the conditions in which they live. Such threats as chronic food shortages and epidemic violence, poor government provision of security and social services, and high infant mortality may require powerful kinship bonds and strongly pronatal norms. Gender-specific rituals may contribute to these. The rate and severity of medical complications may be within the bounds of what members of these societies consider tolerable (Obermayer 1999). Western intervention may be counterproductive. Residents of FGA-practicing nations that are recipients of Western attention may consider outsiders to be arrogant and hypocritical, especially inasmuch as they permit clitoral hood resection and labial reduction for sexual enhancement and aesthetic improvement (Conroy 2006). Even opponents of FGA in places where it is common may perceive outside intervention as patronizing, and as an attempt at cultural domination (Nnamuchi 2012). Citizens of each nation, then, should decide what should be tolerated under their own domestic laws, leaving other nations to cope with FGA without overt pressure, but aiding states as requested in formulating and achieving reproductive policies.

The domestic standards that these same Europeans and North Americans establish should be guided by the State Intervention Test. State interest in harm to the child should be guided by the Direct Effects Basis. Assessing the extent of physical harm would require clinical investigation of the sequelae of each relevant procedure, as performed by trained operators in a medical (or comparable) environment. This currently cannot be done because all forms of ritual FGA are illegal. We must therefore use reasonable estimates. Vulvar nicks or tattoos rarely cause physical harm, though piercings occasionally may. Labium minus reduction and clitoral hood incision performed on physically mature women are probably safe enough to escape being forbidden by the Direct Effects Basis. Were this not the case, North American and European women with ample disposable income would not seek these procedures as aesthetic enhancement. At the other extreme, the harm from infibulation is great enough that infibulation should not be permitted. Decades of experience with resection of precancerous vulvar lesions, and a brief (but large) experience with cosmetic labiaplasty suggest that labiaplasty and clitoral hood retraction can be can be performed safely in adults by experienced surgeons. However, rare claims from a credible source that most women can experience orgasms after partial clitoral removal (Catania et al. 2007), is insufficient evidence to recommend that any part of the clitoris be removed for non-medical reasons. There are many isolated reports of chronic vulvar pain, hypersensitivity to touch or dyspareunia, and sexual dysfunction following amputation of the clitoral head (Abdulcadir et al. 2017). Even though these are usually resolved by clitoral reconstruction in a multidisciplinary setting (De Schrijver et al. 2016), there is enough evidence that clitoral amputation often causes chronic health problems to allow it to occur. As better evidence emerges from nations where clitoral amputation is conducted in medicalized settings (Van Eekert et al. 2021), such evidence will be dispositive.

But genital, sexual, and reproductive health are not the whole story. While there is no physical effect on non-participants, FGA may challenge opinions as to appropriate and enforceable norms. One involves the questions of consent, autonomy, and bodily integrity discussed in the previous chapter. The second is the widespread acceptance among many scholars, NGO's, and national governments that gender identification extends beyond male/female and can be a matter of choice. Ritual FGA celebrates and reinforces binary gender norms based on sexual identity. These binary norms are embedded in the canonical works of the three major Abrahamic religions.[6] A state may view reproductive freedom as permitting behavior outside these traditional norms. Such a state must determine to what extent it will allow religious advocacy, education, or practice to challenge its non-binary norms.

Finally, there is strong revulsion in the Western world toward FGA. Such revulsion need not have a rational basis. As with sale of horse meat in Illinois (*Cavel International, Inc. v. Madigan*, 500 F3d 551, 7th Circuit, 2007), or public nudity in most of the world, local disgust may mandate that a procedure not be permitted, regardless of absence of tangibly detrimental effects. This, of course, is a departure from liberalism. A *modus vivendi* may result in such restrictions, however, if the restriction is sufficiently important to powerful groups that feel strongly about the matter.

Abolition of some less invasive forms of FGA might be challenged under the Likelihood Constraint, on grounds that injury is too unusual to warrant government interference. This is an empiric matter, and I would not permit total or partial clitoral resection under present circumstances. I look to objective physicians who regularly treat women who have had FGA, and to scholars in medicine and other fields, for conclusive evidence. Vulvar nicks and tattoos seem acceptable. Labia minora reduction and clitoral hood incision in uncoerced adolescents seem to be protected under this constraint as well. Any procedure that is acceptable in young women for aesthetic indications should be comparably acceptable for religious reasons.

The Comparability of Effect Constraint deals with unfair discrimination, and demands that the same objective criteria be applied to all groups. Punishment for performing a vulvar nick does not meet this criterion (Arora and Jacobs 2016). It is hard to see how a procedure lasting a second or two, with no lasting effects, should be criminalized. It is more benign than ear piercing, which is frequently performed on infants, and predominantly on girls. Munzer (2018) likely would disapprove of

[6] This is not necessarily true of some offshoots from Judaism, Christianity, and Islam, such as Unitarian-Universalists and Baha'i, who do not take the Hebrew Bible, New Testament, or Quran to be canonical. Some progressive adherents to the three principal Abrahamic religious traditions also reject binary gender norms.

all FGA in minors on the basis of what he regards as a unique saliency of genitalia.[7] But the idea that there is such a saliency requiring abolition is itself a cultural norm. Furthermore, such saliency does not necessarily require that genitalia should be left untouched. Advocates of ritual genital procedures regard those procedures as perfecting or consecrating the genitalia or, generally, the body of the person receiving the procedure. One could argue that particularly salient structures such as female (or male) genitalia are more appropriate to intervention that ignores individual choice because of their importance. Furthermore, one could conclude that any structure that is a widespread target for alteration must have some special saliency, or people would not want to modify it. Perhaps some scholars familiar with the willingness of parents to subject their children to costly orthodontia, subjecting their children to the pain and inconvenience of orthodontic procedures, might favor abolishing aesthetic orthodontia on minors because of the special salience of teeth.

Finally, the Harm/Benefit Constraint also precludes sanctions for the less invasive forms of FGA. Attempts to ban the vulvar nick by punishment are likely to cause more harm than good. Punishment may be administered for utilitarian (Tadros 2011), retributional (Zaibert 2013), or expressive (Wringe 2017) reasons. Expressive (also called communicative) punishment is not primarily concerned with the violator or even the victim, but is directed toward affirming something that is important to the state. If the only basis for suppressing a vulvar nick is public distaste, then the goal of punishment must be primarily expressive. Imposing a punishment sufficient to deter action may cause so much more harm than the action that it would violate the principle of proportionality, a key principle in European and Canadian law (Sweet and Matthews 2008).[8] Utilitarian punishment does not require proportionality (von Hirsch 1992), but it is questionable how much utility would accrue through elimination of ritual circumcision and vulvar nicks. European jurisprudence regards the use of punishment as *ultima ratio* (last resort), appropriate only when private and administrative measures fail (Jareborg 2005). Tuori (2013) equates *ultima ratio* with proportionality. Punishment should then be proportional to a crime. Unjust infliction of harm, of which punishment disproportionate to an offense is an example, exceeds the appropriate power of a liberal state (Ristroph 2005). Both imprisonment and restriction of parental rights are forms of punishment. Consider the effects of imprisonment or family disruption as punishment for a brief, one-time vulvar nick. The family is stigmatized, split up, and often impoverished. The relationship between the child and the imprisoned parent is disrupted. The child is removed from the family unit, and may be exposed to the vicissitudes of the foster care system. It is unlikely that many people will find this punishment to meet a proportionality standard. We should not sacrifice the needs of children to the imperatives of ideology.

---

[7] Munzer does not believe that circumcision in children is warranted for non-medical reasons. He did not address FGA.

[8] Most nations have embraced proportionality analysis in their constitutional jurisprudence, but the United States has not. Rather, American constitutional law employs three levels of scrutiny—rational, intermediate, and strict bases, described by Galloway (1988).

The Harm/Benefit Constraint, then, clearly prohibits interference with *de minimis* procedures performed under conditions that do not cause undue psychological stress. While I do not advocate any sort of FGA, I do not believe it is justified to punish parents who authorize procedures whose harm is *de minimis*. This includes the vulvar nick, and may expand to other procedures. It seems that mature adolescents who can legally consent to widely tolerated aesthetic vulvar procedures also may consent to the same procedures performed to satisfy religious mandates or minority cultural norms. Again, this view does not reflect approval on my part. Rather, it reflects a need for restraint in imposing my will on others. On the other hand, restriction on clitoral amputation, labia majora removal, and surgical reduction of the size of the vulvar orifice seems highly justified. Reasonable and proportionate measures to prevent such procedures are warranted.

15.2 Conclusion

FGA is not as prevalent as male circumcision in the West. It is illegal, and therefore difficult to study. The range of procedures is heterogeneous, ranging from a simple needle prick to removal of the entire external genitalia with narrowing of the vaginal opening. Data regarding actual harm would be most preferable as a basis for regulating ritual FGA. Such data are not available, and are unlikely to become available soon. Absent such information, we must rely on information about analogous procedures. Most FGA is performed in Africa and Asia. There is ample evidence that attitudes toward FGA become more negative following migration from Africa to Scandinavian nations. In Africa itself, there has been a decrease in FGA, but nations differ in the extent to which prevalence has declined. Furthermore, even some nations with stable FGA incidence have experienced a shift toward less destructive procedures (Powell et al. 2020). In Somaliland,[9] the vast majority of men and women of reproductive age want FGC to continue. However, they want to see 'Sunni circumcision'—either a vulvar nick or removal of the clitoral prepuce (Powell et al. 2020)—replace the traditional infibulation. This replacement actually appears to be happening (Powell and Yussuf 2018).

Reduction of FGA requires indigenous motivation. This can be created through local informal social interaction (Nam 2020), community leadership (Hernlund and Shell-Duncan 2007), indigenous health care workers (Asekun-Olarinmoye and Amusan 2008), and even through law (Wouango et al. 2020). Urbanization, education, and prosperity play a role in changing attitudes (Glover et al. 2018). Religion and ethnicity are important in determining whether people favor FGA. Men increasingly are becoming more opposed to extensive FGA procedures (Abathun et al. 2016),

[9] Somaliland is former British Somalia and is the northern part of Somalia. It is self-governing and considers itself independent, but the international community considers it part of the nation of Somalia, so it will not be found on political maps.

both for reasons of beneficence toward women and the belief that marriage to an uncut woman enhances their own sexual experience.

Vulvar nicks on female infants should be permitted. Labial reduction and retraction of the clitoral hood are sufficiently safe to be performed for aesthetic reasons, and so should be available for reasons of conscience if performed on physically mature, uncoerced, decisionally capable females. Procedures more extensive than reduction of the size of labia minora are not appropriately performed on minors. The vulvar nick might even be welcomed as a harm reduction procedure in groups that will accept this ritual but are otherwise likely to obtain more extensive procedures for their minor girls. Members of an immigrant Somali population in Seattle, and a local hospital agreed to perform vulvar nicks on children as an alternative to non-medical infibulation (Coleman 1998). Under pressure from activists who opposed all female genital cutting, the hospital reversed its decision to perform vulvar nick as a harm-reducing procedure to prevent more radical forms of FGA from being performed outside the health care system. Somali women stated that they would instead take their daughters to Somalia or to Somali practitioners in the United States for infibulation. It is not known how many girls actually underwent vulvar infibulation, and how many of those were done under sterile conditions, with adequate anesthesia. Years later, in 2010, the American Academy of Pediatrics (AAP) (2010a) deemed that such a nick was an ethically acceptable compromise with communities that were otherwise likely to subject their daughters to extensive genital cutting, possibly overseas. However, the AAP retracted this opinion under pressure from activists and reissued the original language that opposed all forms of FGA including the nick (American Academy of Pediatrics 2010b). Latham (2016) describes the successful adoption in Khuzistan (a southwestern, predominantly Arabic-speaking, province of Iran) of a clitoral procedure as an intermediate step to eliminating FGA altogether. However, use of vulvar nick as a means of reducing the harm of FGA has been thwarted by activists not only in the United States, but in Italy (Galeotti 2007) and the Netherlands (Obiora 1997).

But let us imagine an endogamous, self-identifying cultural group known as the Arhob. They mostly live as a minority in Tarajug, where they are socially egalitarian, well-educated, and prosperous. Most adults have graduate degrees and work in business and the professions, though they form the bulk of the officer corps in the Tarajug armed forces. Their religion is committed to identification as a man or woman based on anatomy. One year after demonstration of physical maturity (menstruation in females and ejaculation in males) they perform a gender-affirming ritual. The prepuce is removed in all adolescents under favorable medical conditions. Complication rate is minimal. Prior to the procedure, Arhob children receive years of religious instruction. Almost all young Arhobs look forward to the ritual with joy tinged with some apprehension. A month after the procedure the child is honored by a celebration equivalent to a Jewish Bar/Bat Mitzvah or a Latino quinceañera celebration. A large majority of adult Arhobs express satisfaction with their sexual experience. However, those adolescents who refuse to undergo the prepuce resection are unmarriageable and are ultimately ostracized from the Arhob community.

A reasonable person might ask why any government would want to disrupt this state of affairs. Why alienate a group of people whose way of life makes them successful, and who are happy with their prepuce removal? Why stop them in the name of some outside conception of rights that are not part of the Arhob consciousness, let alone part of their ethical framework? If the Tarajug government cannot tolerate this custom of a productive minority—a custom that does not cause tangible harm to recipients of the procedure or to the general society, then that government is the blameworthy party. If they do tolerate the ritual, it should not be the concern of foreigners.

This vignette epitomizes the theme of this book. Relational liberty should be maximized. It even applies to things people do that offend or disgust us, as long as no great tangible harm is done.

References

Abathun, Asresash Demissie, Johanne Sundby, and Abdi A. Gele. 2016. Attitude toward female genital mutilation among Somali and Harari People, Eastern Ethiopia. *International Journal of Women's Health* 8: 557–569. https://doi.org/10.2147/IJWH.S112226.

Abdulcadir, Jasmine, Omar Abdulcadir, Martin Caillet, Lucrezia Catania, Béatrice Cuzin, Birgitta Essén, Pierre Foldès, et al. 2017. Clitoral surgery after female genital mutilation/cutting. *Aesthetic Surgery Journal* 37 (9): NP113–NP115. https://doi.org/10.1093/asj/sjx095.

Abrol, Somya. 2018. Yes, female genital mutilation happens in India; Here's everything you need to know. *India Today* [Online]. February 6, 2018. https://www.indiatoday.in/lifestyle/people/story/female-genital-mutilation-india-clitoris-pleasure-muslim-bohra-community-1162510-2018-02-06.

Ahmadu, Fuambai. 2017. *Equality, Not Special Protection: Multiculturalism, Feminism, and Female Circumcision in Western Liberal Democracies*. In *Universalism Without Uniformity: Explorations in Mind and Culture*, ed. Julia L. Cassaniti and Usha Menon. Chicago: University of Chicago Press, 214–36.

Ahmed Magdy, R., Mohamed M. Shaaban, Heba K. Meky, Mohamed E. Amin Arafa, Tamer Y. Mohamed, Waleed F. Gharib and Abeer B. Ahmed. 2017. Psychological impact of female genital mutilation among adolescent Egyptian girls: A cross-sectional study. *European Journal of Contraception and Reproductive Health Care* 22 (4): 280–5. https://doi.org/10.1080/13625187.2017.1355454.

Alsibiani, Sharifa A., and Abdulrahim A. Rouzi. 2010. Sexual function in women with female genital mutilation. *Fertility and Sterility* 93 (3): 722–724. https://doi.org/10.1016/j.fertnstert.2008.10.035.

American Academy of Pediatrics. 2010a. Ritual genital cutting of female minors. *Pediatrics* 125: 1088–1093. https://doi.org/10.1542/peds.2010-0187.

American Academy of Pediatrics. 2010b. Ritual genital cutting of female minors. *Pediatrics* 126: 191. https://doi.org/10.1542/peds.2010-1568.

Arora, Kavita Shah, and Allan J. Jacobs. 2016. Female genital alteration: A compromise solution. *Journal of Medical Ethics* 42 (3): 148–154.

Asekun-Olarinmoye, Esther O., and Oluwatoyin A. Amusan. 2008. The impact of health education on attitudes towards Female Genital Mutilation (FGM) in a rural Nigerian community. *European Journal of Contraception and Reproductive Health Care* 13 (3): 289–297. https://doi.org/10.1080/13625180802075174.

Askew, Ian, Ted Chaiban, Benoit Kalasa, and Purna Sen. 2016. A repeat call for complete abandonment of FGM. *Journal of Medical Ethics* 42 (9): 619–620.

Bendiksen, Bothild, Trond Heir, Fabakary Minteh, Mai Mahgoub Ziyada, Rex A. Kuye, and Inger-Lise Lien. 2021. The association between physical complications following female genital cutting and the mental health of 12-year-old Gambian girls: A community-based cross-sectional study. *PLoS One* 16 (1): e0245723. https://doi.org/10.1371/journal.pone.0245723.

Bengali, S., and M.N. Parth. 2016. A rebellion inside a Small Indian sect seeks to end a brutal custom: Female genital mutilation. *Los Angeles Times*. June 12, 2016. http://www.latimes.com/world/asia/la-fg-india-genital-mutilation-20160612-snap-story.html.

Berg, Rigmor C., and Eva Denison. 2013. A tradition in transition: Factors perpetuating and hindering the continuance of Female Genital Mutilation/Cutting (FGM/C) summarized in a systematic review. *Health Care for Women International* 34 (10): 837–859.

Berg, Rigmor C., and Vigdis Underland. 2013. The obstetric consequences of female genital mutilation/cutting: A systematic review and meta-analysis. *Obstetrics and Gynecology International* 2013. Article ID 496564. https://doi.org/10.1155/2013/496564.

Berg, Rigmor C., Vigdis Underland, Jan Odgaard-Jensen, Atle Fretheim and Gunn E. Vist. 2014. Effects of female genital cutting on physical health outcomes: A systematic review and meta-analysis. *BMJ Open* 4: e006316. https://doi.org/10.1136/bmjopen-2014-006316

Berg, Rigmor C., Sølvi Taraldsen, Maryan A. Said, Ingvil Krarup Sørbye, and Siri Vangen. 2017. Reasons for and experiences with surgical interventions for Female Genital Mutilation/Cutting (FGM/C): A systematic review. *The Journal of Sexual Medicine* 14 (8): 977–90.

Bočko, Vesna. 2016. Khitan Perempuan: Who speaks for the Indonesian female circumcision? *Ethnologia Actualis* 16 (2): 43–65. https://doi.org/10.1515/eas-2017-0004.

Boddy, Janice. 2020. Re-thinking the zero tolerance approach to FGM/C: The debate around female genital cosmetic surgery. *Current Sexual Health Reports* 12 (4): 302–313. https://doi.org/10.1007/s11930-020-00293-1.

Brown, Elizabeth, Jennifer Carroll, Colleen Fogarty, and Cristina Holt. 2010. 'They Get a C-Section They Gonna Die': Somali women's fears of obstetrical interventions in the United States. *Journal of Transcultural Nursing* 21 (3): 220–227.

Buss, David M., and William von Hippel. 2018. Psychological barriers to evolutionary psychology: Ideological bias and coalitional adaptations. *Archives of Scientific Psychology* 6 (1): 148–158. https://doi.org/10.1037/arc0000049).

Catania, Lucrezia, Omar Abdulcadir, Vincenzo Puppo, Jole Baldaro Verde, Jasmine Abdulcadir, and Dalmar Abdulcadir. 2007. Pleasure and orgasm in women with female genital mutilation/cutting (FGM/C). *Journal of Sexual Medicine* 4 (6): 1666–1678. https://doi.org/10.1111/j.1743-6109.2007.00620.x.

Coleman, Dorianne. L. (1998) The seattle compromise: Multicultural sensitivity and americanization. *Duke Law Journal* 47 (4): 717-783.

Conroy, Ronán M. 2006. Female genital mutilation: Whose problem, whose solution? *BMJ* 333 (7559): 106–107. https://doi.org/10.1136/bmj.333.7559.106.

Davis, Dena S. 2001. Male and female genital alteration: A collision course with the law? *Health Matrix* 11 (3): 487–687.

Lotte, De Schrijver, Els Leyea, and Mireille Merckx. 2016. A multidisciplinary approach to clitoral reconstruction after female genital mutilation: The crucial role of counselling. *European Journal of Contraception and Reproductive Health Care* 21 (4): 269–275. https://doi.org/10.3109/13625187.2016.1172063.

Earp, Brian D. 2020. Zero tolerance for genital mutilation: A review of moral justifications. *Current Sexual Health Reports* 12 (4): 276–288. https://doi.org/10.1007/s11930-020-00286-0.

Earp, Brian D. 2021. Male or female genital cutting: Why 'Health Benefits' are morally irrelevant. *Journal of Medical Ethics* Online ahead of print. https://doi.org/10.1136/medethics-2020-106782.

Earp, Brian D., and Sara Johnsdotter. 2021. Current critiques of the WHO policy on female genital mutilation. *International Journal of Impotence Research*. 33 (2): 196-209. https://doi.org/10.1038/s41443-020-0302-0.

Engelsma, Brian, Gerry Mackie, and Brandon Merrell. 2020. Unprogrammed abandonment of female genital mutilation/cutting. *World Development* 129 (3). Article 104845. https://doi.org/10.1016/j.worlddev.2019.104845. http://www.brandonmerrell.com/papers/Merrell%20-%20Unprogrammed%20Abandonment.pdf. Accessed 12 Apr 2020.

Essén, Birgitta, N.-O. Birgit Bödker, Saemundur Gudmundsson Sjöberg, P.-O. Östergren, and Jens Langhoff-Roos. 2002. Is there an association between female circumcision and perinatal death? *Bulletin of the World Health Organization* 80 (8): 629–632.

Essén, Birgitta, Nils-Otto Sjöberg, Saemundur Gudmundsson, P.-O. Östergren, and Pelle G. Lindqvist. 2005. No association between female circumcision and prolonged labor: A case control study of immigrant women giving birth in Sweden. *European Journal of Obstetrics and Gynecology and Reproductive Biology* 121 (2): 182–85.

Finkel, Michelle A. 2002. Traumatic injuries caused by hazing practices. *American Journal of Emergency Medicine* 20 (3): 228–233.

Frega, Antonio, Giuliana Puzio, Paolo Maniglio, Angelica Catalano, Giusi Natalia Milazzo, Danila Lombardi, Henri Nitiema, and Paola Bianchi. 2013. Obstetric and neonatal outcomes of women with FGM I and II in San Camillo Hospital, Burkina Faso. *Archives of Gynecology and Obstetrics* 288 (3): 513-519. https://doi.org/10.1007/s00404-013-2779-y.

Galeotti, Anna Elisabetta. 2007. Relativism, universalism, and applied ethics: The case of female circumcision. *Constellations* 14: 91-111.

Galloway, Russell W. 1988. Means-end scrutiny in American Constitutional Law. *Loyola of Los Angeles Law Review.* 21 (2): 449–496.

Glover, Jennifer, Helen Liebling, Simon Goodman, and Hazel Barrett. 2018. Persistence and resistance of harmful traditional practices (HTPs) perpetuated against girls in Africa and Asia. *Journal of International Women's Studies* 19 (2): 44–64.

Goodwin, Jo-Ann and David Jones. 2008. The unspeakable practice of female circumcision that's destroying young women's lives in Britain. *Daily Mail.* January 3, 2008. https://www.dailymail.co.uk/femail/article-505796/The-unspeakable-practice-female-circumcision-thats-destroying-young-womens-lives-Britain.html.

Grisaru, Nimrod, M. Simcha Lezer, and R.H. Belmaker. 1997. Ritual female genital surgery among Ethiopian Jews. *Archives of Sexual Behavior* 26 (2): 211–215.

Henrich, Joseph. 2004. Cultural group selection, coevolutionary processes, and large-scale cooperation. *Journal of Economic Behavior and Organization* 53 (1): 3–35.

Henrich, Joseph. 2016. *The Secret of Our Success*. Princeton: Princeton University Press.

Henrich, Joseph. 2020. *The WIERDest People in the World*. New York: Farrar, Giroux, Straus.

Hernlund, Ylva, and Bettina Shell-Duncan. 2007. Contingency, context, and change: Negotiating female genital cutting in the Gambia and Senegal". *Africa Today* 53 (4): 43–57.

Hosken, Fran. 1979. *The Hosken Report: Genital and Sexual Mutilation of Females*. Lexington, Massachusetts: Women's International Network News.

Hunter, John G. 2016. Labia Minora, Labia Majora, and Clitoral Hood Alteration: Experience-based recommendations. *Aesthetic Surgery Journal* 36 (1): 71–79. https://doi.org/10.1093/asj/sjv092.

Jacobs, Allan J., and Kavita Shah Arora. 2017. Punishment of minor female genital ritual procedures: Is the perfect the enemy of the good? *Developing World Bioethics* 17 (2): 134–140.

Jareborg, Nils. 2005. Criminalization as last resort (Ultima Ratio). *Ohio State Journal of Criminal Law* 2 (2): 521–534.

Johnsdotter. Sara. 2013. Discourses on sexual pleasure after genital modifications: The fallacy of genital determinism (A Response to J. Steven Svoboda). *Global Discourse* 3 (2): 256–65. https://doi.org/10.1080/23269995.2013.805530.

Johnsdotter, Sara. 2018. The impact of migration on attitudes to female genital cutting and experiences of sexual dysfunction among migrant women with FGC. *Current Sexual Health Reports* 10 (1): 18–24. https://doi.org/10.1007/s11930-018-0139-4.

Kizilhan, Jan Ilhan. 2011. Impact of psychological disorders after female genital mutilation among Kurdish girls in Northern Iraq. *European Journal of Psychiatry* 25 (2): 92–100. https://doi.org/10.4321/S0213-61632011000200004.

Kremelberg, David, and Arnold Dashefsky. 2016. Targets of out-group hostility in the contemporary United States: Individual- and community-level factors associated with the experience of anti-semitism among American Jews. *Contemporary Jewry* 36 (2): 243–264.

Latham, Susie. 2016. The campaign against female genital cutting: Empowering women or reinforcing global inequity? *Ethics and Social Welfare* 10 (1): 1–14.

Lurie, Jacob, M., Alessandra Weidman, Samantha Huynh, Diana Delgado, Imaani Easthausen, & Gunisha Kaur. 2020. Painful gynecologic and obstetric complications of female genital mutilation/cutting: A systematic review and meta-analysis. *PLoS Medicine* 17 (3): e1003088. https://doi.org/10.1371/journal.pmed.1003088.

Macklin, Ruth. 2016. Not all cultural traditions deserve respect. *Journal of Medical Ethics* 42 (3): 155.

Morison, Linda, Caroline Scherf, Gloria Ekno, Katie Paine, Beryl West, Rosalind Coleman, and Gijs Walraven. 2001. The long-term reproductive health consequences of female genital cutting in rural Gambia: A community-based survey. *Tropical Medicine and International Health* 6 (8): 643–653. https://doi.org/10.1046/j.1365-3156.2001.00749.x.

Munzer, Stephen R. 2018. Examining nontherapeutic circumcision. *Health Matrix* 28 (1): 1–77.

Mutua, Makau. 2007. Standard setting in human rights: Critique and progress. *Human Rights Quarterly* 29 (7): 547–629.

Nam, Youngeun. 2020. Learning through social interaction: Kenyan women against female genital cutting in Kenya. *Culture, Health and Sexuality* 23 (6): 840–853. https://doi.org/10.1080/13691058.2020.1734662.

Niedzwiadek, Nick and Cain Twyman. Branded for Life. *The Daily Tar Heel*, 26 February 2015. https://www.dailytarheel.com/article/2015/02/national-pan-hellenic-fraternities-branding-ritual-is-rooted-in-history.

Nnamuchi, Obijulu. 2012. Circumcision or mutilation—voluntary or forced excision—extricating the ethical and legal issues in female genital ritual. *Journal of Law and Health* 25 (1): 85–121.

Obaid, Zakaria Mahran, Ahmed Wahhed-Allah. Amer, Mohammed Abdel Fatah El. Mahdy, and Amira Elmaadawy Barakat. Mohammed. 2019. Evaluation of psychological and sexual effects of female genital mutilation (Circumcision). *Egyptian Journal of Hospital Medicine* 74 (4): 726–734.

Obermeyer, Carla Makhlouf. 1999. Female genital surgeries: The known, the unknown, and the unknowable. *Medical Anthropology Quarterly* 13 (1): 79–106.

Obiora, L. Amede. 1997. Bridges and barricades: rethinking polemics and intransigence in the campaign against female circumcision. *Case Western Reserve Law Review* 47: 275–378.

Özer, Müjde, Indiana Mortimore, Elise P. Jansma, and Margriet G. Mullender. 2018. Labiaplasty: Motivation, techniques, and ethics. *Nature Reviews: Urology* 15 (2): 175–89.

Piroozi, Bakhtiar, Cyrus Alinia, Hossein Safari, Ali Kazemi-Karyani, Ghobad Moradi, Fariba Farhadifar, Fayegh Yousefi, Amjad Mohamadi Bolbanabad, and Arian Azadnia. 2020. Effect of female genital mutilation on mental health: A case-control study. *European Journal of Contraception and Reproductive Health Care* 25 (1): 33–36. https://doi.org/10.1080/13625187.2019.1709815.

Powell, Richard A., and Mohamed Yussuf. 2018. Changes in FGM/C in Somaliland: Medical narrative driving shift in types of cutting. Evidence to end FGM/C: Research to help women thrive. New York: Population Council.

Powell, Richard A., Mohamed Yussuf, Bettina Shell-Duncan, and Caroline W. Kabiru. 2020. Exploring the nature and extent of normative change in FGM/C in Somaliland. In: *Evidence to End FGM/C: Research to Help Girls and Women Thrive*. New York: Population Council. https://knowledgecommons.popcouncil.org/cgi/viewcontent.cgi?article=2058&context=departments_sbsr-rh.

Public Policy Advisory Network on Female Genital Surgeries in Africa. 2012. Seven things to know about female genital surgeries in Africa. *Hastings Center Report* 42 (6): 19–27.

Ramos, Samuel and Gregory J. Boyle. 2000. Ritual and medical circumcision among Filipino boys: Evidence of post-traumatic stress disorder. In *Understanding Circumcision: A Multi-Disciplinary Approach to a Multi-Dimensional Problem*, ed. George C. Denniston, Frederick Mansfield Hodges, and Marilyn Fayre Milos. Cham, Switzerland: Springer, 253–70.

Rashid, Abdul and Yufu Iguchi. 2019. Female genital cutting in Malaysia: A mixed-methods study. *BMJ Open* 9 (4). https://doi.org/10.1136/bmjopen-2018-025078.

Ristroph, Alice. 2005. Proportionality as a principle of limited government. *Duke Law Journal* 55 (2): 263–331.

Salinas, Cristóbal Jr., and Michelle L. Boettcher, eds. 2018. *Critical Perspectives on Hazing in Colleges and Universities: A Guide to Disrupting Hazing Culture*. New York: Routledge.
Shabila, Nazar P., Abubakir M. Saleh, and Rojan K. Jawad. 2014. Women's perspectives of female genital cutting: Q-methodology. *BMC Women's Health* 14: 11. https://doi.org/10.1186/1472-6874-14-11.
Shaw, Dorothy, and Wendy V. Norman. 2020. When there are no abortion laws: A case study of Canada. *Clinical Obstetrics and Gynaecology* 62 (1): 49–62.
Shay, Thewodros Zewde, Jemal Haidar, and Wambui Kogi-Makau. 2012. Magnitude of and driving factors for female genital cutting in schoolgirls in Addis Ababa, Ethiopia: A crosssectional study. *South Africa Journal of Child Health* 4 (3): 78–82.
Small, R., A. Gagnon, M. Gissler, J. Zeitlin, M. Bennis, R.H. Glazier, E. Haelterman, G. Martens, S. McDermott, M. Urquia, and S. Vangen. 2008. Somali women and their pregnancy outcomes postmigration: Data from six receiving countries. *BJOG: An International Journal of Obstetrics and Gynaecology* 115 (13): 1630–40.
Sweet, Alec Stone, and Jud Matthews. 2008. Proportionality balancing and global constitutionalism. *Columbia Journal of International Law* 47 (1): 72–164.
Tadros, Victor. 2011. *The ends of harm*. Oxford: Oxford University Press.
Tuori, Kaarlo. 2013. Ultima ratio as a constitutional principle. *Oñati Socio-Legal Series* 3 (1): 6–20.
Utz-Billing, Isabell, and Heribert Kentinich. 2008. Female genital mutilation: An injury, physical and mental harm. *Journal of Psychosomatic Obstetrics and Gynecology* 29 (4): 225–229.
Van Eekert, Nina, Veerle Buffel, Sara De Bruyn, and Sarah Van de Velde. 2021. The medicalisation of female genital cutting: Harm reduction or social norm? *Sociology of Health and Illness* 43 (2): 263-280. https://doi.org/10.1111/1467-9566.13153.
von Hirsch, Andrew. 1992. Proportionality in the philosophy of punishment. *Crime and Justice* 16 (1): 55–98.
Wen, Nicole J., Aiyana K. Willard, Michaela Caughy, and Cristine H. Legare. 2020. Watch me, watch you: Ritual participation increases in-group displays and out-group monitoring in children. *Philosophical Transactions of the Royal Society B, Biological Science* 375 (1805): 20190437. https://doi.org/10.1098/rstb.2019.0437.
Whitehouse, Harvey. 1996. Rites of terror: Emotion, metaphor and memory in Melanesian initiation cults. *Journal of the Royal Anthropological Institute* 2 (4): 703–715.
Whitehouse, Harvey. 2018. Dying for the group: Towards a general theory of extreme self-sacrifice. *Behavioral and Brain Sciences* 41 (e192): 1–62. https://doi.org/10.1017/S0140525X1800024910.1017/s0140525x18000249.
Whitman, James O. 2017. *Hitler's American Model: The United States and The Making of Nazi Race Law*. Princeton: Princeton University Press.
Wood, Paul L. 2018. Cosmetic genital surgery in children and adolescents. *Best Practice and Research Clinical Obstetrics and Gynaecology* 48 (2): 137-146. https://doi.org/10.1016/j.bpobgyn.2017.08.003.
World Health Organization. 1998. *Female Genital Mutilation: An Overview*. Geneva: World Health Organization.
World Health Organization. 2014. Female genital mutilation and other harmful practices: Prevalence of FGM. http://www.who.int/reproductivehealth/topics/fgm/prevalence/en/. Accessed 25 Oct 2014.
Wouango, Josephine, Susan L. Ostermann, and Daniel Mwanga. 2020. *When and How Does Law Effectively Reduce the Practice of Female Genital Mutilation/Cutting? Evidence to End FGM/C: Research to Help Girls and Women Thrive*. New York: Population Council.
Wringe, Bill. 2017. Rethinking expressive theories of punishment: Why denunciation is a better bet than communication or pure expression. *Philosophical Studies* 174 (3): 681–708. https://doi.org/10.1007/s11098-016-0703-6.
Zaibert, Leo. 2013. The instruments of abolition, or why retributivism is the only real justification of punishment. *Law and Philosophy* 32 (1): 33–58.

Part IV
Conclusion

Chapter 16
Conclusion

Abstract This chapter summarizes the reasons for adopting a liberal pluralist approach. It reviews ethics as a simple combinatorial system. Much as with the alphabet or musical notation, a few building blocks can be combined to yield an almost infinite number of products. Different social roles, modes of cooperation, ethical concepts, interests, values, political goals, and groups with which we identify form the core units of this system. Finding principled solutions to real-world problems involves a complexity difficult for the human mind to grasp, and impossible to solve definitively. Furthermore, the preferred solutions change as external circumstances change. The formal rules necessary to bind us together into a society that can allow flourishing should allow for the greatest possible freedom for individuals, their kinship groups, and their chosen associations all to find their own solutions. In this regard, the chapter reprises the State Intervention Test to protect children against frank parental malfeasance. I speculate that the way forward will be based on better empiric understanding of what contributes to individual and societal flourishing. Finally, I admonish physicians and state officials to remember that a child is part of a family, and will continue to be part of a family after physicians and officials are no longer active participants in the child's life.

Mary Ann Glendon notes a paradox of liberalism. Individual liberty is a necessary feature of liberalism. An effective government, free markets, and a vibrant civil society are all in tension with one another, and with individual liberty (Glendon 1991), I would add that human flourishing and personal liberty are also mutually necessary and mutually in tension. These paradoxes are individual instances of value pluralism. We have seen that roles (Ross 1930), modes of cooperation (Curry et al. 2020) ethical concepts, interests, values, political goals, and groups with which we identify form an intricate combinatorial system (or intersecting group of combinatorial systems). Finding principled solutions to real-world problems often involves a complexity difficult for the human mind to grasp, and impossible to solve definitively. Furthermore, changing circumstances may change the balance that is best applied to competing demands of interest, desire, and principle. The correct balance among individuals with interests, individuals with roles, individuals with power, abstract principles and

A. J. Jacobs, *Assigning Responsibility for Children's Health When Parents and Authorities Disagree: Whose Child?*, The International Library of Bioethics 90,
https://doi.org/10.1007/978-3-030-87698-2_16

values, and groups must come from wisdom, and not from clever systems-building. Aristotle (1976, Book 1 Chap. 1) asserted long ago (possibly in reaction to Plato) that politics and ethics were matters of judgment, and not of rigorous reason.

My starting point is that the state ought to tolerate a wide variety of beliefs and practices, even if offensive to the majority (Jacobs 2013).

First, changing circumstances might render disfavored practices beneficial, or might warrant a change in dominant mores and laws. Consider family size. I stated that current overpopulation can render pronatal policies obsolete. Conversely, the Paraguayan War of 1864–1870,[1] which exterminated most adult Paraguayan men, led to patriarchal norms (Boggiano 2020) and to polygyny (Economist 2012). These were necessary to repopulate the nation and to accommodate the needs of surviving women. A second reason for mutual toleration is that it protects all. What is favored today may be disfavored tomorrow. A general practice of 'live and let live' provides security for all of us to live as we wish. In this spirit, American.

> law affords constitutional protection to personal decisions relating to marriage, procreation, contraception, family relationships, child rearing, and education... Our precedents have respected the private realm of family life which the state cannot enter. (*Planned Parenthood of Southeastern Pa. v. Casey,* 505 U.S. 833, Supreme Court, 1992, 851; internal quotation marks and citations omitted).

In short, allowing freedom to others tends to protect our own freedom. One of the liberties guaranteed in the US is the liberty to perpetuate one's values and ways of life through one's family. So, as a third point, limiting parental discretion may have antinatal effects. If potential parents cannot propagate their values and ways of life through child-rearing, and their actions are under intense state scrutiny, there is less motivation for them to have children. Fourth, policies that limit minority practices may result in loss of government legitimacy, with withdrawal or active rebellion by minorities (Jackson et al. 2012; Trinkner et al. 2018).

Fifth, the contingency of our beliefs should make us humble. Our views are heavily influenced by our circumstances. Mahmoud Ahmadinejad and Volker Zotz were born the same day, 28 October, 1956. Ahmadinejad is a Shiite populist who, as president of Iran, was noted for his confrontational policies. Zotz is a Buddhist pacifist professor (see http://www.volkerzotz.eu/) Had Ahmadinejad and Zotz been switched at birth, their ultimate beliefs, values, and ideas would have been different. The baby who was born Zotz but who grew up as Ahmadinejad likely would have been a Farsi-speaking Shiite Muslim. The other baby may not have become a Buddhist, but probably would have come to appreciate the fine wines of the Landau-in-der-Pfalz region in which he was raised. It is a commonplace that children are likely to adopt the viewpoints of their parents and contemporaries on matters such as politics and religion. This positionality does not imply a radical relativism. But it should make us skeptical enough of our own views, mores, and behavior that we mostly tolerate others'.

[1] Paraguay simultaneously fought against Brazil, Argentina, and Uruguay. Its opponents' population outnumbered Paraguay's by over 20:1, with an even greater economic disparity. Up to 90% of adult Paraguayan men died as a result of the war, leaving a sex ratio of men to women of no more than 0.5.

Shklar observed that it is easier to recognize clear injustice than to characterize what is just (Shklar 1984). The limit of tolerance, then, is the point where others create conditions of danger or seriously infringe on others' relationships.

Sixth, parents are more concerned for their children than are NGO activists or government officials. They bear the brunt of both the good and bad consequences of family life (Buchanan and Brock 1989). We should ordinarily defer to parents' judgments, then. Seventh, it is a liberal axiom that freedom of expression of ideas allows the best ideas to prevail. This notion may have been first defended in the modern Western world by John Milton in the 17th century:

> Let [Truth] and Falsehood grapple; who ever knew Truth put to the worse, in a free and open encounter? ... Give her but room, and do not bind her when she sleeps, for then she speaks not true, as the old Proteus did, who spake oracles only when he was caught and bound, but then rather she turns herself into all shapes, except her own, and perhaps tunes her voice according to the time. (Milton 1644).

This notion that the best ideas will prevail in the competition among ideas is frequently called the principle of the 'marketplace of ideas.' The phrase, "free trade" in ideas appeared in *Abrams vs. US,* 250 US 616, Supreme Court, 1919, Holmes, J, *dissenting*, 630. The actual designation of competition of ideas as a "marketplace"[2] has been attributed to William Douglas (*US vs. Rumely*, 345 US 41, Supreme Court, 1953, Douglas, J, *concurring*, 56).[3] I argue that a marketplace of practices, of ways of life, and of ways of relating to other people is just as important. As with speech, there are limits. We do not allow fraud[4] or defamation. We cannot allow cultures that regard some of their members as chattel slaves. Similarly, actions should not create severe harms to others.

Eighth, finally—and also attributable to Milton (1644)—the sort of people who would judiciously interfere with individual liberty would not agree to serve as censors or as regulators of our private behavior, leaving such work to people interested in wielding power over others and likely to abuse it.

One reason it is harder to achieve a vision of good than to recognize evil is that differences frequently arise over how to prioritize competing goods. Liberty, order, equality of opportunity, equality of distribution, and prosperity may all require different programs or policies. Rather than reinforcing one another, important principles and goals often have to be balanced *against* each other. I have argued that the

---

[2] The analogy is to an economic model of pure competition. A problem with the idea of a marketplace of ideas is that the marketplace is more like monopolistic competition or, in an age of dominance of dissemination of ideas by vast media companies, oligopoly. Mill and Holmes did not have in mind the manipulation of large populations by a limited number of large media companies that exerted great control over the ideas to which people may be exposed. A discussion of the four common models of market structure—pure competition, monopolistic competition, oligopoly, and monopoly—can be found in any introductory economics text. An online text that describes these four models is OpenStax. (2020). *Principles of Economics* Houston: Rice University, Chaps. 8, 9 and 10. Available at https://opentextbc.ca/principlesofeconomics/#main.

[3] Neither of these judicial opinions advocating a 'market' of ideas was a precedential majority opinion. One was a dissent and the other a concurrence.

[4] Fraud, in this context is a deliberate or reckless misrepresentation that a statement is factual, and made to another person with the hope or intention that this person would rely on its factual nature.

emphasis on autonomy and choice in current law and ethical thought gives short shrift to the factors that appear to be most important in human flourishing. These consist of relational capabilities, physical security, and various tangible capabilities such as health and material resources. Relational goods include membership in a family and in groups with strong norms of belief and behavior. Families, and these larger groups, are attractive and personally enriching in part because of the interpersonal bonds among their members. Thus, autonomy itself is to a large extent relational, as people choose their goals and values in the context of their environments and associates. To cite an intellectually trivial but personally important example, the snack that people are likely to reach for differs from state to state in the US (Ben-Yehuda 2020); this undoubtedly is largely due to mutual influence. There seems to be no principled reason why the favorite snack in North Dakota is sunflower seeds, but South Dakotans prefer Milky Way. Both are readily available in each state, and both are imported from other states.

Parents are the default decision-makers for children. They know their children best. Furthermore, what happens to a child in the family usually affects other family members more than it affects others outside the family. Parents are better situated to understand the position of the child relative to other family members and to other acquaintances than are professionals. Sometimes, deliberately or not, parents make decisions that create or threaten great harm to a child. In such cases, the state should intervene based on the *parens patriae* doctrine or its European equivalents. The decision to intervene should be based on avoidable failure of parents to meet a child's needs, which I called parental malfeasance. The resolution of the problem should be based not on maximizing fulfillment of the child's interests (let alone maximizing the child's health to the exclusion of all other interests), but should maximize the needs and legitimate interests both of the child and of other stakeholders in the parental decision.

Family-oriented ethical theorists have reached broad accord on the existence of three zones of parental behavior. A parental act or choice may conform with a reasonable concept of what is unexceptionable. An act might also be unacceptable, inviting or demanding state action to compel change. Between these extremes is an area of parental action that is debatable or suboptimal but tolerable. Much recent literature has used Gillam's terminology for this intermediate zone, calling it the *parental zone of discretion* (Gillam 2016). I have further divided the middle zone into two. I did this in order to match the nomenclature describing the parental behavior with one of four possible classes of state response. The state should not interfere with parental action or behavior that lies within the *zone of acceptability*. The *zone of state attention* comprises parental behavior that invites education of parents, or provision of facilities for voluntary parental use. If parental behavior threatens children's interests to an extent that merits nudges, opt-out programs, or incentivization of parents to participate in a program, that action is included in the *zone of concern*. Finally, the *zone of unacceptability* is the area of parental action that calls for state coercive intervention to prevent or reverse the parental action, and possibly to punish the parents. There are two phases of any state intervention. The first is the decision that intervention is warranted. I term this the *identification phase*. Second, the state must decide what to do. I term this the *resolution* phase.

This identification phase is based on a needs principle—the requirement that parents meet certain fundamental child interests that are termed needs. The definition of these needs as legal rules is political, determined in a democratic society through a *modus vivendi*. I propose that the framework for the *modus vivendi* should be based on a sufficientarian process (Saunders 2021). Sufficientarianism requires that the state grant all relevant individuals a sufficient amount of each *currency* (defined as a person's interest that can somehow be measured or estimated) before any surplus is distributed. In the case of state interference with parents the currency is *protection from parental malfeasance*. Such malfeasance need not be intentional; rather, I would apply a strict liability standard; i.e., a person's liability for damage that she caused without regard to her state of mind (Shavell 1980).[5] Again, the level of sufficiency is always a political decision. There is no principled way to establish a sufficiency threshold.

I propose as a standard for sufficiency in the area of parental care through the Direct Effects Basis of my State Intervention Test:

> It is warranted for a state to overturn a parental decision if, as a consequence of the decision, unreasonable burdens are likely to be created… for children to whom the decision applies, by: creating a substantial chance of death or of major disruption of a physiological function, or creating other objectively severe harmful effects, such as malnutrition or major psychological morbidity. (In situations where both a disease and a proposed treatment carry such risk of harmful effects, intervention is permissible if parents seek care whose risk/benefit ratio greatly exceeds the risk/benefit ratio expected from the management choice proposed by health care professionals.)

But the question of overriding parents' decisions does not end with harm to their children. When there are important public health (or other major political) objectives, the state may constrain the liberty of parents to make decisions for children. One commonly discussed issue is vaccination. Another is minors' decisional capacity in accessing reproductive medicine. Diekema (2020) implies that the most important reason for carving out this immunity from the consent rule is the burden on society of birth of unwanted babies to adolescents. Compulsory physical education, exclusion of a child with head lice from school, involuntary psychiatric hospitalization of a suicidal or violent minor, and supervised administration of anti-tuberculosis drugs are other possible examples of government requirements that might be imposed against the wishes of parents. There has been insufficient attention to the ethics of overriding parental decisions to promote public goods, common goods, or the safety of individuals and society as a whole. I emphasize these public reasons for overriding parents in the Indirect Effects Basis of the Test:

> It is warranted for a state to overturn a parental decision if, as a consequence of the decision, unreasonable burdens are likely to be created either for Society as a whole or members of society besides the involved child.

---

[5] For example, a parent rendered quadriplegic through no fault of her own may no longer be able to care for a small child.

The resolution phase of state intervention is based on maximizing the needs and legitimate interests of the child and his family—of the child, the child's parents, and those close to the child's parents. It involves not only health considerations, but all aspects of life, including material resources, education, core beliefs, and behavior dictated by those core beliefs. Health care workers and institutions have far more competence in addressing health interests than in balancing their patients' health interests against other interests not related to health. Furthermore, they may be unsympathetic to patients' and families' priorities.

Any state-imposed restriction can be used as a pretext to disadvantage or injure members of disfavored minorities or other people who run afoul of common beliefs and norms, even if their behavior nominally falls within legal bounds. Therefore, I proposed some constraints on government action that would prevent states from interfering with parental decisions even if one of the Bases for action is satisfied. These constraints include:

1. The supposed harm underlying the restriction is actual, rather than hypothetical; and likely, rather than rare; this is the *Likelihood of Effect Constraint.*
2. The harm that the restriction seeks to avoid must be of a magnitude greater than harms typically tolerated for comparable practices; this is the *Comparability of Effect Constraint.*
3. Benefits of the restriction to all parties concerned should foreseeably exceed overall harms. This is the *Benefit/Harm Constraint.*

The harms that form the basis for restriction must be actual, empirically demonstrable, tangible harms, and must be sufficiently common to reasonably justify action. Possible harms befalling children of mainstream parents and those from minority cultures (or of idiosyncratic parents) must be treated similarly. Finally, governments should not be so assiduous in stamping out harm that the governmental action causes more harm than the reprehensible practice that the government is trying to suppress.

Supposed autonomy and open future considerations are superseded by considerations relating to the child's flourishing. Whether the standard for decisions relates to interests, harms or, (as I propose) needs, parents are to make decisions based on beneficence. The fact that individuals possess conflicting values, and that even people with similar values may be so situated as to have different needs, means that parents will differ in their decisions. We should not try to supersede decisions unless the conditions of the Test apply. It follows that parents may authorize enhancement procedures at their discretion, with assent of an older minor being a reasonable requirement. Parents have a better understanding of requirements for flourishing than a younger minor might have. Furthermore, many enhancement procedures are safer and more effective in children than in adults. Efficacy may be greater when procedures are done at a young age. This is especially true if one considers the effects of enhancement procedures on psychosocial development. This includes dominance/submissiveness parameters and sexual image and self-image. Many of the calls to delay procedures until maturity seem pretextual. Delaying ritual circumcision until the age of consent allows the individual to make a choice, but after almost two decades of conditioning to an uncircumcised body image, and, in Europe, exposure to societal messages largely disapproving of circumcision, based partially on a strong tradition of philosophical opposition to Judaism (Jacobs 2013).[6] Objecting to ritual childhood circumcision seems inconsistent with endorsement of medicating or operating on children for purposes of furthering gender affirmation. If one opposes circumcision on deontic grounds, it would seem that consistency would require opposing administration of puberty-blocking hormones on deontic grounds. Those who oppose childhood circumcision (Brussels Collaboration 2019), or even ear piercing (Sarajlic 2020) of children should oppose programs of medical and psychological intervention whose effects are greater than those of *de minimis* physical intervention.[7] Those actually participating in clinical investigation and treatment of gender incongruous minors justify their positions based on traditional pediatric beneficence grounds (de Vries et al 2014; Rafferty 2018).

There are at least four possible bases for respect for patient autonomy in medicine. First is the Kantian belief that respect for autonomy is required *a priori* (Gillon 1985). This belief does not comprise a consensus in society or even in academia. From feminists to communitarians, many scholars and writers reject autonomy as a value with overarching priority outside the limited arena of consent to medical intervention. Even within the medical arena, many patients prefer to make decisions in conjunction with others, such as family and friends, known as relational autonomy (Dove et al. 2017).

Second, autonomy stands as a bulwark against physicians' having too much power, which is subject to abuse without some checks (*Schloendorff vs. Soc. of New York Hosp.*, 105 N.E. 92, 94, New York Court of Appeals, 1914). This view of autonomy is the legal basis for parental decision-making on behalf of the child (Katz et al. 2016; Feudtner et al. 2018), which empowers children vis-à-vis the physician, albeit through their parental surrogates.

Third, the physician is an expert with regard to health, but is not expert at helping patients balance health priorities against other priorities. An adult patient was once referred to me just before her retirement for early endometrial cancer. She asked me if she should postpone a long-planned six-week trip around the world. I told her that the delay might reduce her chance of cure by a few percent. I could not tell her whether prompt treatment was more important than the trip she had planned with her family. This basis for autonomy—that the patient (or his surrogate) has a better understanding of the patient's needs and interests than physicians do (Buchanan &

[6] This philosophical trend does not necessarily demonize Jews as individuals, although we see this in Schmitt's work and in his actions against Jewish scholars in Germany (Caldwell 2005). Writers may criticize Jewish theology, following the example of Marcion in the 2nd century (Tyson 2006). It may also play on anti-Jewish tropes (Frosh 2011), or simply criticize Jews for their particularism (Kant 1793).

[7] The physical consequences of puberty-blocking hormones are said to be at least partially reversible if the hormones are discontinued. Hormonal treatment has a negative effect on fertility, which the circumcision and vulvar nick do not. And the social and psychological effects of marked delay of puberty are not as easily altered as the bodily changes, independent of whether puberty-blocking is likely to be associated with social affirmation of an atypical gender.

Brock 1989; Iltis 2010), also weakens the moral authority of physicians vis-à-vis parents. Fourth and finally, in a pluralistic society, social harmony is best served if people give each other room to make their own decisions, unless those decisions are likely to cause great harm to others.

We should be humble enough to appreciate that we may not fully appreciate the impact of (for example) transgender identification in circumstances very different from our own. Such circumstances might include (1) a self-contained agricultural religious community in which heterosexual marriage is an intrinsic part of life; (2) a family in which athletic performance is the most important determinant of a person' sense of worth; (3) a family whose adults are two feminist women married to each other, and (4) a family committed to non-interference in its children's development of gender identity (Compton 2018). We must understand that physical appearance may be overwhelmingly important in some families, academic or athletic success in others, and spending time with a large extended family in still others. A wise and sensitive therapeutic team will approach every child differently, depending on the child's circumstances. Sometimes, as with enhancements solicited by parents, there may be discordance between family values, a child's values, and a child's capabilities. At other times, parental desires may be dangerous to the child (as in refusal of life-saving transfusion) or to others in society (as in vaccine refusal).

Shared decision-making is the ideal for a child receiving evaluation or treatment within the health care system. When there is an impasse, the parents should have the final word unless they are malfeasant in their decision, as defined by the State Intervention Test. Regardless of the clinical issue, physicians unable to reach accommodation with parents should defer to the parents unless one of the Bases of the Test applies.

On a personal note, this book was written in the shadow of the pandemic of Covid-19, which afflicted me as I was revising this book. This has reinforced my belief that biomedical ethics must accept a more communitarian ethos. We must face disasters by focusing on how to stabilize and right the vessel of society, rather than concentrating on exalting individual autonomy or granular fairness of resource distribution. Application of the Indirect Effects Prong is an area that is wide open for future research.

In preparing this book, I frequently was enticed down numerous rabbit holes, and learned many interesting details that I cannot share because of space. I wish I could talk about tribes in which children are frequently born with polydactyly, and it is considered normal. I've become familiar with the evil genius, Carl Schmitt, whose work seems to anticipate critical social justice theory.

What has struck me, and worked its way into this book at many levels, is the sophistication of much social science. Empirical work performed across many societies, leading to papers with scores of authors, are elucidating human needs as they are. This work should, and will, supplement and replace much speculation on this subject. As I have noted, work by noted thinkers has disregarded the revelations of social science. Focus on a parent–child dyad is important in solving individual problems, but ignores the greater stage on which conflicts arise and are played out.

Neurobiology is in its infancy with regard to its ability to contribute to our knowledge of human needs and motivation, and this may be the case for quite a while.

I conclude with an admonition and plea to healthcare professionals and another to government officials.

To healthcare workers: You must always realize that the child in your care got where he was as part of a family, and will return to the family of which he is an important part after you have cared for him. You, on the other hand, are someone the child sees intermittently for health-related services.

To government officials, including judges: I related a story about a government official who told a senator that she cared for the senator's children as much as the senator did. The senator responded by asking her to tell him their names. Any particular child is more important to his parents than to you. The child will continue to live with his parents. You should defer to parents' decisions except in threatening or exigent circumstances.

References

Anonymous. 2012. The never-ending war. *The Economist*, Dec 22, 2012. ISSN 0013–0613.

Aristotle. 1976. *Ethics* (trans: Thomson). London: Penguin Books.

Ben-Yehuda, Anna. 2020. Here is each state's favorite snack according to google. *Time Out*, Jul 21, 2020. https://www.timeout.com/usa/news/here-is-each-states-favorite-snack-according-to-google-072120.

Boggiano, Barbara. 2020. Long-Term effects of the Paraguayan war (1864–1870): From male scarcity to intimate partner violence. *HCHE Research Paper, No. 2020/21*, University of Hamburg, Hamburg Center for Health Economics (HCHE), Hamburg.

Brussels Collaboration. (2019). Medically unnecessary genital cutting and the rights of the child: Moving Toward consensus. *American Journal of Bioethics* 19(10):17–28. https://doi.org/10.1080/15265161.2019.1643945.

Buchanan. Allen E., and Dan W. Brock. 1989. *Deciding for others: The ethics of surrogate decision making*. Cambridge: Cambridge University Press.

Caldwell, Peter C. 2005. Controversies over carl schmitt: A review of recent literature. *Journal of Modern History*. 77 (2): 357–387. https://doi.org/10.1086/431819.

Compton, Julie. 2018. 'Boy or Girl?' Parents raising 'Theybies' let kids decide. *NBC News*, Jul 19. https://www.nbcnews.com/feature/nbc-out/boy-or-girl-parents-raising-theybies-let-kids-decide-n891836.

Curry, Oliver S., Mark Alfano, Mark J. Brandt, and Christine Pelican. 2020. Moral molecules: Morality as a combinatorial system. *OSF Preprints*. https://doi.org/10.31219/osf.io/xnstk.

de Vries, Annelou L. C,. Jenifer K McGuire, Thomas D. Steensma, Eva C. F. Wagenaar, Theo A. H. Doreleijers, and Peggy T. Cohen-Kettenis. 2014. Young adult psychological outcome after puberty suppression and gender reassignment. *Pediatrics* 134(4):696–704. https://doi.org/10.1542/peds.2013-2958.

Diekema, Douglas S. 2020. Adolescent brain development and medical decision-making. *Pediatrics* 146 (1): S18-24. https://doi.org/10.1542/peds.2020-0818F.

Dove, Edward S, Susan E, Kelly, Federica Lucivero, Mavis Machirori, Sandi Dheensa, and Barbara Prainsack. 2017. Beyond individualism: is there a place for relational autonomy in clinical practice and research? *Clinical Ethics* 12(3):150–65. https://doi.org/10.1177/1477750917704156.

Feudtner, Chris, Theodore Schall, and Douglas Hill. 2018. Parental personal sense of duty as a foundation of pediatric medical decision-making. *Pediatrics* 142 (Supplement 3): S133–S141. https://doi.org/10.1542/peds.2018-0516C.

Frosh, Stephen. 2011. Psychoanalysis, antisemitism and the miser. *New Formations* 72: 94–106. https://doi.org/10.3898/NEWF.72.07.2011.

Gillam, Lynn. 2016. The zone of parental disc: An ethical tool for dealing with disagreement between parents and doctors about medical treatment for a child. *Clinical Ethics* 11 (1): 1–8.

Gillon, Raanan. 1985. Philosophical medical ethics: Rights. *British Medical Journal* 290 (6485): 1890–1891. https://doi.org/10.1136/bmj.290.6485.1890.

Glendon, Mary Ann. 1991. *Rights talk: The impoverishment of political discourse.* New York: Free Press.

Iltis, Ana S . 2010. Toward a coherent account of pediatric decision making. *Journal of Medicine and Philosophy* 35 (5): 526–552.

Jackson, Jonathan, Ben Bradford, Mike Hough, Andy Myhill, Paul Quinton, and Tom R. Tyler. 2012. Why do people comply with the law? Legitimacy and the influence of legal institutions. *British Journal of Criminology* 52 (6): 1051–1071.

Jacobs, Allan J. 2013. The ethics of circumcision of male infants. *Israel Medical Association. Journal: IMAJ* 15 (1): 60–64.

Kant, Immanuel. 1793. *Religion within the limits of reason* alone (trans: Theodore M. Greene and Hoyt H. Hudson). New York: Harper Torchbooks.

Katz, Aviva L., Sally A. Webb, and Committee on Bioethics, American Academy of Pediatrics. 2016. Informed consent in decision-making in pediatric practice. *Pediatrics* 138(2):e20161485.

Milton, John. 1644. *Areopagitica.* http://www.gutenberg.org/ebooks/608.

Rafferty, Jason, and Committee on Psychosocial Aspects of Child and Family Health, Committee on Adolescence and Section on Lesbian, Gay, Bisexual, and Transgender Health and Wellness. 2018. Ensuring comprehensive care and support for transgender and gender-diverse children and adolescents. *Pediatrics* 142(4):e20182162. https://doi.org/10.1542/peds.2018-2162.

Ross, David W. 1930. *The right and the good.* Oxford: Oxford University Press.

Sarajlic, Eldar. 2020. Children, culture, and body modification. *Kennedy Institute of Ethics Journal* 30 (2): 167–190. https://doi.org/10.1353/ken.2020.0005.

Saunders, Ben. 2021. A sufficiency threshold is not a harm principle: A better alternative to best interests for overriding parental decisions. *Bioethics* 35 (1): 90–97. https://doi.org/10.1111/bioe.12796.

Shavell, Steven. 1980. Strict liability versus negligence. *Journal of Legal Studies* 9 (1): 1–25.

Shklar, Judith N. 1984. *Ordinary vices.* Cambridge Massachusetts: Belknap Press.

Trinkner, Rick, Jonathan Jackson, and Tom R. Tyler. 2018. Bounded authority: expanding "Appropriate" police behavior beyond procedural justice.*Law and Human Behavior* 42(3):280–93.

Tyson, Joseph B. 2006. Anti-Judaism in Marcion and his opponents. *Studies in Christian-Jewish Relations* 1 (1): 196–208.

Index

A. J. Jacobs, *Assigning Responsibility for Children's Health When Parents and Authorities Disagree: Whose Child?*, The International Library of Bioethics 90,
https://doi.org/10.1007/978-3-030-87698-2

The manufacturer's authorised representative in the EU is Springer
Nature Customer Service Centre GmbH, Europaplatz 3, 69115 Heidelberg,
Germany. If you have any concerns regarding our products, please
contact ProductSafety@springernature.com

Printed and bound by CPI Group (UK) Ltd, Croydon, CR0 4YY
30/09/2026
02225246-0012